SURGERY

A Complete Guide for Patients and their Families

SURGERY

The University of Toronto
Department of Surgery

VELUT ARBOR ÆVO

A Complete Guide for Patients and their Families

Editors:

Allan Gross, M.D.
Latner Professor and Chairman
Division of Orthopedic Surgery
Department of Surgery
University of Toronto

Penny Gross, Ph.D.
Senior Research and
Program Evaluation Analyst
Ministry of Community and Social Services
Government of Ontario

Bernard Langer, M.D.
R.S. McLaughlin Professor and Chairman
Department of Surgery
University of Toronto

Medical Art Editors:

Linda Wilson-Pauwels, A.O.C.A., B.Sc., A.A.M., M.Ed.
Assistant Professor and Acting Chairman
Department of Art as Applied to Medicine
Faculty of Medicine
University of Toronto

Margot Mackay, A.N.S.C.A.D., B.Sc., A.A.M.
Associate Professor and Course Director
Department of Art as Applied to Medicine
Faculty of Medicine
University of Toronto

Harper & Collins
TORONTO

First published in 1989
by Harper & Collins Publishers Ltd.
Suite 2900, Hazelton Lanes
55 Avenue Road,
Toronto, Ontario M5R 3L2
Canada

Publisher's Note: The contents of this book are not intended to be used as a substitute for consultation with your physician. All matters pertaining to your health should be directed to a health care professional.

Canadian Cataloguing in Publication Data
Main entry under title:

Surgery: a complete guide for patients and their families

Includes index.
ISBN 0-00-217905-9

1. Surgery - Popular works. I. Gross, Allan.
II. Gross, Penny. III. Langer, Bernard.

RD31.3.S87 1989 617 C89-093049-X

Printed and bound in Canada

Editors: Shelley Tanaka, Margaret McCaffery
Production Editor: Kathryn Schroeder
Designer: Scott Richardson
Typesetter: Jay Tee Graphics Ltd.

Contents

Acknowledgements

Our special thanks to our editors, Shelley Tanaka and Margaret McCaffery.

Thanks to Professor Alex Wright, of the Department of Art as Applied to Medicine, for his support and enthusiasm that helped get the project off the ground.

Also, thanks to Professor Betty Akesson, of the Department of Anatomy, whose critical eye was of great help in ensuring the accuracy of the illustrations.

We would also like to thank the following people who contributed in the preparation of this book: Sophie Gaida, Maureen Glaab, Jeremy Gross, Robyn Gross, Celia King, Judy Levy, David Rubinoff, Rachael Rubinoff, Robert Rubinoff, Robina Salter, Martina Santangelo, and Betty Webster.

Foreword

The average life expectancy of a North American is now well over 70 years; about 50 percent of these individuals will require an operation some time in their lives. From the point of view of the surgeon, most operations are straightforward procedures like tonsillectomies, hernia repairs, cataract operations and D & C's — operations that surgeons describe as "routine" or "low risk."

This assessment is based on our accumulated knowledge about the risks and benefits of specific procedures, our familiarity with modern methods of anesthesia, pain relief and methods of reducing the risks of infection and other complications. It also brings into bearing our confidence in the capability of the professionals, both medical and non-medical, to bring patients smoothly through their operations.

From the patient's point of view, however, every operation represents a major life event — possibly a life-threatening one. Patients are not reassured by an operation being "routine;" their situation is unique, and as far as they are concerned, a complication or mortality rate is either 100 percent or zero. The same technology that provides reassurance to surgeons and anesthetists may be itself unnerving and threatening to the patient. And the fact that most operations take place in a hospital — which tends to diminish the patients' individuality and removes them from their usual sources of comfort and support — adds to the trepidation with which most people approach the prospect of surgery.

Physicians and surgeons have a responsibility to give patients information about their disease, the various options available for treatment, and some understanding of what is involved in the recommended operative procedures. In a sophisticated, educated society, this involves a considerable amount of explanation and detail, and it is often not possible for a surgeon to provide sufficient information in the time available or, indeed, for patients to know what questions to ask to gain a better understanding of their situation.

Surgery: A Complete Guide for Patients and Their Families is the brainchild of Allan and Penny Gross, and was developed to fill the gap between the busy surgeon and the patient who needs a clear, non-technical source of information. It is not an exhaustive textbook of surgery for the layman, but is rather an introduction to the world of surgery, aimed primarily at the patient who will be undergoing a specific operation.

This book is a collaborative effort. The authors are from the Faculty of Medicine at the University of Toronto, and are well-recognized authorities in their fields. The artwork has been provided by faculty and students in the Department of Art as Applied to Medicine. All editors, authors and artists have donated their time freely in the preparation of this book, and any proceeds from its sale will go to the University of Toronto Surgical Alumni Association and to the Department of Art as Applied to Medicine to further research and education at the University of Toronto.

Bernard Langer
R.S. McLaughlin Professor and Chairman
Department of Surgery
University of Toronto

Introduction

This book is intended to bridge the gap between the surgeon, who perceives surgery as an everyday event, and the patient—for whom it may be a life crisis. Knowing what to expect from surgery removes the mystery and helps to alleviate anxiety experienced not only by the patient but also by the patient's family. It may also help the patient along to a speedier recovery.

We hope to provide answers to questions patients and their families usually ask before surgery is done. Surgeons from the teaching hospitals of the University of Toronto describe the most commonly performed operations. Case histories illustrate typical situations that might well be similar to those in which the readers find themselves.

This book has also been written for all those who may be involved in the caring of patients: allied health care personnel, social workers, family physicians and surgeons. We hope that the book will in some way assist these professionals in understanding what patients and their families are going through, and enable them to provide better care.

Surgery: A Complete Guide for Patients and Their Families takes the patient step-by-step through many surgical operations, describing the diagnostic procedures, alternative non-surgical treatment, the actual operation, possible complications, and recent advances that have been made in the field.

If you have been told you need surgery, you should find out the name of the operation and the type of surgeon (thoracic, cardiac, etc.) who will perform it. You can then look up the surgical specialty in this book. This book does not describe every operation, but it does describe in detail the most commonly performed surgical procedures in each specialty. In addition, there are chapters focusing on broader topics such as anesthesia, cancer surgery, transplant surgery and the complications of surgery in general.

You may find that after reading about the operation you have more questions. Take those concerns to your surgeon or family physician. *Surgery* is meant to be a supplement to, not a substitute for, your doctor's advice.

Chapter 1

The Practice of Surgery

Robert D. Henderson

Former Professor of Surgery
University of Toronto

Former Surgeon-in-Chief
Women's College Hospital, Toronto

For most people, entering a hospital for surgery is both novel and frightening. Concerns about their health are magnified by the unfamiliar surroundings, the many different staff members, the thought of anesthesia and the anticipation of pain. In some circumstances the disease necessitating surgery is a major life threat.

For others the disease has produced disability, and their hope is that surgery will bring relief. In all cases an awareness of what is going to happen and what the expected effects will be can relieve anxiety and help both the patient and family become part of the recovery process.

Going into a hospital can be an intimidating experience for patients and their friends and families — the noise, the smells, the lights, the bustle. It's often hard to know just what all those people in the white coats do. Are they lab technicians, nurses, medical students, interns, residents or surgeons, and what's the difference?

Hospital Staff: Teaching Hospital vs. Community Hospital

A teaching hospital is affiliated with a medical school, and one of its functions is to help train physicians. As a result, there are a number of different professionals involved in a patient's care.

The patient's first line of communication is with the nurses who provide day-to-day care. In addition to nurses, you will likely come in contact with medical students, who may accompany staff or examine patients on their own. Medical students are not yet qualified physicians — they are in the hospital to observe and learn. They cannot write orders or take responsibility for patients' treatment.

A final-year medical student (a student in the fourth year of medical school training) is often called a "clinical clerk." Clinical clerks are part of the hospital team; they may examine patients, perform minor procedures with the help of a resident and write orders, but report to a supervising staff member at all times.

Interns have passed their basic medical school examinations and are allowed to examine patients and write orders as fully qualified doctors. They are, however, still supervised, and are not granted a licence to practice (e.g., as a family practitioner or general practitioner) until their one-year internship is over.

After internship, those physicians who want to specialize in a certain field of medicine, such as surgery, internal medicine, obstetrics and gynecology, must take a residency training program which takes a further four or five years. Residents are sometimes referred to as R1, R2, R3 and R4, depending on their year of training.

The first year or two of a surgical residency involves learning about diagnosis and care for surgical patients. In the operating room, the resident learns basic surgical skills as a surgical assistant. In the third and fourth years, and possibly fifth, the resident becomes more independent in caring for surgical patients. He or she will perform some operations independently. By the final year, the surgical resident is able to make independent decisions about patient care and perform routine surgery on his or her own.

After resident training, further exams must be taken before a physician can become a full-fledged surgeon. Surgeons who are going to work in large teaching hospitals may spend one or two additional years training in a highly specialized unit to learn new methods or techniques that will complement the surgical expertise available in their hospital. Many surgeons embark on further years of research or specialty training — the average surgeon, before going into practice, has spent 10 to 12 years in training, including medical school.

Patients in teaching hospitals have many sources of care and information. If medical attention is needed, the nurse may consult a clinical clerk or an intern. If more authoritative advice is required, a resident is called and, if necessary, the resident will communicate with the staff surgeon.

While patients sometimes feel uncomfortable about the parade of people in a teaching hospital, one of the benefits is that experienced residents are available to supply care around the clock. Each day, the surgical team, consisting of a nurse, clinical clerk, intern and surgical resident, will make routine daily rounds, visiting all surgical patients. The staff surgeon may also visit the patient daily.

Community hospitals do not take part in teaching; therefore, they have no students or residents. In a community hospital, a surgery patient deals with a nurse, possibly an intern, and the surgeon. The surgeon is responsible for the patient's daily care. Although the surgeon is the principal medical contact, the patient's family physician will also play a major role.

A community hospital tailors the complexity of surgery to its facilities. A small hospital in a remote community will concentrate on routine general surgery and emergencies that require instant attention. Large community hospitals can offer an extensive range of surgical specialties, lacking only the most complex, highly specialized, or rare and costly areas of expertise. The larger community hospitals will usually have interns. One advantage for patients in a community hospital is that their family doctor may be on staff there, to perform certain procedures or assist at others, and also participate in their daily care. Patients often find this familiar face very reassuring.

What happens in the hospital?

Surgical operations are often spoken of as being emergencies, urgent operations or elective operations. A patient brought into the emergency department with a major hemorrhage or other life-threatening condition is taken immediately for emergency surgery, which is carried out just as soon as the patient and the operating room can be made ready. If cancer is diagnosed and a tumor must be removed as soon as possible, that is considered urgent surgery, which usually takes place within a few days. Elective surgery is scheduled for conditions that are not life-threatening and can be done at a mutually convenient time for the patient and the surgeon. The wait can be from several days to several months.

Patients are generally referred to a particular surgeon, either by their family physician or another specialist. The choice of surgeon is ultimately up to the patient, but is usually made in consultation with the referring physician, who will likely recommend a surgeon in the hospital where the referring physician works (most physicians are affiliated with a hospital). This provides continuity of care between the two doctors. A patient can, however, choose to be referred to a surgeon in another hospital.

In an emergency, patients will be referred to the staff surgeon on call, but even then they can request another surgeon, should that surgeon be available. In elective or even urgent surgery, the patient may ask for a second surgical opinion.

When you enter the hospital, a nurse will usually review your chart, check your identity, ask about known allergies, make dietary arrangements and help you settle in your room. A clinical clerk or intern will arrive, obtain a detailed history and do a general physical examination. A resident will review this history and do a physical examination. Each day a resident and/or the staff surgeon will make rounds, review your status, prepare you for surgery or check your postoperative progress. They should be made aware of any concerns or unexpected symptoms you may have. One should never hesitate to ask questions.

Before or immediately after admission, each patient will have tests done to determine the exact cause of symptoms and to assess general health. The diagnostic tests vary, depending on the problem, and their results will be used to decide whether surgery is necessary and, if so, what surgery should be performed. A basic physical examination and blood, urine, ECG (electrocardiogram) and other tests determine the patient's level of general health. If problems are found, they are either corrected before surgery, or additional safeguards are taken.

Every hospital requires surgical patients to sign a consent form which states that they understand the procedure and its complications and are willing to go ahead and have the surgery. If the patient cannot sign for any reason, the closest relative signs the consent. All surgery, from the removal of a toenail to a heart transplant, carries a risk to life and health. For minor procedures the risk to life is exceedingly small — the risk for uncomplicated removal of a gall bladder, for example, would be less than 1 percent. Other risks to health are rare, but must be considered. (See chapter 4.)

Specific risks vary with each operation. Their frequency depends on the type of surgery and the patient's physical condition. However, the success rate associated with operations is generally high, or the operation would have been previously discarded.

Before surgery, the anesthetist will evaluate the patient. (See chapter 3.) Usually mild sedation is given the night before surgery to allay anxiety. Once in the operating room, the patient is put to sleep in minutes — the next conscious moment will occur after the operation in the operating room or recovery room once the operation is completed. During the operation vital signs (breathing rate, pulse, blood pressure) are constantly checked, and blood and fluid replacement are maintained.

Each operation requires a surgeon and an anesthetist. In a teaching hospital, the surgeon usually has two assistants — a surgical resident and an intern. Routine operations can be done with one resident assisting. A scrub nurse is in charge of the instruments. A circulating nurse performs various duties for the surgeon and anesthetist such as getting additional instruments, blood or drugs. The operating room is also in voice contact with the head nurse at the central operating-room desk.

In a community hospital, the assistant is a general practitioner or intern. Some general practitioners become specialized in assisting, and this becomes a major part of their work.

After the operation, pain can be controlled with medication, but some discomfort must be tolerated. The patients who do well are usually those who can tolerate pain and become physically active early. If you can sit up, breathe deeply, move your legs and get on your feet promptly, your body functions return more rapidly, and your recovery will likely be greatly accelerated.

Recovery time varies with the operation and the patient. Some procedures can be done as day surgery, and the patient goes home the same day and returns to work within a few days. Other patients may spend several weeks in hospital, not returning to work for several months. In either case, follow-up by the surgeon is important to ensure complete recovery. The surgeon checks wound healing, improvement in preoperative symptoms and any signs of complications. In some cases periodic follow-up and further testing may be necessary for several years.

Chapter 2

Surgical Research

Steven M. Strasberg

Professor of Surgery
University of Toronto

Head, Division of General Surgery
Mount Sinai Hospital, Toronto

The practice of surgery in the twentieth century has been changed dramatically by surgical research. Some spectacular changes have been introduced: transplanting organs, such as the kidney, heart, liver and lung; replacing damaged tissues and organs with artificial devices, such as artifical joints and heart valves; and reimplanting amputated limbs and fingers.

Many other developments such as diagnostic, operative and postoperative techniques are less likely to make the headlines, but are just as important and have made surgery much safer.

Surgical research often begins with the observation of a clinical problem for which there is no solution. Possible solutions may be developed in the laboratory and then tested on animals. Once a reasonable degree of safety has been reached, the method will be tested on patients.

Organ transplantation is a good example of such a problem. For each organ, particular techniques had to be developed. These techniques were tested on animals until the best one was found. Only then was the operation applied to humans. Organ transplantation is a particularly difficult problem. Not only must the best way be found to remove the old organ and sew in the new one, but more complex problems must be solved — how to prevent the body from rejecting the new organ, how best to preserve the new organ until transplantation, and how to replace the function of the diseased organ by artificial means until a human organ is available.

In such research, surgeons, internists, biochemists, immunologists, engineers and many other types of researchers may combine forces, each asking very different kinds of questions. To control rejection we must understand how the body recognizes tissue that has come from another individual. For artificial organs, complex engineering problems must be overcome. As new drugs or techniques are developed, they, too, must be tested to determine their value.

Aside from the spectacular developments that one reads about in the daily news, members of the public are most likely to come into contact with surgical research when confronted by those opposed to the use of animals in research or if, as patients, they are asked to participate in testing a new procedure.

Surgical research would be impossible without the use of animals. Many of the medical advances in this century would simply not have occurred without animal research. Researchers have obligations to use as few animals as possible, to minimize their suffering and to be certain that the studies are potentially important in developing new knowledge. To make sure these obligations are fulfilled, universities have special committees to examine each proposed study, and university and government inspectors continually supervise animal housing and study conditions.

As a hospital patient, you may be asked to participate in a medical research study. Your participation may lead to new knowledge which may eventually benefit many others.

The most common type of study a patient may be asked to participate in is called a *clinical trial*. When a new technique or drug is developed in the laboratory, its benefit may be obvious, as with the discovery of penicillin. In most cases, however, it is not immediately clear that a new discovery will lead to better results than the standard treatment already available. In other words, while the treatment may be new, it may not be better than the old treatment, and unless it is put to the test, we will never know. Using unproven new discoveries could actually lead to a lessening rather than an improvement in medical care.

Clinical trials must be approved by university committees and the committees of agencies supporting the research. These committees decide whether the new discovery is ready for testing in humans, if the testing procedure takes proper account of patient safety, and if the information to be given to patients about the trial is clear and complete.

To get an objective answer to the question whether the new treatment is better than the current one, there must be no bias. To avoid bias, neither patient nor doctor must be able to choose a particular treatment. Patients are randomly assigned to receive one treatment or the other. In studies of new drugs, this process of avoiding bias is taken further by not permitting either the doctor or the patient to know whether the drug to be received is the new or the standard treatment. This is, of course, not possible in trials of surgical operations.

A good example of surgical clinical trials and the issues they raise is in the treatment of breast cancer. A trial was set up to determine whether less breast tissue could be removed in a limited mastectomy, with the same benefit as total mastectomy. Some patients believed that removal of the entire breast was necessary to cure cancer and refused to enter the trial because they were afraid they would be selected to receive the other treatment. Others, hearing of the new approach, decided that it was better and refused to enter the trial in case they were selected to receive a total mastectomy. As it turned out, the trial showed that limited mastectomy was as good for some groups of patients. If the trial had not been done, total mastectomy would still be the only treatment available today.

If you think those who refused to enter in case they were chosen to have a total mastectomy chose wisely, think again. No one knew the answer to the question: what if complete mastectomy had provided better results? There are times when a random choice is as good as any. If you need somewhat more selfish reasons to participate in a clinical trial, there are at least two. First, many diseases have a hereditary component. Answers today may mean better treatment for the next generation. Second, if the new treatment is found to be beneficial, patients in the trial and receiving the old treatment can be switched to the new treatment as soon as a difference is found.

Another type of research in which patients are asked to participate is the donation of body fluids or tissues for research. Animal tissues are not identical to human tissues; once research gets to a certain point, it may be necessary to study human tissue. For instance, you may be asked to give a small amount of blood or other body fluid such as urine or bile. If you are having an operation, you may be asked for a small amount of tissue such as fat or skin. These are usually minute pieces of tissue whose absence is not noticeable, but whose importance in studies is great. Sometimes the tissues requested are diseased and are to be removed as part of the operation. Sometimes, however, small portions of normal tissues are needed for comparison with diseased tissues. Like clinical trials, these studies are always reviewed before approval to ensure that they are important and safe.

No patient is obligated to participate in these studies, but without patient participation, medical research would be impossible. There is immense satisfaction in knowing that you have contributed to the advancement of medical care.

If any practitioner gives testimonial type evidence only — "Look what my drug or my operation did for this particular patient" — you know that his or her claims are not scientifically sound and have a good chance of being incorrect. What may occur in one patient may not occur in another, and must be tested on many patients before it can be said to work.

As a citizen, you have a right to know what your government is doing to support medical research. You may also wish to support agencies which fund specific types of research. By doing so, you can help to ensure that there is adequate funding for medical research, so that the health care available to you and future generations will be the best possible.

Chapter 3

Anesthesia

Ernest Hew
Associate Professor
Department of Anesthesia
University of Toronto
Staff Anesthetist and Co-Director
Intensive Care Unit
Mount Sinai Hospital,
Toronto

Sari O'Sullivan
Illustrator

Pain is both a sensation (a conscious awareness of a noxious stimulus) and an emotional experience (an intense feeling of displeasure resulting in certain behavior).

When tissues are injured in any way, chemicals from the injured cells leak into the fluid surrounding the nerve endings.

The nerve endings stimulate and/or sensitize pain receptors to generate electric impulses. These impulses are transmitted via sensory nerves to the spinal cord and the brain. Pain is experienced only when the impulse arrives at the brain.

The Prevention of Pain

Pain can be treated (or blocked) at different points in the pain pathway (Fig. 3.1). With local anesthesia, the patient is awake, but the part being operated on is "frozen." This can be achieved in a number of ways. First, the pain receptors may be blocked by a local anesthetic agent, like the one a dentist might use for freezing before dental work. Second, transmission of the electrical impulses carrying the information about pain may be interrupted anywhere along the length of the sensory nerve before it reaches the spinal cord. This can be done by injecting an anesthetic that blocks nerve

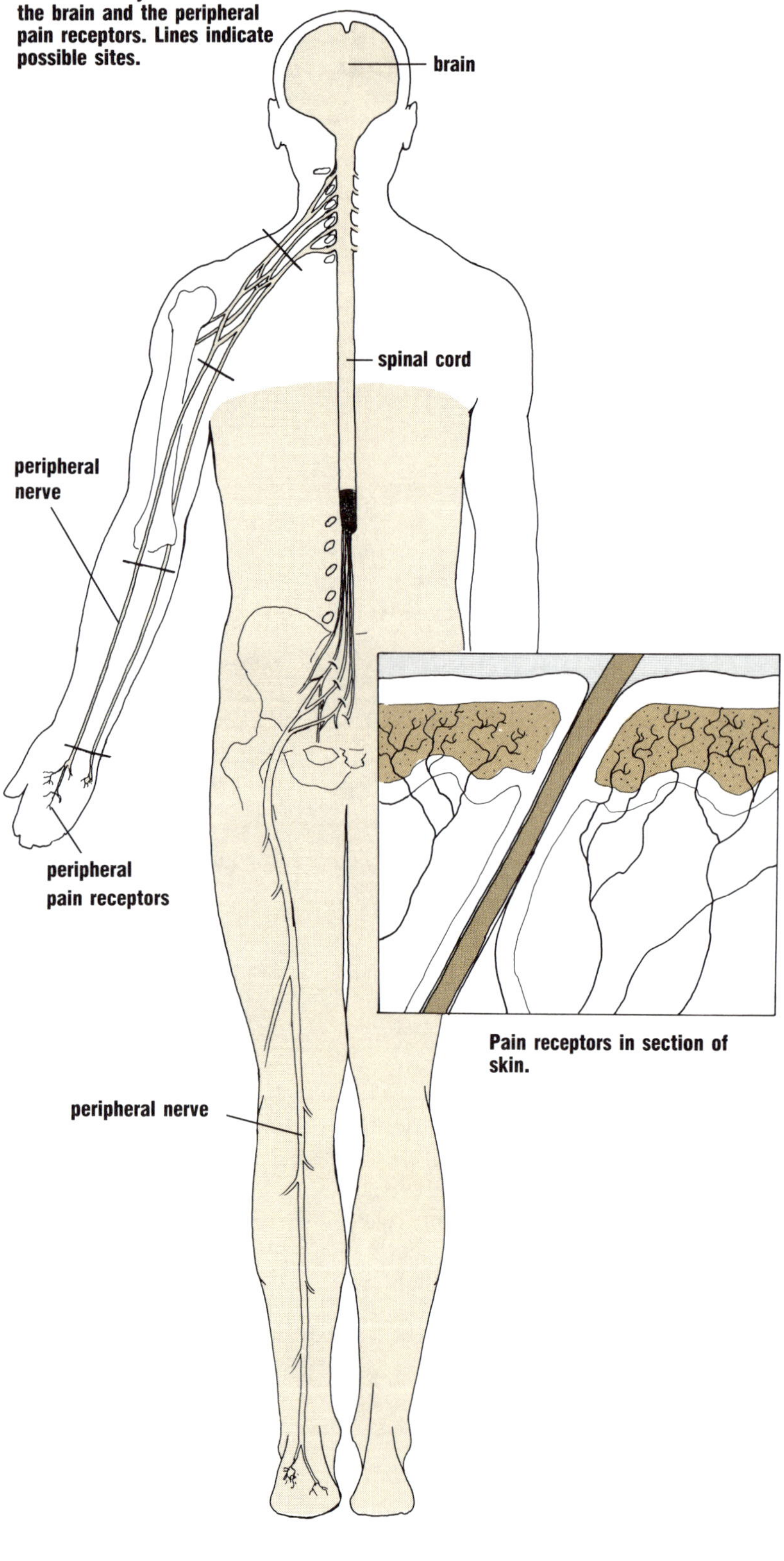

Figure 3.1
Pain pathway. Pain may be "blocked" anywhere between the brain and the peripheral pain receptors. Lines indicate possible sites.

Pain receptors in section of skin.

impulse transmission; the block can be peripheral (usually involving one nerve) or regional (involving one area but often more than one nerve).

The third point at which the transmission of a nerve impulse may be interrupted is in the spinal cord itself. Two methods, the epidural block and the spinal block, are commonly used today.

Epidural Block

In an epidural block, the local anesthetic solution is injected in the lower back, into the epidural space surrounding the spinal cord (Fig. 3.2). The solution diffuses through the coverings of the spinal cord to enter the subarachnoid space which contains cerebrospinal fluid. This fluid bathes the spinal cord, and drugs entering this space invariably have a rapid and direct effect on the spinal cord and its coverings. Sensation is lost below the level of the block — usually, but not necessarily, on both sides of the body.

An epidural block may be used as the sole anesthetic for any operation below the level of the diaphragm, which is the main muscle of respiration. With this anesthetic the patient may be sedated or may be wide awake. The epidural block is the most commonly recommended method of preventing pain during childbirth and for cesarean sections, because the blood flow to the fetus is maintained.

Spinal Block

In a spinal block, the local anesthetic is injected directly into the cerebrospinal fluid (Fig. 3.3). It takes effect usually within one minute, while an epidural block often takes 10 to 20 minutes. The dose of anesthetic used for a spinal block is about 10 percent of the dose required to produce the same level of block via the epidural space, because the anesthetic does not have to diffuse through the spinal cord coverings.

The spinal block has one significant disadvantage which the epidural block does not have: the risk of headache, believed to be due to leakage of cerebrospinal fluid through the hole made in the coverings of the cord by the needle. The headache usually disappears by the sixth day, or earlier.

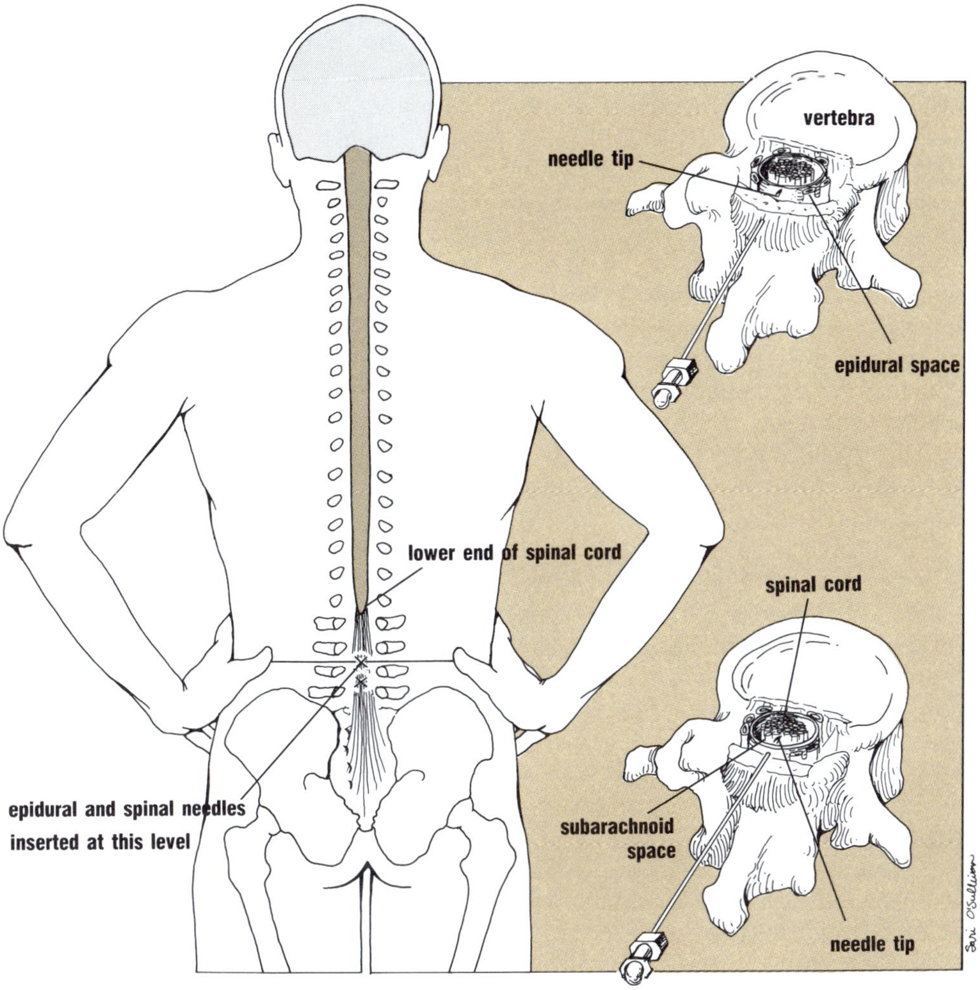

Figure 3.2
Spinal and epidural anesthesia. In an epidural block (top detail), the anesthetic is injected into the epidural space surrounding the spinal cord. In a spinal block (bottom detail), the anesthetic is injected directly into the subarachnoid space containing cerebrospinal fluid (CSF).

Other potential complications of spinal and epidural anesthesia include a decrease in blood pressure and difficulty in emptying the bladder. Backache, if it occurs, is shortlived and is not severe. A history of chronic back pain does not prevent the use of spinal or epidural anesthesia.

More serious complications, such as convulsions, infection of the covering of the spinal cord (meningitis) and death have been reported, but they are very rare.

For a spinal or epidural block, the patient may be asked to assume one of two postures: sitting up while leaning forward, or lying on one side, curled up like a cat (Fig. 3.3). These positions facilitate the placement of the needle into the lower back.

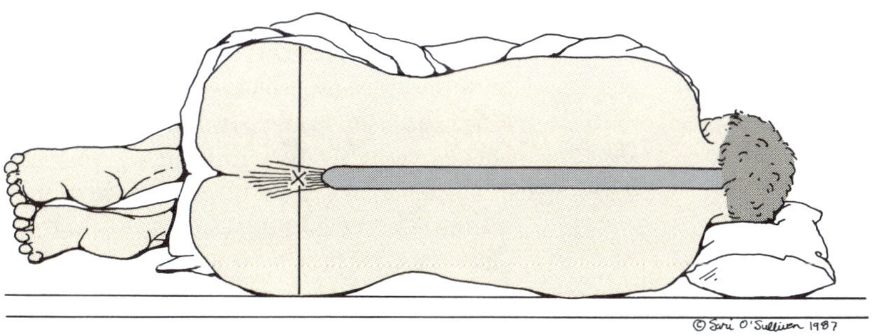

Figure 3.3
Position for spinal and epidural anesthesia.

General Anesthetic

In addition to local anesthetic, the transmission of nerve impulses and the sensation of pain can be blocked at the brain level by general anesthetics and narcotics.

Modern anesthesia started with the use of diethyl ether by a dentist, William Thomas Green Morton, in 1846. Before this, patients were given narcotics and/or alcohol, or were simply held down or knocked unconscious. Nitrous oxide (laughing gas) had been tried, but it was too weak to induce surgical depths of anesthesia safely.

Chloroform was introduced in 1847 by Sir James Young Simpson, a Scottish obstetrician. It had several advantages over ether. It was more rapid-acting, had a more pleasant smell, was cheaper and was not explosive. Its major disadvantage was that it damaged the liver. It is therefore no longer used.

Ether and chloroform dominated the "rag and bottle" era of anesthesia, but there were many complications. Induction of anesthesia (the time taken to reach the level of unconsciousness necessary to allow surgery) was often difficult (patients often fought and had to be physically restrained), prolonged (up to 30 minutes) and frightening (for both patients and doctors). Usually there was excessive salivation, which was sometimes inhaled into the lungs, causing pneumonia. It was also common for patients to have nausea and vomiting after the operation. And occasionally it was impossible to induce deep enough anesthesia solely by inhalation, because if the patient had lung disease (tuberculosis was common in those days), this prevented transfer of the anesthetic vapors in the inhaled gases to the bloodstream.

During a general anesthetic, a patient must first be induced, or brought to a level of unconsciousness. No one route of induction is appropriate in all patients. The method of induction chosen will depend on the patient, the type of surgery and the surgeon, as well as the anesthetist and the equipment and drugs available. If the patient has a preference, this should be discussed with the anesthetist. Most anesthetists will cater to the patient's wishes if the risks are not increased and the surgeon is not opposed to the choice. An intravenous is commonly started in the back of the hand or somewhere on the forearm. If you are very frightened of needles, you can ask to be anesthetized by inhaling gas via a mask.

Sodium thiopentone (Pentothal) is still the most commonly used intravenous induction agent because it is easy to use and is always effective. Onset of action is 10 to 60 seconds. Occasionally it is given rectally via a small hollow plastic tube so that sleep is induced gradually, over 10 to 20 minutes. This technique may be useful in people (especially children) who are afraid of needles and masks.

Once the general anesthetic state has been induced, it must be maintained for the duration of the operation. This is usually done using one or a combination of drugs. There are a number of agents that maintain the general anesthetic state, although we still have no idea how and why they do so.

Halothane (Fluothane) was developed in Britain in 1951, and by 1958 it was the main inhalational anesthetic agent in the western world. It has a relatively pleasant smell and is very safe, with few disadvantages. It is a rare cause of hepatitis, and in adults should not be used at the same time that the surgeon is injecting adrenalin, since the combination may cause irregular heart beats and even cardiac arrest.

Enflurane (Ethrane) was introduced in North America in about 1972. It soon replaced halothane as the main inhalational anesthetic, since it had all the advantages of halothane and none of its disadvantages. However, enflurane lowers a patient's seizure threshold and is therefore not used in epileptic patients.

Isoflurane (Forane) was introduced

around 1981, and has virtually replaced halothane and enflurane. Currently it is the most commonly used potent inhalational agent in North America. So far it does not appear to have any major disadvantages.

Today, most surgery cannot be performed without anesthesia. In Canada, all anesthetists are medical doctors with extra training in anesthesia. A general practitioner anesthetist will have had six months to two years of specific training in anesthesia, while a specialist must have completed three to four years, including one year of internal medicine or intensive care unit (ICU) work.

In the United States, there are also "nurse anesthetists" with two or three extra years of specific training, who may practice independently or may work under the supervision of the physician specialist.

Anesthesia care falls into three parts: the preoperative visit, the care during the operation, and the postoperative management in the recovery room or the intensive care unit.

Preoperative Visit

Unless you and/or your surgeon have requested an anesthetic consultation beforehand, the first time you will likely meet an anesthetist (anesthesiologist in the United States) is the night before or the day of your surgery.

The anesthetist will want to know about any allergies, drugs currently or recently (within the past six months) taken, any personal or family history of a bad experience with anesthesia, any history of chest pain, shortness of breath, heartburn, excess smoking, alcohol, narcotics or other medical problems. It is very important to be honest about the use of drugs and alcohol, because of the potential problems with the anesthetic and surgery.

The ideal patient for anesthesia is not excessively overweight or underweight, is pink (well oxygenated), has a normal regular heartbeat, normal exercise tolerance (i.e., no chest pain or shortness of breath), and is conscious and able to move arms and legs appropriately.

Lab tests before anesthetic and the surgery include blood and urine, chest X-rays, and an electrocardiogram (ECG) if the patient is over 45, or if the need is otherwise indicated.

For some complicated medical conditions, or in cases of major anesthetic risk, it is wise to consult the anesthetist even before making the decision to have surgery.

Many patients' worst fears about surgery relate to anesthesia:

- "Must I have a needle?"
- "I hate masks, or anything on my face!"
- "Will the tube damage my teeth when I've just paid my dentist a fortune for them?"
- "Do I have to remove my nail polish and take out my false teeth?"
- "If I have a local anesthetic, what happens if I want to scratch or go to the bathroom in the middle?"
- "I'm a singer . . . I don't want any tubes down my throat!"
- "Why do I have to take my underwear off when they are going to operate on my hand?"
- "Don't give me any blood transfusions . . . I don't want AIDS!"

It is very important if you have questions like these to talk to your anesthetist.

For elective patients, the anesthetist who sees you before surgery may not be the one who eventually gives you your anesthetic. In most hospitals, the anesthetists work as a team, and the cases are assigned randomly. It is, however, possible for the patient to request a specific anesthetist.

For emergencies, or for outpatients who arrive at the hospital on the day of the operation, the anesthetist will likely see you just before you enter the operating room or, sometimes, in the operating room itself.

Some anesthetists will allow you into the operating room wearing nail polish or false teeth, but many won't. The reasons are that they need to look at your nails to check your color, and there is a fear you could swallow false teeth. Hospitals do not wish to be liable for any misadventure that could occur through wearing nail polish or not removing false teeth.

Sometimes elective surgery is cancelled or delayed because the patient forgot instructions not to eat or drink anything the night before, or has just developed a cold. A full stomach makes vomiting and inhaling stomach contents into the lungs more likely; a cold may lead to pneumonia in the postoperative period. Surgery is best postponed in these situations if there is no emergency.

Drugs are often given orally or by injection before anesthesia and surgery, to relieve pain, calm anxious nerves, and to prevent excessive salivation which may be a nuisance during operations like teeth extractions.

One real fear, hardly mentioned, is the risk of anesthesia. It is difficult, perhaps impossible, to determine this risk accurately. There are many factors to take into account: the patient's condition, the surgeon and the type of surgery, the anesthetist and the anesthetic.

The risks of anesthesia are similar to those of driving a car, or walking along the street. We all accept that there are car accidents and that people do get mugged, but we still drive and walk every day. If the risks of anesthesia are major, I tell patients that it is similar to the roads being treacherous, or the neighborhood being a tough one, with poorly lit streets. If the risks are really high and outweigh the potential benefits of the surgery, I tell patients to stay home if at all possible!

Anesthetic-related deaths are of great concern to us all. Exact figures are difficult to obtain; they differ from country to country, and hospital to hospital, but generally the odds of a healthy person dying from anesthesia is approximately one in 15,000.

During the Operation

During the operation, the anesthetist's main role is to prevent pain and monitor all aspects of the patient's oxygenation and ventilation, and circulation. In special cases, such as brain, heart and transplant surgery, the anesthetist may help the surgeon even more by controlling the patient's blood pressure, heart rate, intracranial pressure and body temperature. (Lowering the blood pressure decreases bleeding and improves the surgeon's view of the operative field.)

If relaxing the muscles is required to improve the surgeon's operative field, a specific muscle relaxant drug is used during general anesthetic. If muscle relaxants are used, the patient should be artificially ventilated, since normal spontaneous breathing may not be adequate if the diaphragm (the main breathing muscle) is weak or paralyzed.

If the patient is being artificially ventilated, the breathing passage is secured open by inserting a plastic endotracheal tube (Fig. 3.4) via the mouth into the windpipe. This tube is then connected to the anesthetic breathing circuit.

If oral surgery is to be performed and the tube obstructs surgical vision and access to the mouth, the tube may be inserted via the nose. Because the gases inhaled are absolutely dry and the tube itself is an irritant, patients frequently have hoarseness, sore throat, cough and sometimes nose bleeds. Fortunately, none of these is prolonged or serious.

A general anesthetic is similar to an airplane flight. The dangerous times are take-off and landing; in between is cruising or maintenance of the anesthetic while the surgeon operates. The anesthetist's job is to give the surgeon the best possible operating conditions compatible with patient safety. This involves preventing pain (analgesia), putting you to sleep (anesthesia), and providing muscle relaxation, if necessary.

If you are awake when you are taken to the operating room, do not be alarmed by all the equipment in the room. You will be transferred to the operating table and attached to the necessary equipment for monitoring your heart rate, blood pressure and pulse. None of these is painful (Fig. 3.5).

Oxygenation and Ventilation

A prime responsibility of the anesthetist is to ensure that the brain, heart, lungs, kidneys, liver and spinal cord are being adequately supplied with oxygen. Oxygenation is assessed by skin color, heart rate and the patient's level of consciousness. Ventilation is assessed by respiratory rate, volume of each breath and the inhaled and exhaled carbon dioxide concentration.

The anesthetic gas and oxygen are delivered together via a mask or an endotracheal tube. If a mask is used, the patient usually breathes on his or her

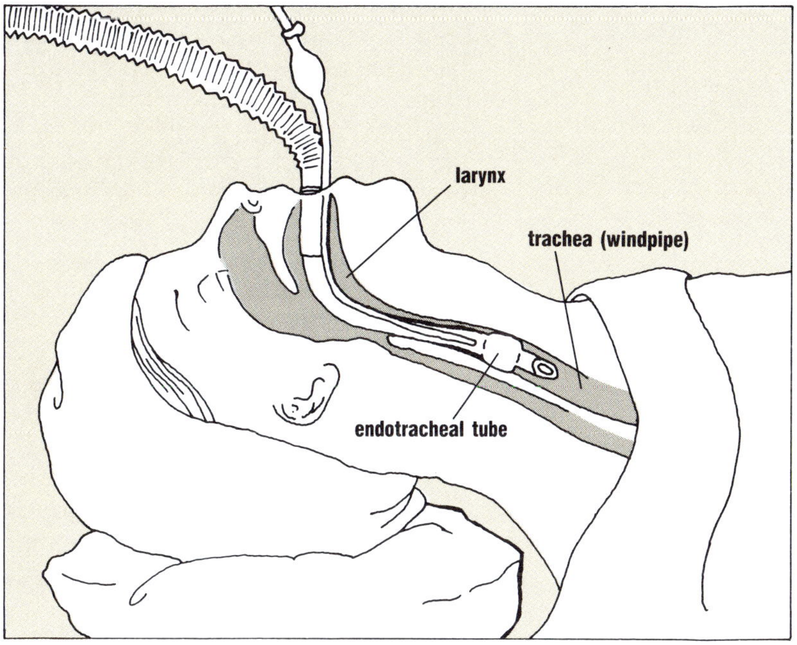

Figure 3.4
Endotracheal tube.

Figure 3.5
Operating room equipment.

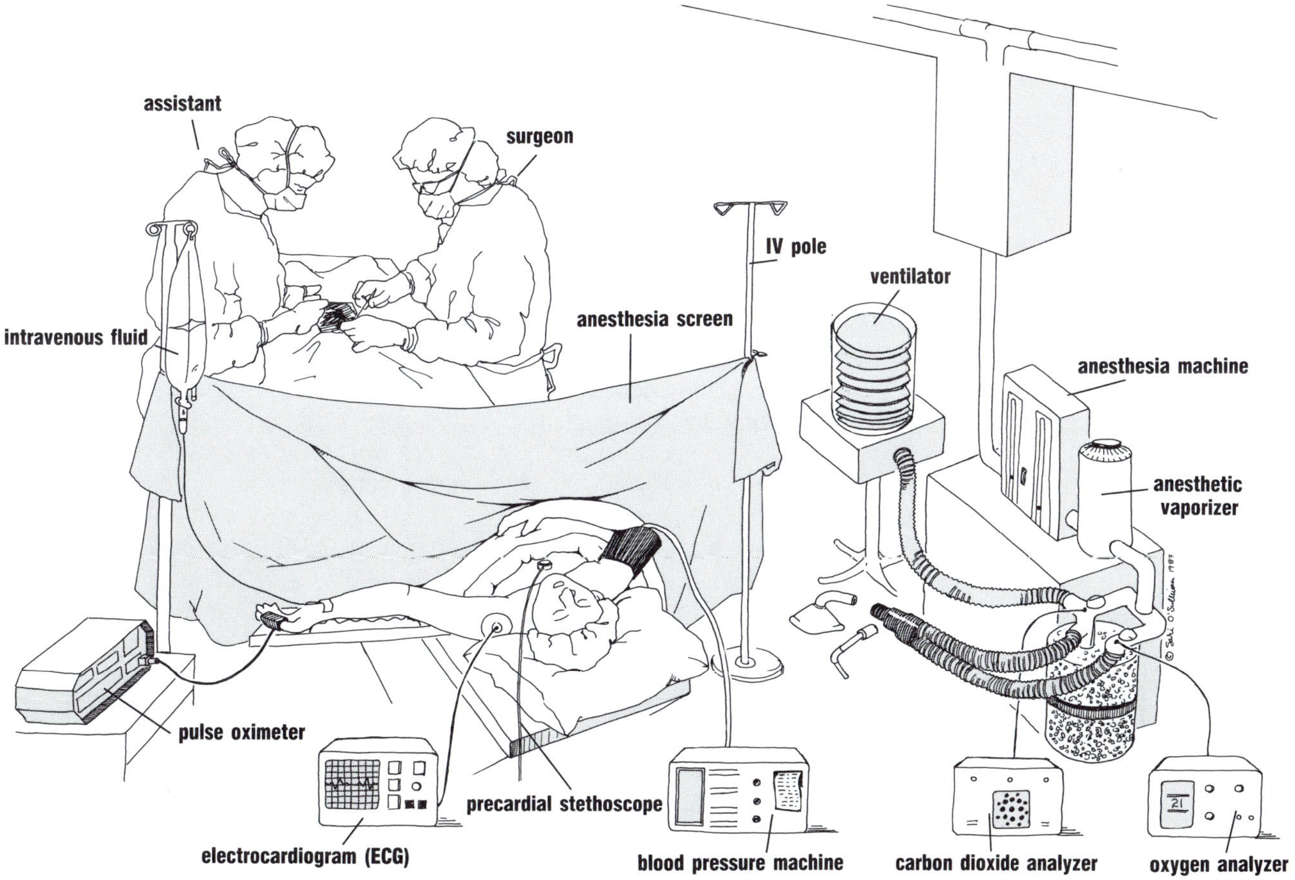

own. If the tube is used, the patient may breathe spontaneously, or be mechanically ventilated using an artificial ventilator.

Oxygen reaches the blood by first being inhaled in normal breathing, or blown into the lungs using an artificial ventilator. The lung consists of millions of tiny air sacs called alveoli (Fig. 3.6). Each alveolar sac is separated from a tiny blood vessel (capillary) by an extremely thin membrane which allows oxygen and carbon dioxide to pass through. Oxygen becomes bound to hemoglobin in the red blood cells, and is transported via the circulation to the body tissues. In exchange, carbon dioxide and water are taken up by the circulation and subsequently excreted. Carbon dioxide is excreted by the lungs, and water, in the form of urine, is excreted by the kidneys.

Circulation

During the operation, the anesthetist also monitors the patient's circulation and administers blood transfusions, if necessary. Circulation is assessed by blood pressure, urine output and skin temperature.

Blood transfusions may be done as whole blood, containing all the components. A special request may be required for this. Most commonly, stored blood that provides only red blood cells is used. This is called red cell concentrate or "packed cells." Red blood cells contain hemoglobin, the compound that combines with oxygen and transports it. The amount of oxygen in the blood will depend on the hemoglobin content.

Blood donations are screened for hepatitis B and AIDS. The screening test for AIDS is approximately 95 percent accurate. It is possible for a donor to have contracted the virus without yet having a positive blood test, which takes about six weeks to three months to show up. However, the possibility of getting AIDS through blood transfusions is very low.

Many hospitals have started autotransfusion programs. This means the patients donate their own blood once a week for one month before the scheduled surgery. Then if a blood transfusion is required during surgery, they are given their own blood. Estimating the amount of blood that might be needed is based on previous blood requirements during specific operations. For example, for a hip replacement, two units of blood are provided, based on previous experience of blood loss during that operation.

Normal individuals may lose 10 percent of their blood volume with no risk. During surgery and anesthesia, we commonly allow a blood loss of 25 to 30 percent of the patient's estimated blood volume before transfusing blood, since the oxygenation of the tissues is unaffected even when this level is reached. The decision to give a transfusion is made by the anesthetist and the surgeon. The anesthetist administers the blood through an intravenous line.

Postoperative Care

After surgery, you are taken to the recovery room, usually breathing on your own. The anesthetic is usually allowed to wear off naturally. The time taken to excrete the anesthetic drugs varies with different patients and with the same patient at different times, depending partly on the drugs given, and how well the kidneys, liver and heart are functioning. The duration of the after-effects of general anesthesia is entirely unpredictable.

It is common to wake up with an oxygen mask on your face. The added oxygen helps to maintain adequate oxygenation while you are still drowsy.

Your vital signs (pulse, respiration, blood pressure and, if necessary, temperature) are monitored closely in the recovery room, since your stay here is an extension of the anesthetic period. You will remain in the recovery room until your vital signs are stable — usually about one to two hours.

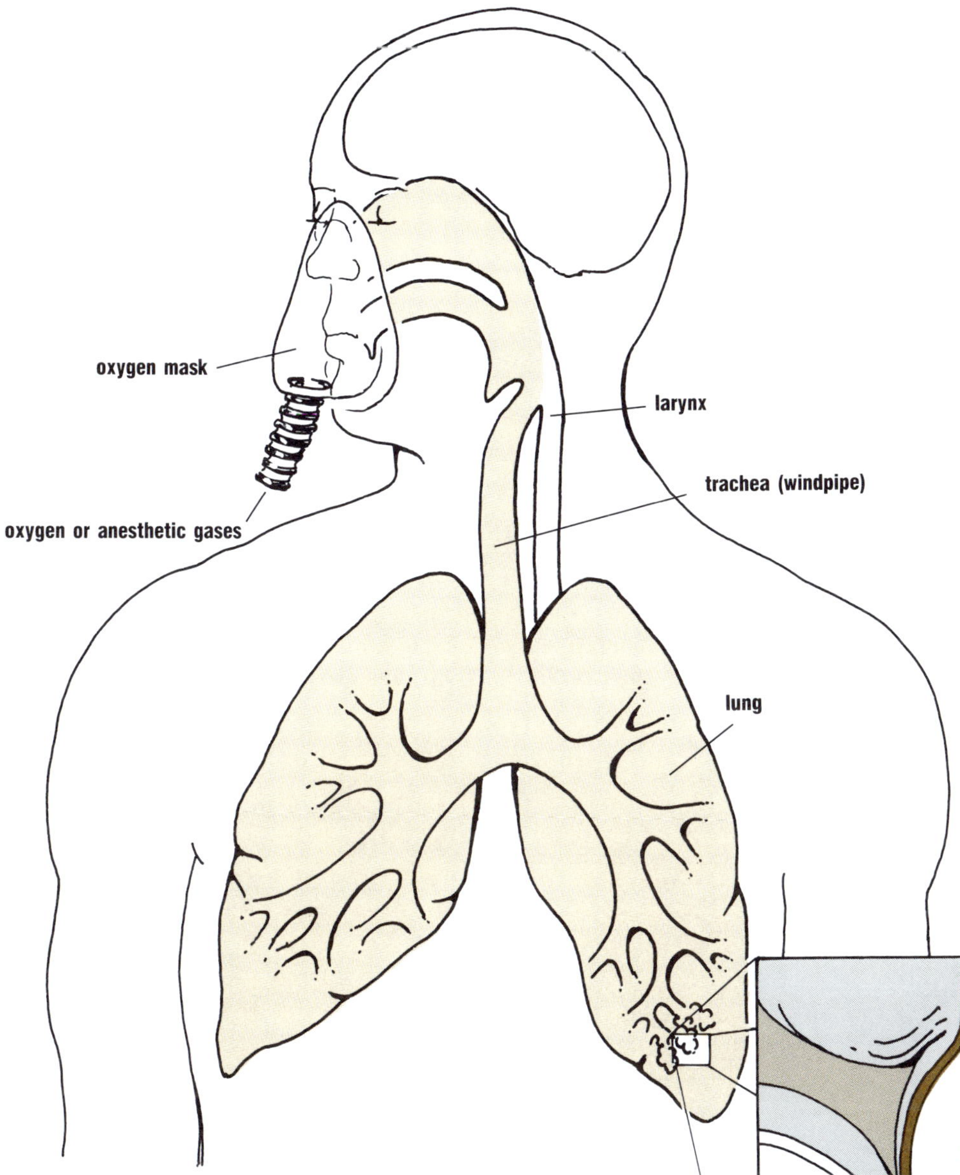

Figure 3.6
Gas exchange in the lungs. Oxygen is inhaled into the lungs, where it passes into the bloodstream in exchange for carbon dioxide, which is excreted by the lungs.

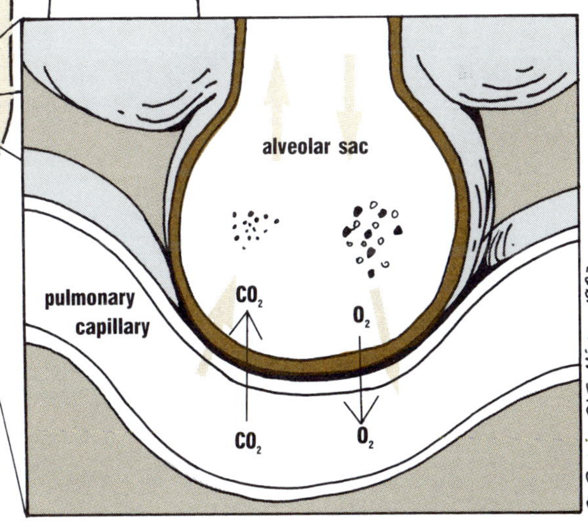

Enlargement of alveolar sac to show O_2-CO_2 exchange.

A major problem in the immediate postoperative period is the control of pain. When you awake in a strange environment, you become anxious, your heart rate speeds up, your blood pressure increases and there is a gradual (sometimes not so gradual) awareness of pain. You may need narcotics for pain relief, but these drugs can make you drowsier and may depress your breathing further, even to the point of causing a respiratory arrest.

The alternative to narcotics is nerve blocks using local anesthetics. Unfortunately, these blocks do not last long — usually two to 12 hours, depending on the specific nerve blocked and the anesthetic injected. But pain from an incision may continue for days. Repeating the blocks can be uncomfortable for patients and time-consuming for the nurses and doctors, so only patients with bad lung disease, whose breathing we cannot risk depressing by narcotics or other drugs, usually receive nerve blocks, even though most postoperative patients would benefit from their use. The pain relief and general well-being of a properly nerve-blocked patient is often better than can be obtained using narcotics.

Narcotics are sometimes injected into the epidural space. This method is safe and effective, provided precautions are taken, often including monitoring in an intensive care unit. For this reason, the technique is not used in most patients. There simply are not enough intensive care beds available.

Recent Advances

As the cost of in-hospital stay increases, it makes better economic sense to do more outpatient surgery. Anesthesia for outpatients demands drugs that act and wear off rapidly. Patients must be fit for street traffic as soon as possible after their surgery. For this reason, a new intravenous anesthetic called propofol (Diprivan) may replace Pentothal.

Chapter 4

General Complications of Surgery

Alan W. Harrison
Professor of Surgery
University of Toronto
Vice-President, Medical Affairs
Sunnybrook Medical Centre, Toronto

Megan Welsh
Illustrator

All surgical procedures, whether major (requiring general anesthesia and/or more than one hour of surgery) or minor (with or without general anesthesia) carry some risk. After all, surgery is a form of trauma; the more extensive the surgery, the greater the trauma, both psychologically and physically.

It is the surgeon's job to weigh the risk of possible complications from surgery against the potential benefits of the surgery for the individual patient. In order for the surgeon to decide that the procedure is warranted, the potential benefits should outweigh the potential complications.

Complications are medically described in terms of "morbidity" and "mortality" rates. The latter is self-explanatory. Any death in hospital within one month of surgery is considered a complication of the surgery, even when the cause of death is a seemingly unrelated disease process, such as a stroke or heart attack. "Morbidity" is any complication that injures but doesn't kill. This could be wound infection, thrombophlebitis or pneumonia.

Complications of surgery have four major causes: those related to the patient's mental and physical health, those related to the anesthesia (see chapter 3), those related to the specific surgery performed, and those complications related to operations in general or to other treatment the patient receives while in the hospital.

Patient Factors

The patient's age, preexisting diseases, nutritional status, drugs (including alcohol and tobacco) and infections all influence the risks of surgery. Other factors are more unpredictable. Good mental attitude, tolerance to pain and discomfort, and the ability to cooperate and participate in the convalescence are vital for a smooth recovery, whether the patient is having his or her appendix out or a lung removed. The patient who refuses to move, to take deep breaths, or to cough because it hurts too much, is often a more likely candidate for complications — or at least a more prolonged recovery period. A good mental attitude and a will to recover is particularly beneficial for patients undergoing extensive cancer surgery.

Age

Age alone is no contraindication to surgery. In elective surgery, such as hip replacement or gallbladder removal, the patient over age 60 has a 5 times greater chance of dying from the operation in comparison to a younger patient. However, in the case of major emergency surgery, such as for bowel obstruction or perforated ulcer, the risk is 20 times greater for the patient over 60.

The compounding factor in the elderly is their higher incidence of coexisting diseases, particularly heart disease, lung disease and diabetes. Adding the morbidity and mortality rate of these diseases to the risk of surgery can make elderly patients "poor" risks for surgery.

Older patients generally have higher thresholds for pain and are often more likely to cooperate and accept instructions. Consequently, many older patients will do very well after surgery, unless a major complication or setback occurs. However, their recuperative powers are diminished as a natural consequence of aging.

Preexisting Disease

Coronary Artery Disease

Patients who have had a previous heart attack or who have angina (caused by insufficient blood supply to the heart muscle) have a higher risk of heart attack after surgery.

The incidence of heart attack as a complication of surgery is approximately 0.15 percent overall. In patients who have had a heart attack more than six months before surgery, the incidence is 5 percent. The incidence of heart attack increases proportionally to the interval of time between a previous heart attack and the surgery (the risk of a new heart attack is 33 percent if the surgery is done within three months of a previous heart attack).

High Blood Pressure (Hypertension)

If high blood pressure is lowered with medication before surgery, the patient is at no increased risk for surgery. If high blood pressure is not lowered, the risk of heart attack or stroke is significant. In general, hypertension medication is continued up until and including the day of surgery.

Heart Failure

Heart failure (when the heart is unable to pump blood at an adequate rate) may cause shortness of breath, inability to lie flat at night or leg swelling. Heart failure must be treated before surgery, because

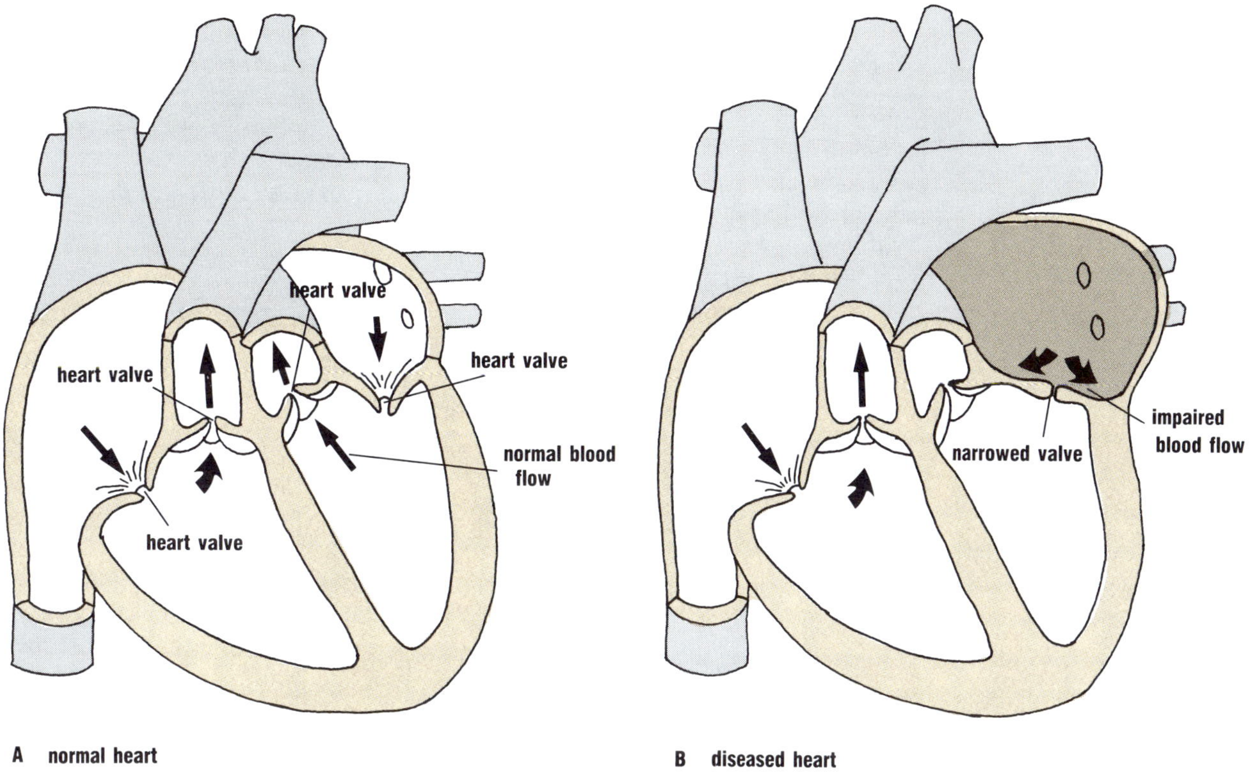

Figure 4.1
Heart valve disease. In a normal heart (A), blood flows freely through the valves. When the valves are narrowed (stenosis) from disease, the blood flow is impaired (B).

a diseased heart may respond poorly to the extra demands placed on it by surgery.

Heart Valve Disease

Diseased heart valves impair normal heart function and limit the heart's reserve, increasing the risk of surgery (Fig. 4.1). These patients are given antibiotics before, during and after the operation to prevent infection on the diseased valves.

Patients who have had previous valve replacement surgery must stop taking anticoagulants (blood thinners) before surgery, and resume taking them after the operation.

Changes in Heart Rate and Rhythm

Drugs can take care of this condition which, when treated, does not significantly increase the risk of surgery as long as the underlying heart condition is under control.

Pacemakers

The presence of these devices alone (see chapter 14) does not increase the risk of surgery. However, a cardiologist's assessment is important, and both the surgeon and the anesthetist must know the type of pacemaker the patient has and whether it is functioning properly. Electrocautery (a metal cauterizing instrument heated by electricity) must not be used in the vicinity of the pacemaker because it can cause electromagnetic interference, blocking the normal function of the pacemaker.

Lung Disease

A lung disease such as emphysema causes the lungs to lose their elasticity.

This interferes with breathing and the condition can worsen after an operation. The individual's lung disability must be completely evaluated before the operation, and lung function must be stabilized before surgery. Such patients may have to be on a respirator after surgery, because weakness, pain and discomfort may inhibit chest movement.

All lung diseases should be properly treated before surgery, because complications such as lung collapse and pneumonia are an increased risk. This also applies to the common cold; patients booked for surgery should notify their surgeon if they have a cold.

Diabetes and Other Metabolic Diseases

Well-controlled diabetes does not increase the risk of surgery. Naturally, specific precautions must be taken to maintain control of the diabetes and other metabolic diseases (such as Addison's disease and gout) before, during and immediately after surgery — when the patient is unable to eat or to take medications by mouth.

Vascular Disease

Patients with varicose veins (see chapter 13) commonly ask if they are in danger of "throwing off" clots to their lungs. If they have superficial varicose veins and have good postoperative care, their chances of suffering a pulmonary embolism (blood clot in the lung) are no greater than normal. The risk of pulmonary embolism is greater, however, in patients who have had previous deep venous thrombophlebitis (clotting in the deeper veins in the legs). These patients may have a long history of a chronic swollen leg and may have had problems with ankle ulcerations.

Hardening of the arteries (arteriosclerosis) causes narrowing of the arteries, which increases the risk of strokes, heart attacks and circulation problems in the legs as a complication of surgery.

Allergies and Drug Sensitivities

Both the surgeon and the anesthetist must be aware of any known allergies that the patient may have. Some patients will have reactions to certain pain medication, antibiotics or certain anesthetics and sedatives. Knowledge of such allergies can prevent an unnecessary complication.

Blood Disorders

Anemia, the most common blood disorder, occurs when the blood's oxygen-carrying capacity is decreased. Provided the anemia has been treated, and the patient's hemoglobin is at acceptable levels, the risk of surgery is not increased. Sometimes a transfusion is required before the operation.

Some relatively rare disorders of blood clotting can cause severe postoperative bleeding. Most of these are inherited diseases, so the patient is usually aware of the problem. Properly treated before, during and after surgery, these disorders will not significantly increase the risk of complications. Patients who are aware of abnormal bruising or bleeding in the past should report this to their surgeon so that proper treatment can be instituted if necessary.

Certain drugs, other than traditional anticoagulants (blood thinners) such as heparin and coumadin, can cause increased bleeding. Aspirin is the most common. It lowers the blood's ability to clot. Such drugs should not be taken for at least one week before surgery.

Kidney and Other Urinary Tract Disease

Patients with impaired kidney function accumulate waste products and cannot maintain normal levels of body fluids and electrolytes. This places them at increased risk after surgery, which involves further losses of body fluids and electrolytes. Patients with kidney impairment must often take smaller doses of drugs, since the kidneys can no longer break down and eliminate the full dose, which would then accumulate in the body, potentially reaching toxic levels.

For surgery such as hernia repair, prostate obstruction should be treated first. Otherwise the hernia will likely recur because of the pressure exerted each time the patient has to urinate.

Liver Disease

The liver is responsible for many important body functions, such as protein production for body repair, manufacture of blood clotting factors, storage of sugar for body energy and detoxification of drugs. Significant liver disease greatly increases the risk of surgery, because any major surgery will temporarily decrease liver function even further and could precipitate liver failure.

Although alcoholic cirrhosis is the most common form of liver disease seen in North America, hepatitis B is on the increase. It can be transmitted to the surgeon in body fluid via a cut, contaminated needle or a mucous membrane. Because jaundice is a symptom of hepatitis B, it is important that anyone who has had jaundice (not due to gallstones) be tested before surgery. Once the risk is known, the necessary precautions can be taken to decrease the danger.

Nutrition

Malnutrition

This has three major causes: inadequate food intake, inability of the intestine to absorb the food, or loss of nutrients due to chronic intestinal problems.

Malnutrition interferes with normal healing and increases the body's susceptibility to infection. Malnourished patients experience a greater incidence of incision separation, incision infection and breakdown of tissue repairs.

The biggest medical advance in treating malnutrition has been the ability to feed patients totally through an intravenous line. Nutritional problems can now be corrected before surgery, so that patients have fewer complications and a shorter convalescence.

Obesity

Patients who are 15 percent or more over their ideal weight have more postoperative complications such as pulmonary embolism, pneumonia, heart attack and stroke. Also, some operations (abdominal and pelvic surgery) can be technically much more difficult, or even impossible, because of the obesity.

Infectious Diseases

Infectious diseases such as AIDS, hepatitis B and tuberculosis all increase the risk of surgery for the patient. They may also put health care personnel at risk. An awareness of these conditions allows precautions to be taken to ensure the best treatment for the patient and the safety of those providing care.

Drugs and Surgery

Medications

The anesthetist and the surgeon must be aware of all medications a patient is taking, since some may alter the normal response to anesthesia and to the stress of surgery (See chapter 3.)

Non-Medicinal Chemicals

The three most habitually used chemicals are alcohol, tranquilizers and tobacco. Patients who stop taking these drugs may suffer withdrawal symptoms. Delirium following alcohol withdrawal, for example, significantly increases the mortality rate after surgery. In addition, chronic use of alcohol interferes with healing, so that incision separation is much more common in the alcoholic.

Addictive drugs such as morphine and cocaine are all associated with severe withdrawal symptoms. They may also be associated with malnutrition, other diseases and an impaired body immune system, all of which increase the risk of complications from surgery.

Habitual smokers have a higher incidence of emphysema, bronchitis and vascular disease, all of which increase the risk of surgery.

Possible Complications for all Surgery

Incision Complications

Infection

Infection is caused by bacteria entering the operative site. Fortunately, not all wounds that are contaminated with bacteria develop infections; it depends on the amount of bacteria and the patient's resistance, or ability to kill the bacteria. However, even in operations such as hernia repair, there is an infection rate of 1 to 3 percent. Certain diseases or drugs, obesity, malignancy, age or malnutrition all reduce the body's defenses and predispose it to infection.

Sources of infection from the patient may be bacteria on the patient's skin or normal bacterial inhabitants of the gastrointestinal, respiratory or genitourinary tract, which can contaminate the area of surgery. The type of surgery and the circumstances surrounding the operation are also factors. In emergency surgery, circumstances may not be ideal. The bowel may not have been emptied in the case of bowel surgery, or there may be acute inflammation or infection at the site of the operation, as in the case of a ruptured appendix. Infection of the wound in uncomplicated, acute appendicitis occurs in 15 percent of cases. That rate doubles if the appendix ruptures.

Wounds from injuries occurring in road accidents, industrial accidents or sports also have a high infection rate because dirt is often introduced with the injury. Generally, the surgery should be done as soon as possible. The patient's skin should be shaved and painted with a surface disinfectant (prepped) in the operating room immediately before the procedure so that the skin will be as free of bacteria as possible.

Wound infections become apparent about four or five days after surgery, with pain, swelling, redness and fever. The usual treatment is surgical drainage; antibiotics are generally reserved for those cases that do not respond to simple drainage.

The surgeon and operating-room staff can also take steps to decrease the infection rate. This means good preoperative preparation, including improving the patient's nutrition, using antibiotics, handling tissues as little as possible, using as few sutures as possible, using closed suction drains well away from the site of the incision and practicing good sterile technique.

Wound Separation

Wound separation (dehiscence) generally refers to separation of an abdominal wound. The incidence is approximately 2.5 percent and increases with age, malignancy, protein malnutrition, vitamin C deficiency (scurvy), coughing, obesity, hemorrhage, infection and excessive use of sutures. Usually the disruption occurs around the fifth day after the operation and is preceded by some bloody discharge. Treatment consists of closing the wound again.

Incision Hernia

If the muscle and tendinous layers of the abdomen do not heal properly after abdominal surgery, an incisional hernia can result. Infection and/or obesity are predisposing factors. Since the hernia is usually quite large, strangulation (cutting off the blood supply) is rare. The hernia can generally be repaired surgically, depending on the patient's overall disability.

Keloid

A keloid is a distorted, raised and extended incisional scar. It is an exaggeration of the normal healing process. Some people, particularly those with dark skin, are genetically predisposed to form keloids. Unfortunately, it is often difficult to predict which patients have this predisposition. Keloids occur more often with incisions in areas such as the abdomen. Besides the disfiguration, the keloid is often itchy and sensitive. In some cases actual bone is deposited in the deeper areas of the incision. Many efforts have been made to prevent keloids, including radiation and cortisone both in the incision and via the bloodstream, but to date there is no absolute way of predicting, preventing or curing keloid formation. It can, however, often be minimized by choice of incision, prevention of wound infection and by the use of cortisone.

Respiratory Complications

Respiratory problems are the prime cause of postoperative mortality, accounting for 25 percent of deaths following surgery. They are a major contributing factor to another 25 percent.

Atelectasis

Collapse of the lung, or atelectasis, accounts for 90 percent of all postoperative lung complications. It occurs when a bronchial tube becomes blocked by mucous secretions and there is no air flow to the air sacs in the lungs (Fig. 4.2). Fever and increased heart rate are early signs.

Atelectasis will occur to some degree in 38 percent of patients undergoing chest and abdominal surgery, but in only 3 percent of patients undergoing surgery in other areas such as limbs, neck or brain. Patients who have undergone chest and abdominal surgery are reluctant to breathe deeply or cough, because it hurts. Consequently, the secretions are not coughed up and the bronchial tubes may become blocked. Smoking, chronic bronchitis, asthma, oversedation (which reduces the cough reflex and depth of breathing) and restrictive dressings all predispose the patient to postoperative atelectasis.

The treatment is vigorous physiotherapy to encourage deep breathing and coughing, and antibiotics.

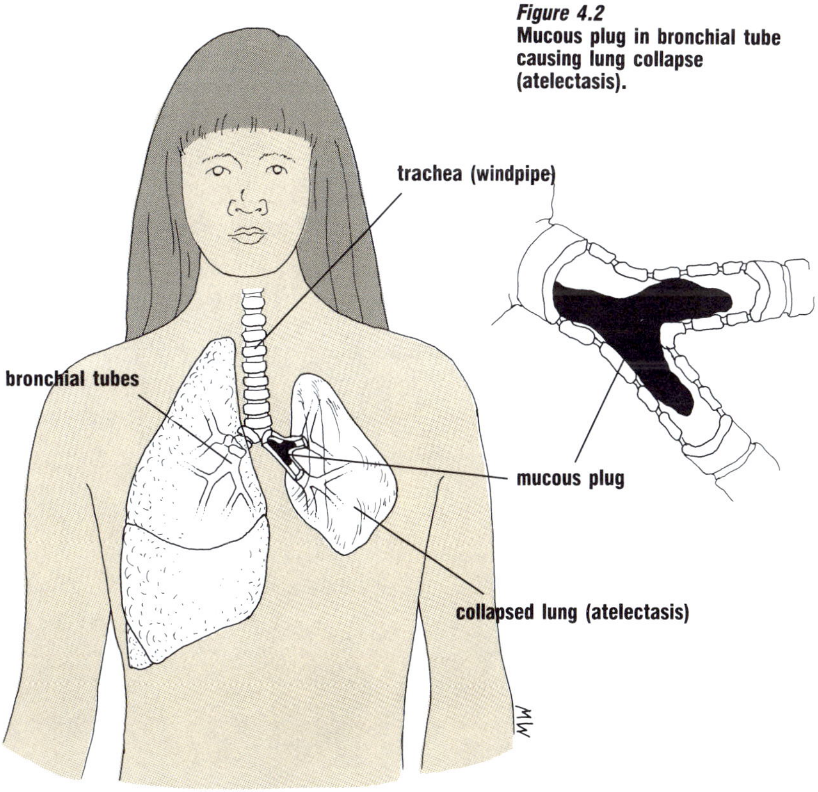

Figure 4.2
Mucous plug in bronchial tube causing lung collapse (atelectasis).

Pneumonia

Pneumonia, an acute lung infection, may complicate persistent or neglected atelectasis, existing lung disease or prolonged tracheal intubation (a breathing tube inserted down the patient's throat).

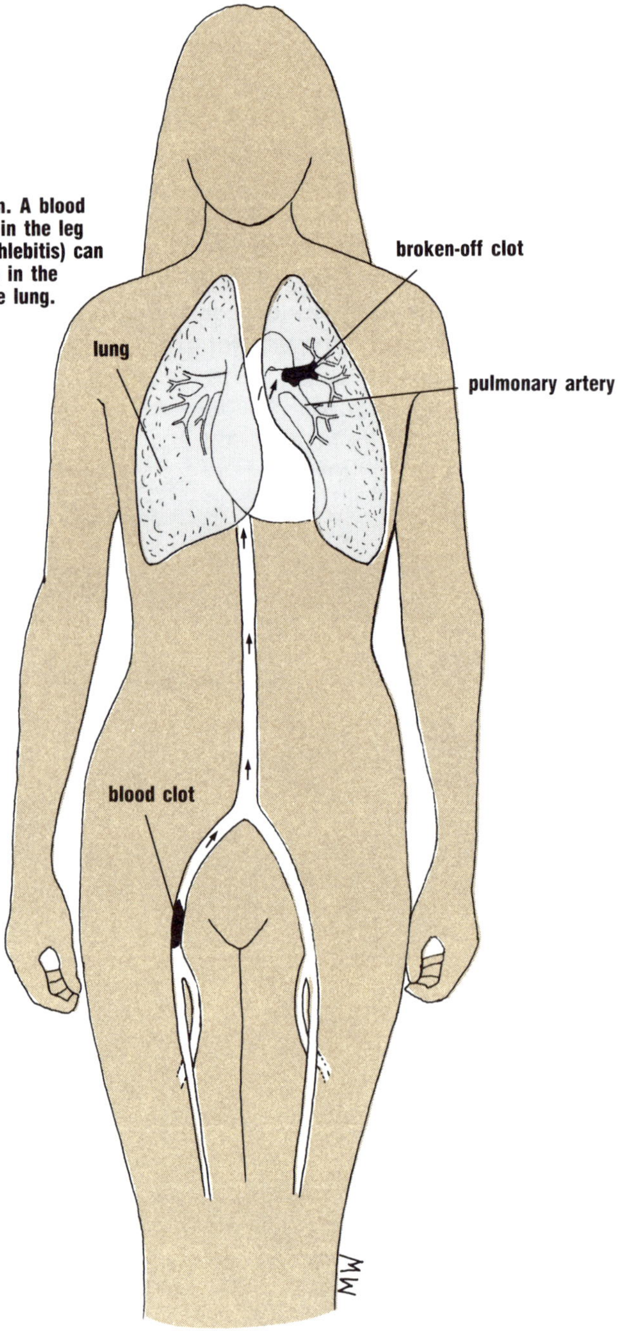

Figure 4.3
Pulmonary embolism. A blood clot in a deep vein in the leg or pelvis (thrombophlebitis) can break off and lodge in the major vessels of the lung.

Pulmonary Edema

Pulmonary edema (fluid in the lungs) may result from a combination of excess intravenous fluid and the heart's inability to function as a satisfactory pump. The lungs then flood from the back-up pressure. Fluid leaks out of the lung capillaries into the air sacs and produces frothy, bloody sputum. Emergency measures to reduce the fluid load, maintain oxygenation and improve heart function must be instituted if the patient is to survive. Maintaining a proper fluid balance can be a major challenge in many patients with severe heart disease.

Pulmonary Embolism

Pulmonary embolism occurs when blood clots from the deep veins in the legs or pelvis (thrombophlebitis, see page 39) break off and lodge in the major vessels of the lung (Fig. 4.3). If the clot is large enough, all circulation to the lungs may be instantly cut off, resulting in immediate death. Fortunately, in most cases the clots are small and produce only transient symptoms of shortness of breath and/or minor chest pain. Some patients may cough up blood.

Pulmonary embolism is the most common cause of sudden unexpected death following surgery. The risk is higher in the elderly, the obese, the immobilized patient and the patient with multiple injuries including fractures. It is a relatively rare complication in the healthy young adult, although the risk does increase with certain types of surgery, such as pelvic and hip operations. Overall, the incidence of pulmonary embolism varies from 0.1 to 0.5 percent, depending on the surgery and the patient's age and state of health.

Pulmonary embolism must be suspected if there is any unusual shortness of breath and/or chest pain. Diagnosis is often made by a lung scan, which is done by injecting a small, safe dose of a radioactive substance intravenously.

The treatment for pulmonary embolism

consists of painkillers, oxygen to reduce breathing difficulties, and bed rest to reduce the possibility of further embolism. Anticoagulants (blood thinners) such as heparin and coumadin are given to prevent further clot formation in the veins of the legs and/or pelvis.

Surgery is rarely done to remove blood clots in the lung, because the mortality rate is high. However, in some situations, such as patients recovering from brain surgery, anticoagulants cannot be used. In this situation it may be necessary to tie off or place a filter in the main vein into which the veins of the legs and pelvis drain.

Cardiovascular Complications

Heart Complications

The two most common postoperative heart complications are heart attack and heart failure (see page 32). The very stress of surgery can precipitate a heart attack in people with coronary artery disease, which may or may not have caused symptoms before the surgery. A heart attack is the second most common cause of sudden unexpected death in the postoperative patient.

Heart failure generally occurs in patients with previously diagnosed heart disease. It can be precipitated by the increased strain put on the heart from the stress of surgery and the subsequent extra load placed on it from the use of intravenous fluids.

Vascular Complications

Arterial Thrombosis

Clotting of the blood in the artery (arterial thrombosis) is almost unknown in healthy young individuals. It usually occurs in patients with hardening of the arteries, where cholesterol builds up on the lining of the artery, causing narrowing of the vessel and eddying of blood flow (blood does not progress normally through the channel, but instead forms little whirlpools). If there is any decrease in blood flow and blood pressure during or following surgery, the blood clotting will likely occur at the narrowed sites. If the clot occurs in the carotid (neck) vessels, stroke may occur; in the coronary arteries of the heart, a heart attack may be the result; if it occurs in the legs, numbness and coldness will likely result.

In the legs, the process may not cause any immediate symptoms, but may become apparent during convalescence when the patient finds walking difficult because of aching and tightening in the calf muscle.

Thrombophlebitis (Phlebitis)

Thrombophlebitis (blood clotting in a vein) is a common postoperative complication. The major cause is immobilization associated with surgery (e.g., surgery of a fractured hip). This is why great emphasis is placed on early mobilization of the patient after surgery.

Previous vein disease increases the incidence of thrombophlebitis. The birth control pill increases the tendency of the blood to coagulate, and therefore can increase the risk of thrombophlebitis. Women should not resume taking the pill until they have recovered from surgery.

The symptoms vary greatly. There may be no symptoms. If the calf veins are affected and there are symptoms, the calf may be tender and firm, aching when the patient is standing. If the larger deep veins of the upper thigh and pelvis are involved and there are symptoms, then the whole leg may swell and ache. It is when thigh and pelvic veins are involved that pulmonary embolism can occur if a piece of the clot breaks away and travels up into the lung vessels. (See page 38.) If the superficial varicose veins clot, there may be local redness and tenderness over the ropy veins that can be felt under the skin, a condition called superficial phlebitis, which rarely causes pulmonary embolism.

Diagnosis can be confirmed by injecting radioactive substances and then scanning the leg, or by injecting contrast material into the veins of the foot, and following the course of the contrast material up the vein by X-ray.

The best treatment is prevention, which is why all patients who can walk are encouraged to do so as soon as they have recovered from the anesthetic. Patients of high risk, such as the patient who has suffered thrombophlebitis previously, are a special concern. Such patients should wear elastic stockings before and after the operation. Early and continued walking is a must. In selected cases mild anticoagulants are given before surgery and continued into the convalescent period.

Once thrombophlebitis has occurred, the treatment is bed rest, full length support stockings and anticoagulants. In most situations, recovery is complete. However, approximately 33 percent of patients who have suffered thrombophlebitis will have recurring episodes. In 5 percent of cases ulcers about the ankle may occur many years later.

Genito-Urinary Complications

Bladder Retention

The inability to urinate is a very common problem following any type of surgery, but is more common after surgery around the pelvic and genital areas. In the older male an enlarged prostrate is generally the cause. The problem is relieved by passing a catheter (tube) into the bladder and draining off the urine. The catheter may be left in place for several days or removed immediately after the bladder has been emptied.

Bladder and/or Kidney Infection

This is usually a complication of catheterization. Even with the best of techniques, occasional bladder infections are inevitable. The source of the infection is often a dormant bacterial organism in the urethra that is stirred up by the catheterization.

Kidney (Renal) Failure

This is fortunately uncommon, but may occur as a complication of very major surgery. The incidence of this complication has been reduced by more sophisticated means of maintaining the body's fluid and chemical balance after surgery.

Gastrointestinal Complications

Nausea

The most common postoperative complication is nausea. Intravenous feeding is generally all that is required. If nausea and vomiting persist, a tube passed through the nose into the stomach will decompress the stomach (Fig. 4.4). A nasogastric tube is used in most major abdominal surgery and removed when the patient is passing gas (flatus). The use of the tube allows the intestine to recover its normal muscle function and prevents abdominal distention, which might otherwise occur from gas trapped in the bowel.

Paralytic Ileus

Distention of the bowel with gas due to a temporary paralysis of the bowel from the surgery is called paralytic ileus. It causes the patient to vomit. A nasogastric tube is both the treatment and the prevention.

Hiccups

Hiccups may occur, particularly after upper abdominal surgery. Insertion of a nasogastric tube may relieve the problem by decompressing the stomach. Unfortunately, hiccups have no specific cause and no sure cure; they will follow their course. Irritation of the diaphragm is generally felt to be the precipitating factor.

Inhaling Vomit

This is a particular risk in the elderly and the sedated. Patients should lie on their side until fully awake or conscious.

Vomiting Blood

The stress of surgery can alter the resistance of the stomach lining to the gastric juices and acid, reactivating an old ulcer or causing a new one. These peptic ulcerations can bleed. This was once a major life-threatening complication, but is seen much less now and is better treated with new anti-ulcer drugs.

Constipation

This is frequently seen in the elderly. It is precipitated by the prolonged bed rest that can follow surgery and by the use of narcotics, which control pain but also depress bowel function. The problem can be prevented by the use of stool softeners and cathartic drugs to increase intestinal activity.

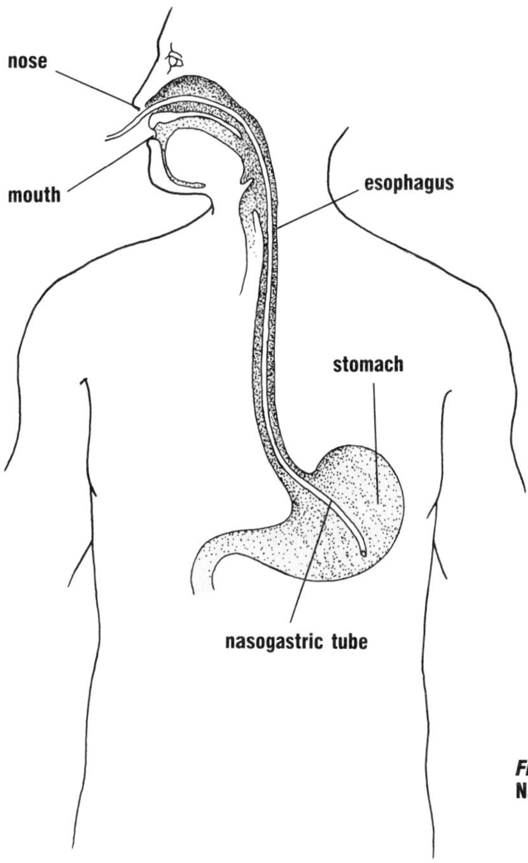

Figure 4.4
Nasogastric tube.

Mental and Neurological Complications

The most common neurological complication of surgery is stroke. Other neurological complications are exceedingly rare, except in surgery dealing directly with the central nervous system.

Postoperative disorientation is quite common in the elderly. It is precipitated by the stress of surgery and compounded by the fact that the patient is in unfamiliar surroundings, often with tubes coming out of various orifices. The condition is often called "moon madness," because the symptoms are worse at night. In most circumstances the patient returns to normal once all the tubes and intravenous lines are removed, but some elderly patients never fully recover. This factor must be weighed against the potential benefits of surgery when considering purely elective surgery in the very elderly.

True psychoses can occur following surgery but are rare. They are primarily due to withdrawal (generally from alcohol), or a serious metabolic or biochemical disorder, such as poorly controlled diabetes.

Sepsis (Infection)

The incidence of infection in surgical patients is approximately 7 percent. It may be limited to the incision (see page 36), or may cause general blood poisoning, with such symptoms as high fever, general toxicity and possibly shock. Sepsis accounts for one-third of all postoperative deaths. In order to decrease the incidence of infection, the surgeon attempts to identify and correct predisposing factors. Timing the operation when the patient is in optimal condition, judicious use of antibiotics where indicated, and containment of potential contamination at surgery are all important.

Factors which predispose patients to develop an infection include malnutrition, age, tissue trauma, diabetes, malignancy, concurrent infection, recent antibiotic therapy (which may allow other organisms not sensitive to the antibiotic to grow), immunosuppressive drugs, inability to mount a response to infection, obesity, indwelling catheters and prolonged preoperative hospital stay (which can expose patients to bacteria).

The infection, once diagnosed, is treated with antibiotics and drainage of pus, if present.

Drug Reactions

Allergic Reactions

These vary from a mild rash to an intense generalized body reaction that can result in sudden death. All other medications must be stopped, and the patient is given antihistamines, perhaps cortisone and, in a severe reaction, an immediate injection of adrenalin. The most common drug sensitivities are to penicillin, sulpha drugs and codeine.

Toxic Reactions

These are more common with certain drugs such as antibiotics or cancer drugs. Drug toxicity may damage the ear, liver, kidney or bone marrow. With the administration of certain intravenous antibiotics, blood levels may be measured daily to ensure that the dose used will fight the infection but won't cause further toxic reactions.

Antibiotic Diarrhea

Certain antibiotics kill the normal intestinal bacteria, which are then replaced with bacteria which can proliferate and produce intestinal inflammation.

Skin Complications

Bed sores result from prolonged pressure on the skin over bony prominences in patients who are severely debilitated and often in a poor state of nutrition. They occur most commonly over the lower spine (sacrum) and over the prominence of the hips. However, they may occur at the back of the heels or elbows. Bed sores are a particular problem in paraplegics. Prevention is the best treatment. This includes special mattresses and seating cushions, a specific nursing routine to encourage mobilization and avoid undue pressure on the target areas, good nutrition and appropriate general skin care.

Preventing Complications

The best treatment is always prevention. The patient, surgeon, nursing staff and hospital all play a role in preventing complications from surgery.

Patient's Responsibility

Patients should make every effort to improve their general health if they know they are to have surgery. This would involve curtailing tobacco and alcohol consumption, improving nutrition, weight loss where required, and a supervised program of physical activity. The patient should make the surgeon aware of any allergies and any medications being taken. The patient and the patient's family should thoroughly understand the reasons for the surgery, its nature, the major complications that could occur, the overall risks of the procedure and, of course, the anticipated benefits.

Following surgery, the patient should make every effort to follow the instructions of the surgeon, nurses, physiotherapists and other health professionals. This isn't always easy, since they may cause pain. Deep breathing and coughing, for example, are very important if the patient has had chest or abdominal surgery. Early walking, if possible, is beneficial in all surgery.

Surgeon's Responsibility

The surgeon should make every effort to maximize the patient's physical health before surgery, including consultation with an internist and anesthetist, particularly in patients with significant heart and/or lung disease.

The surgeon should inquire about any allergies or sensitivity reactions the patient has had in the past, and should be aware of all medications the patient has been taking in the past year. The surgeon must also be satisfied that the patient and interested family have been told the reasons for the surgery, the possible complications and the overall prognosis.

Following surgery, the surgeon should contact the patient's family, unless otherwise requested by the patient, and inform them of the patient's progress. Regular visits by the surgeon are both comforting to the patient and allow the surgeon to monitor the patient's progress. On discharge, the patient should be given instructions about diet, activity and a projected date for return to work. Arrangements should also be made for a follow-up visit if necessary.

Nurses' Responsibility

A good relationship between the nurses and the patient does wonders in overcoming a patient's fears and anxieties. The nurses prepare the patient for the upcoming surgery, including drug administration, enemas and perhaps shaving the site of the incision. After surgery, nurses provide round-the-clock care — getting the patient out of bed, monitoring food and fluid intake, bowel and bladder infection, temperature and pulse, taking care of the incision and recording the patient's complaints and symptoms. The nurse communicates any abnormalities to the surgeon. In this way, possible complications can be recognized early and treated.

Hospital's Responsibility

The hospital's responsibility is to provide caring, competent staff and the proper resources required for good patient care.

Chapter 5

General Surgery Pediatric

Robert M. Filler
Professor of Surgery and Pediatrics
University of Toronto
Surgeon-in-Chief
Hospital for Sick Children, Toronto

Kerri Weller
Illustrator

The first "pediatric surgeons" treated abnormalities of the head and neck, chest, heart, abdominal organs, kidney and urinary tract, bones and nervous system. Now that some of these fields have their own specialists, pediatric surgeons generally treat congenital and acquired problems of the lungs, intestines, liver and endocrine glands of children.

They also repair injuries and abnormalities of body development, such as hernias and abdominal wall defects. This chapter describes three of the most common pediatric surgical problems: appendicitis, pyloric stenosis and inguinal hernia.

Appendicitis

The appendix is a small tube about as thick as a pencil. It is connected to the large intestine in the lower right part of the abdomen (Fig. 5.1). The whole of the appendix may be contained in this portion of the abdomen, or the tip may rest deep in the pelvis or up in the right flank. In humans the appendix no longer has any function.

Appendicitis, or inflammation of the appendix, is the most common reason for emergency abdominal surgery in children and adolescents. Approximately 8,000 Canadian children have this operation annually, and 80,000 in the United States.

Appendicitis is rarely seen in Third World countries; this has been attributed to the high fiber diets eaten in those countries.

Appendicitis is usually caused by obstruction of the appendix, most often by fecal material (Fig. 5.2). Viral infections of the intestinal tract, gastroenteritis, chicken pox or measles can cause the lining of the appendix to swell, also leading to obstruction of the appendix.

When its normal secretions cannot empty because of this blockage, the obstructed portion of the appendix swells, cutting off the blood supply and damaging the wall. The bacteria that are usually found in the appendix can now multiply, invade and destroy the injured wall. The damaged wall eventually disintegrates, and the appendix ruptures or breaks apart so that invading bacteria spills into the abdominal cavity.

Infection in the abdominal cavity is called peritonitis. It is very serious, because it can spread to all parts of the abdomen, liver and blood stream. Before antibiotics, many young people died of ruptured appendix. The time from obstruction of the appendix to perforation is usually 18 to 36 hours, which is why this condition is called ''acute'' appendicitis.

Some patients with long-standing abdominal complaints for which no specific cause can be found have been diagnosed as having ''chronic'' appendicitis, and have had their appendices removed. However, there is little scientific evidence to support the existence of ''chronic'' appendicitis, and most surgeons no longer accept this diagnosis. Occasionally acute appendicitis may subside spontaneously without medical treatment.

Although physicians and surgeons have been well aware of appendicitis for almost one hundred years, it is still quite possible for the diagnosis to be missed or delayed. The number of ''normal'' appendices found at surgery performed for suspected appendicitis ranges from 11 to 32 percent. In 30 percent of children with appendicitis, perforation and peritonitis have already occurred by the time of surgery.

Appendicitis usually starts with pain near the navel. Most patients lose their appetites at this time. About six hours later, when the wall of the appendix becomes inflamed, the pain moves to the right lower abdomen where the appendix is located. Vomiting and fever, usually less than 100°F (39°C), commonly occur at this time.

Unfortunately, the usual symptoms of appendicitis do not always occur. Viral or bacterial infections of the intestinal tract, or an unusually located appendix, may mask or modify the classic symptoms.

When the patient is examined, the physician feels the abdomen to determine if there is any inflammation inside, and whether it is over the appendix. The most significant finding is persistent tenderness in the right lower abdomen. Rectal examination may be necessary to find an inflamed appendix deep in the pelvis.

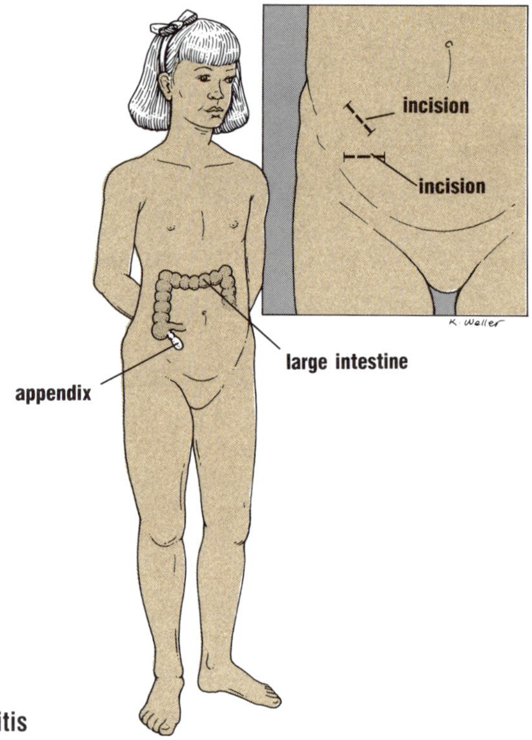

Figure 5.1
Position of appendix and common incisions used to remove it.

Case Study: Appendicitis

It wasn't like Tessa to pick at her food. Usually the active eight-year-old wolfed down whatever was served, asked for more, and was off to play with her friends as soon as she could leave the table. This evening her little brother, Ryan, got most of her dinner. She complained of a tummy ache and went off to watch TV, even though there were two hours of daylight left when she would normally have been playing baseball with her friends.

Two hours later, Tessa began to cry. ''Mom, it hurts down here,'' she wailed, pointing to the lower right side of her abdomen. Her mother thought she might be a little constipated, so she gave her warm apple juice and put her to bed with a hot water bottle. A short time later Tessa suddenly came flying out of her room to the bathroom, where she threw up copiously. ''Oh, Mom, it hurts,'' she sobbed.

Realizing that the child had now been in pain for six hours, her parents called their family doctor. He told them to take her directly to the emergency department at the children's hospital if her symptoms persisted for another two or three hours.

Appendicitis is generally diagnosed by careful evaluation of the patient's symptoms and physical examination. There is no laboratory test or X-ray that will confirm or deny the diagnosis beyond a shadow of a doubt. However, blood tests are usually done to see if any other conditions exist. Many people seem to have heard that the white blood cell count can be used to diagnose appendicitis. This test has about the same significance as fever. Both can be elevated in appendicitis, but they can be elevated for many other reasons as well. Furthermore, both can be normal in appendicitis.

A urinalysis is important, because it can confirm or deny the presence of a urinary tract infection, which can mimic appendicitis. X-rays of the abdomen are usually not particularly helpful in diagnosing appendicitis, but they are occasionally necessary to rule out the possibility of another abdominal abnormality.

Non-Surgical Treatment

Although surgery is required to cure almost all cases of appendicitis, antibiotics are used in conjunction with surgery to reduce the incidence of infection in the incision, to treat peritonitis if the appendix has ruptured before surgery, and to contain infection in those cases for which surgical attention is not immediately available. One or two doses of antibiotic will reduce the incidence of infection in the incision, but a ruptured appendix needs five to seven days of treatment. There are many suitable antibiotics: usually two or three drugs are combined, because the infection is often caused by several different species of bacteria.

Because many patients vomit and have little to eat or drink before surgery, and since this state of poor intake will persist for some time after the operation, patients are given intravenous fluids for a day or two following the surgery. In most cases, a nasogastric tube is passed down the nose into the stomach to prevent further vomiting or choking on vomit.

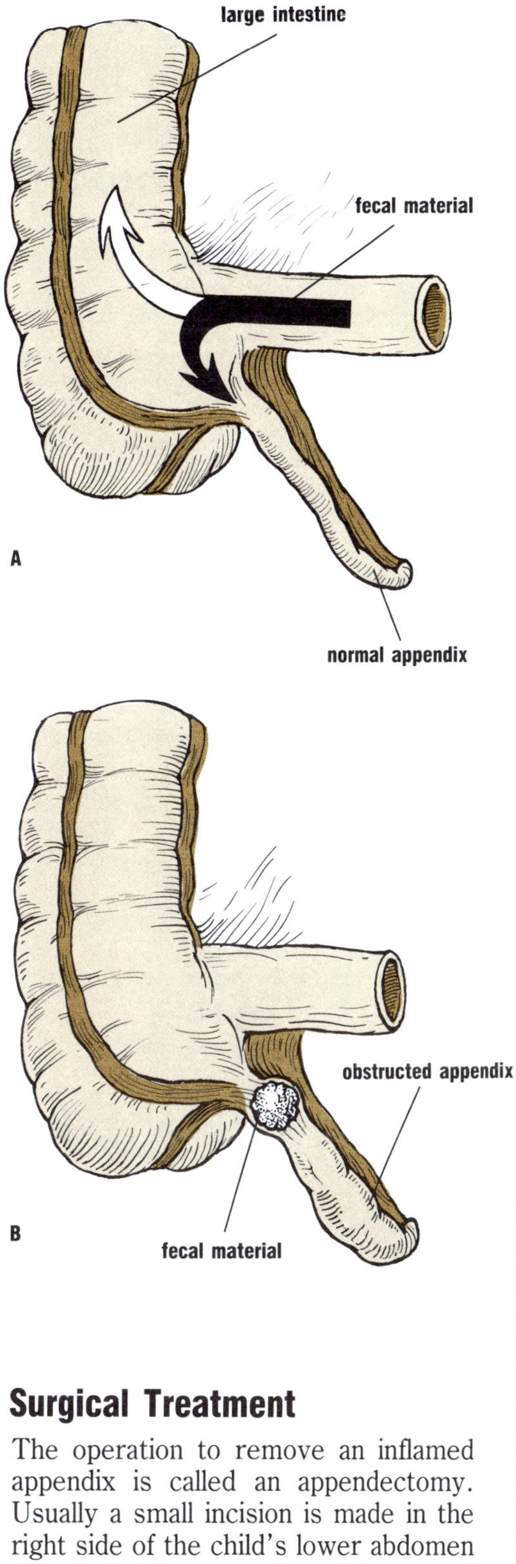

Figurc 5.2
Obstructed appendix. Fecal material can pass by the appendix or enter it (A), causing an obstruction (B).

Surgical Treatment

The operation to remove an inflamed appendix is called an appendectomy. Usually a small incision is made in the right side of the child's lower abdomen (Fig. 5.1). The appendix and the part of the large intestine it is attached to are pulled up into the wound, and the appen-

Three hours later, with Tessa now unable to move for pain, and with a rising temperature, her parents left Ryan in the care of a neighbor and drove to the hospital.

That night Tessa had her appendix removed, and three days later she was back home, very proud of her two-inch scar taped with skin tapes, which the surgeon said would come off on their own. Although her tummy was sore, she was none the worse for wear. Her greatest concern was that her scar would be healed in time for her to take part in her school's swim meet.

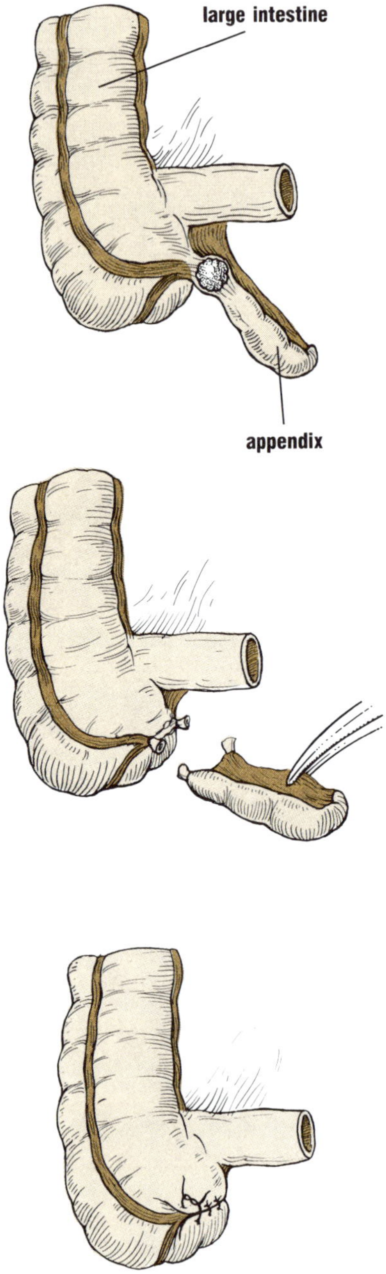

A

B

C

Figure 5.3
Appendectomy. The inflamed appendix (A) is removed (B), and the stump is closed with stitches (C).

dix is amputated. The remaining stump is closed with a stitch (Fig. 5.3).

The operation is more difficult if the appendix has ruptured, because other parts of the intestinal tract may adhere to the infected appendix. Pus in the abdominal cavity is removed by suction.

Some surgeons also irrigate the abdominal cavity with a salt or antibiotic solution before stitching up the abdomen. If there is a large abscess in the abdominal cavity, a soft rubber drain may be inserted to draw pus out through the skin. Drains are usually taken out five to seven days after surgery.

If the appendix appears normal, the surgeon inspects other organs in the abdominal cavity, to see what may have caused the symptoms, but it is rare to find any other serious condition. The symptoms usually turn out to be caused by a viral infection of the intestinal tract and need no further treatment. Although normal, the appendix is usually removed anyway, to prevent appendicitis in the future.

On rare occasions a ruptured appendix is not recognized, and the patient develops a large abdominal abscess. In these cases the abscess is drained, and the appendix is removed six to eight weeks later, after the inflammation has subsided.

Complications

Complications from surgery are relatively rare. The most frequent one is infection in the incision, which occurs in up to 5 percent of cases, most often in those where the appendix has ruptured.

Scar tissue (adhesions) within the abdomen can occur after any abdominal operation, but are much more common after a ruptured appendix. Most adhesions cause no problems, but they obstruct the intestine in about 2 percent of patients (these obstructions can occur even several years later). The adhesions can also block the ends of the fallopian tubes, possibly causing infertility.

Recent Advances

Antibiotics have greatly decreased the mortality and complication rate from appendicitis. In most hospitals today it is very rare to have a child die of a ruptured appendix, whereas even 10 years ago the mortality rate was as high as 5 percent. A special type of bacteria, which grows best in environments without oxygen, used to render antibiotics useless, but there are now new drugs that kill these bacteria.

After surgery, fluids and food are started as soon as the surgeon determines that the patient's intestinal tract is able to tolerate it. In uncomplicated appendicitis this usually occurs within 24 hours, but may be up to five days if the appendix was ruptured.

The site of the incision is painful, but this is usually easy to control with painkillers. Most children can go home three to five days after surgery, but if the appendix was ruptured, the hospital stay can be up to 10 days.

Diagnosis

For reasons we do not yet understand, the muscle surrounding the pyloric canal grows excessively in infants with pyloric stenosis, blocking the outflow channel of the stomach. Thus, as the stomach fills with milk or water, it churns vigorously to overcome the obstruction. When the narrowing is mild, the stomach can still empty, but as the obstruction progresses, the vigorous stomach contractions force the stomach contents back up the esophagus, and the infant may have ''projectile vomiting'' (Fig. 5.5).

The vomiting usually starts between two and four weeks of age, immediately after a feed. Initially the baby may vomit once or twice a day, but as the obstruction increases, the vomiting becomes more frequent and more forceful. Occa-

Pyloric Stenosis

Food and stomach contents leave the stomach by the pyloric canal to enter the first part of the small intestine (duodenum) (Fig. 5.4). The stomach muscle around the pyloric canal can contract and relax to regulate the speed of stomach emptying.

If the outlet of the pyloric canal becomes narrowed (stenosis), food and fluid will not pass and the child will begin vomiting. Pyloric stenosis usually affects infants between two weeks and two months of age.

The incidence of pyloric stenosis is about one in 500 births. It is more common in whites than blacks, and four times more common in males than in females. We do not know the exact cause, although heredity has been implicated, because the incidence of pyloric stenosis in children of affected parents is 7 percent. The female parent who had pyloric stenosis as an infant has a four times greater chance of having affected offspring than a similarly affected male. Five to 10 percent of infants with pyloric stenosis have siblings or close relatives who have had the condition.

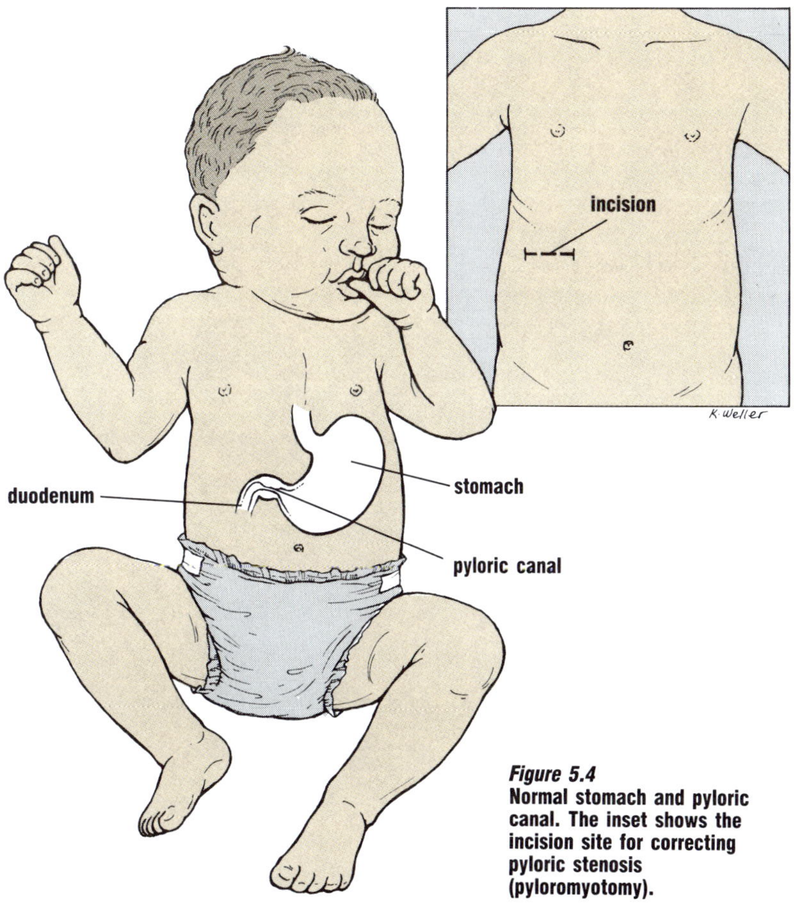

Figure 5.4
Normal stomach and pyloric canal. The inset shows the incision site for correcting pyloric stenosis (pyloromyotomy).

sionally, the vomited fluid may contain brownish material, which is partially digested blood that sometimes oozes from an irritated stomach wall. As the vomiting continues, the infant becomes dehydrated, loses weight and does not grow.

Often a small movable mass about the size of an olive can be felt in the upper abdomen. This is the thickened muscle along the pyloric canal and, if it can be felt, no other diagnostic tests are needed. However, the child may still have pyloric stenosis even if a lump cannot be felt. Then the child would be examined by a barium X-ray or by an ultrasound scan of the abdomen.

Non-Surgical Treatment

Infants who are vomiting a lot become very dehydrated and lose salt, which must be replaced with intravenous fluids before surgery. In the most severe cases, fluids may be needed for several days, but if the diagnosis is made fairly soon after vomiting begins, fluid and salt can be replenished in several hours.

Because the abnormal thickness of the pyloric muscle tends to recede over several months, even without treatment, several European centers have recommended that surgery not be performed. They give small, frequent feedings by mouth and intravenous feedings until the thickening of the muscle disappears. This method of treatment has never gained favor in North America because it requires a prolonged hospital stay, and the long-term evaluation of these patients has suggested that the child's full growth potential may be impaired.

Surgical Treatment

The surgical treatment for pyloric stenosis is called a pyloromyotomy. The infant is given a general anesthetic and a small incision is made in the upper abdomen (Fig. 5.4). The surgeon locates the enlarged pyloric muscle and splits it down to, but not through, the innermost lining of the canal. (Fig. 5.6). This relieves the obstruction so that the stomach can empty.

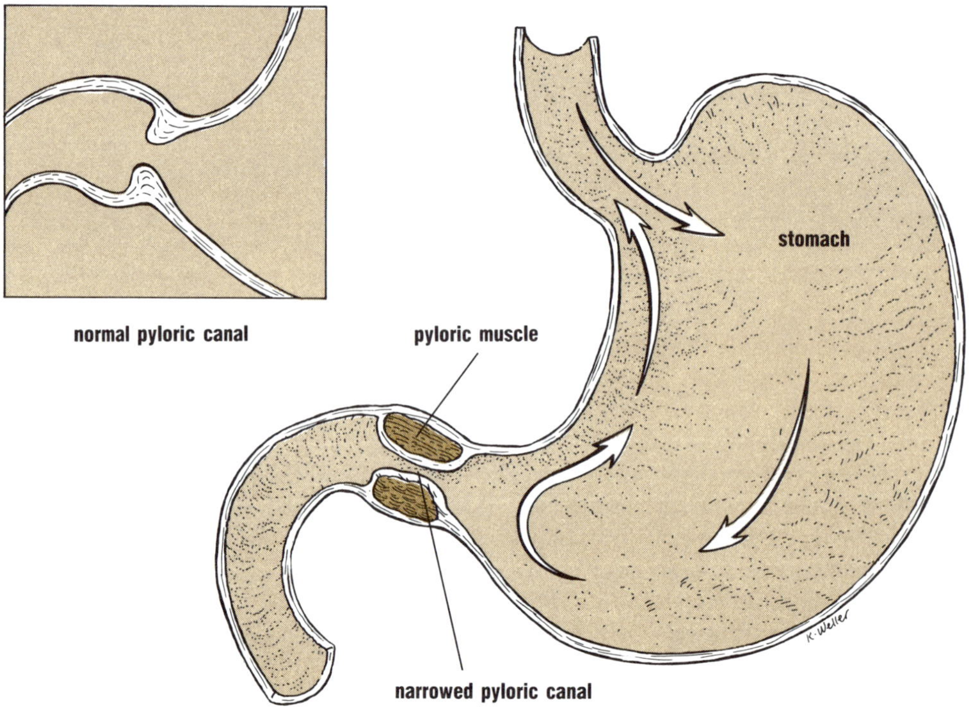

Figure 5.5
Pyloric stenosis. The pyloric muscle becomes enlarged, narrowing the pyloric canal and causing food to become trapped in the stomach.

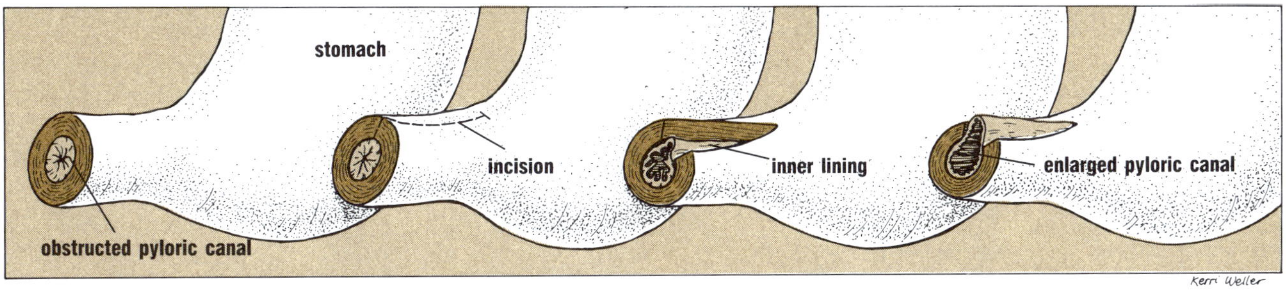

Figure 5.6
Pyloromyotomy. The surgeon cuts through the thickened pyloric muscle to the inner lining of the pyloric canal, thereby relieving the obstruction.

The infant is fed 12 to 24 hours after surgery. The baby may vomit after the first few feeds, but two or three days after the operation most infants are tolerating all their feeds and are ready to leave hospital. Although breast-feeding may have to be interrupted for a day or two during the hospitalization, mothers can pump and store breast milk, which can be given to the infant by bottle for the first few feeds after surgery. Thereafter normal breast-feeding can resume.

Complications

Complications following operation for pyloric stenosis are not common. Failure to split all of the enlarged muscle around the pyloric canal might result in continued vomiting, requiring a second operation, but this is very rare. Some months after surgery, the abnormal thickness of the pyloric muscle disappears, and children with pyloric stenosis are not prone to any other stomach illness in later life.

With modern anesthetic and surgical techniques and careful attention to dehydration and salt loss, the current mortality from pyloric stenosis is well below 1 percent.

Inguinal Hernia and Hydrocele

An inguinal hernia is a protrusion of the small intestine through the abdominal wall into the groin (Fig. 5.7). The protrusion may extend into the scrotum in boys or into the labia in girls. A hydrocele is similar to a hernia, except that fluid rather than intestine flows through the abdominal wall. In North America today, inguinal hernia repair is the most frequent operation performed by a pediatric surgeon.

The incidence of inguinal hernia in children ranges from 0.8 to 4.4 percent.

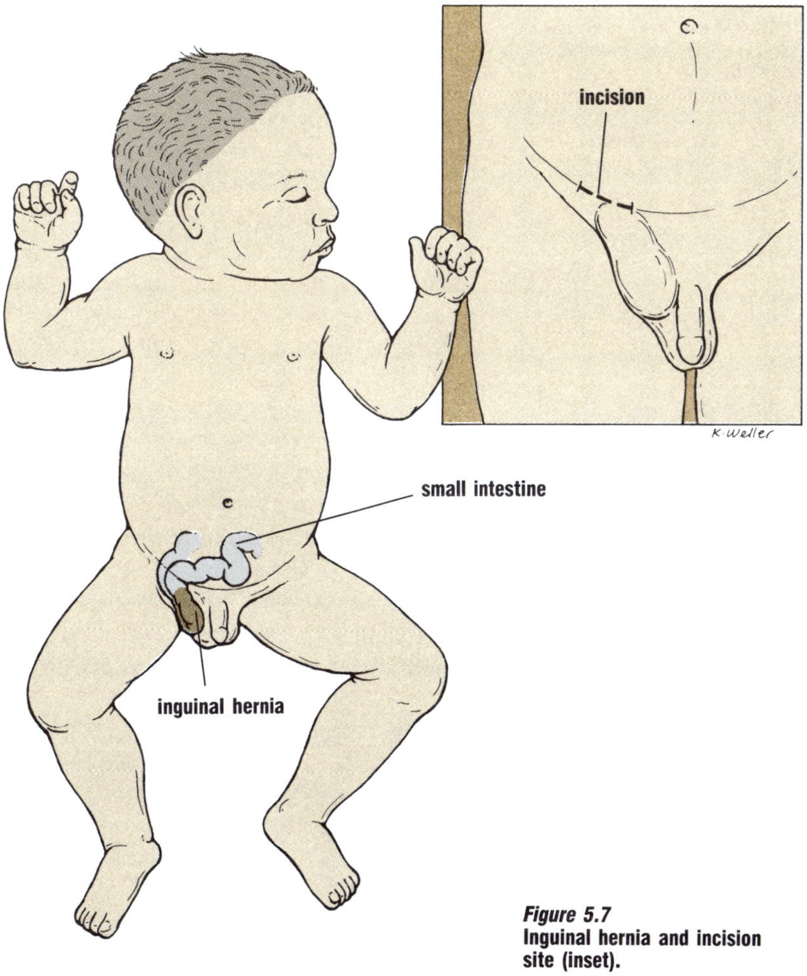

Figure 5.7
Inguinal hernia and incision site (inset).

Case Study: Inguinal Hernia and Hydrocele

At three months, Jason was growing well — "He's got more hair than his old man" was his father's rueful comment — and the family doctor called him a "grade A baby." So Ted was a little disturbed to see a bulge in Jason's groin on the right side as he was washing him. The baby was crying because he'd just had his face washed. When he calmed down, his father took another look — no bulge. Just another anxious parent, — that's me, he thought.

But Ted and Jennie mentioned the bulge to their family doctor at Jason's checkup the following week. Dr. Marks took a look and said, "There's nothing there at the moment, but you could be right. Let's get Jason an appointment with a surgeon at the children's hospital to make sure."

In the surgeon's office Jason screeched lustily because he didn't like the paper on the examining table. "Look, doctor, there it is!" Dr. Weldon needed only a quick look to make the diagnosis: inguinal hernia.

These hernias are found in 30 percent of premature infants, but in less than 1 percent of 10-year-olds. Inguinal hernia is most common during the first year of life, with a peak during the first month. Approximately one-third of children with a hernia are less than six months of age. Boys are affected approximately six times more often than girls. Sixty percent of hernias occur on the right, 30 percent on the left, and in 10 percent of children both sides are affected.

Childhood inguinal hernias and hydroceles usually occur when the process of descent of the testis in boys and migration of the round ligament of the uterus in girls is not fully completed prior to birth. The testicle (round ligament in girls) develops in the abdomen. Before birth it descends through the groin into the scrotum (labia in girls). Its pathway is a finger-like extension of the abdominal cavity called the processus vaginalis. After testicular or round ligament descent, the opening between the abdominal cavity and the processus vaginalis closes.

If this closure does not occur, intestine or abdominal fluid can enter the groin and scrotum through the open processus vaginalis. If the opening between the processus vaginalis and the abdominal cavity is large, a hernia will form (Fig. 5.8). If the opening is small, allowing just abdominal fluid, a hydrocele will form. A child with a hydrocele may eventually develop a hernia if the small opening enlarges.

The size of a hernia or hydrocele bulge varies, depending on the diameter of the sac and the pressure within the abdomen. For example, when standing and coughing or straining, the increased pressure in the abdomen tends to force fluid or intestine into the sac. When reclining and relaxing, the contents of the sac tend to return into the abdominal cavity, and the bulge or lump may completely disappear.

In most hernias the intestine moves freely in and out of the abdomen, causing few symptoms except for the presence of a bulge. These hernias are called "reducible." If the herniated intestine becomes trapped in the sac, such a hernia is said to be "incarcerated." This is a serious complication, because the trapped intestine usually kinks and becomes obstructed. If the incarcerated hernia is not treated, the blood supply to the intestine and/or to the testes can be cut off, causing gangrene (death of tissue) of the intestine and testes. The overall incidence of incarceration is approximately 10 percent. In children up to two months old, it is 25 percent; in the older child or teenager the incidence is 1 percent.

The initial symptoms of incarceration are pain and tenderness over the lump in the groin, severe abdominal cramps, vomiting and lack of bowel movements. If medical attention is not obtained promptly, the incarcerated intestine may rupture, causing a life-threatening infection. The mass of incarcerated intestine may also cause testicular damage by compressing and obstructing the blood vessels to the testicle.

A hydrocele can occur in the groin or more commonly, in the scrotum. The bulge is usually soft, not painful, and feels like a balloon filled with water. The bulge can be very large.

The fluid in a hydrocele may become entrapped because the pathway from the abdominal cavity is so small, especially in newborns. When entrapped, the bulge does not change in size. Unlike an incarcerated hernia, an entrapped hydrocele produces no symptoms except for the swelling. It does not damage the testicle.

The major reason to repair an inguinal hernia is to treat or prevent incarceration of the intestine. The urgency for repair is greatest in the youngest patients. The major reason for treating a hydrocele is to prevent a hernia from forming.

Diagnosis

The diagnosis of an inguinal hernia or hydrocele is made by detecting a lump

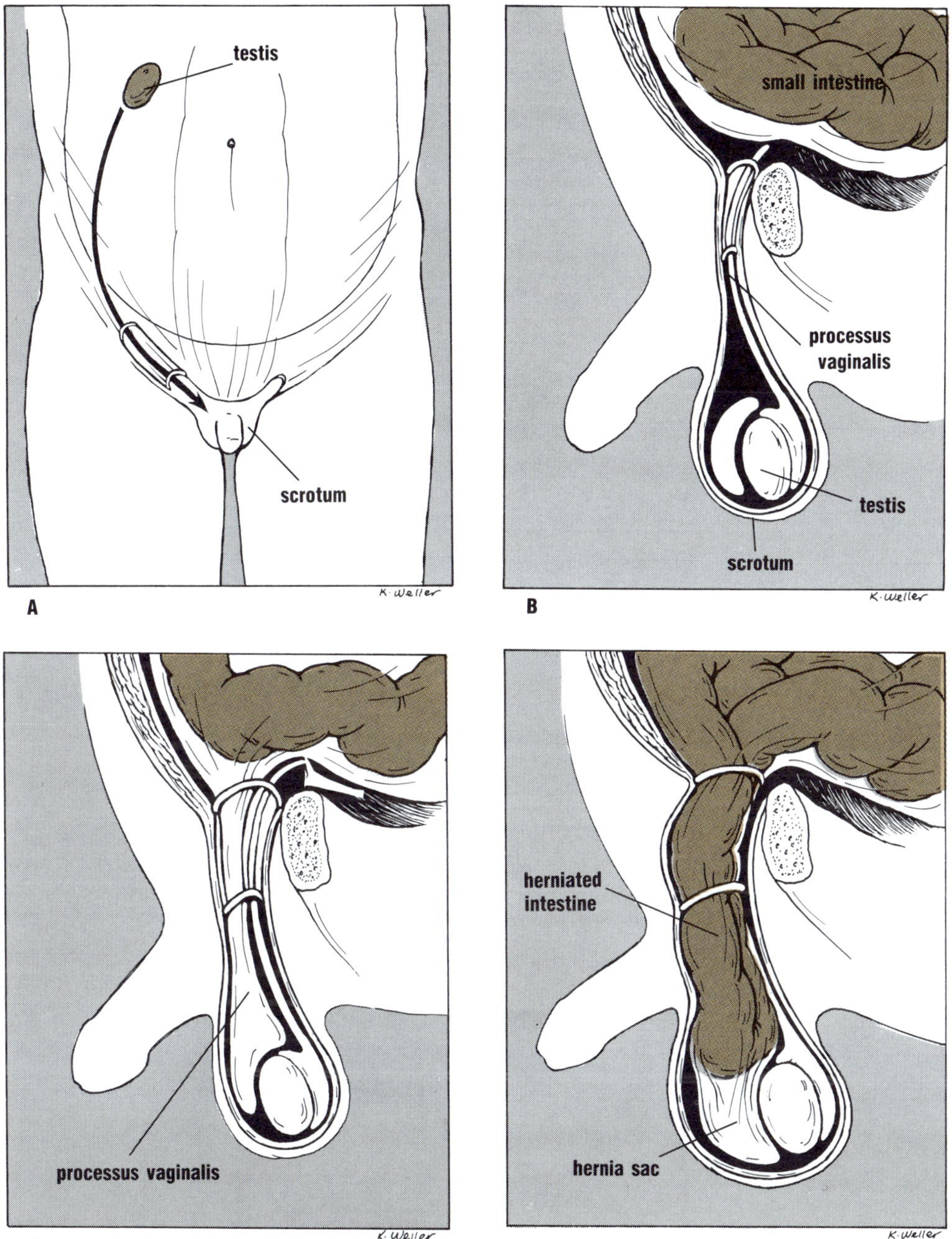

Figure 5.8
Development of inguinal hernia. The testis descends into the scrotum before birth (A). Normally the processus vaginalis closes after this occurs (B). In the formation of a hernia, the processus vaginalis does not close, leaving an open passage from the abdomen to the groin and scrotum (C). A hernia occurs when the small intestine pushes into this open passage (D).

or bulge in the groin or scrotum (labia in girls). Since most hernias are not incarcerated, the lump is not always present when the doctor examines the child, but some thickening of the tissue in the groin may show that a hernia has been present. At other times the surgeon must rely on a referring physician's examination or a parent's description of the abnormality to make the decision to operate.

Non-Surgical Treatment

Hernias do not disappear spontaneously and eventually require surgery, but non-surgical procedures are routinely employed as a first step in treating incarcerated hernias. In many cases, the intestine can simply be pushed back into the abdominal cavity, which eliminates the need for an immediate operation. The

Within a week Jason was in the hospital. Jennie and Ted were glad he wouldn't have to stay overnight. He could go home as soon as he had recovered from the anesthetic. Dr. Weldon said he'd probably be pretty sore for a day or two, but that he'd be fine after that.

All went well during surgery, and Jason soon began to complain as he came around. The staff gave Jennie and Ted some tips on how to keep him comfortable, and they made an appointment with Dr. Weldon for a follow-up checkup.

Jennie and Ted didn't get much sleep the first night, but by the next morning Jason seemed more comfortable. He was back to normal a day later.

child can then be properly prepared for a hernia repair in the next 12 to 24 hours. Trusses are no longer used for hernias in infancy or childhood.

Unlike a hernia, a hydrocele will disappear in over 90 percent of children in the first year of life. In general, only hydroceles that persist beyond the first year are surgically repaired.

Surgical Treatment

The operation is performed through a lower abdominal skin crease in the affected groin (Fig. 5.7). When the intestine is back in its normal position, the opening from the abdominal cavity into the groin is closed, and the sac that enclosed the herniated intestine is removed. (Sometimes a portion of the sac surrounds the testis and is then not removed completely.) In adult hernias, the muscles of the lower abdomen and groin usually need to be repaired, but this is not usually the case with childhood hernias.

Most hernia and hydrocele operations can be done without admitting the child to hospital. Hospitalization is necessary for premature infants, those with other serious medical problems, and when the hernia is incarcerated. Since most children cannot lie still unless completely anesthetized, a general anesthetic is usually used.

Many surgeons surgically explore the other side after repairing a hernia on one side, because they might find another opening in the processus vaginalis, which could be the site of a future hernia. The likelihood of finding an unsuspected abnormality on the ''normal'' side is greatest in children under one year of age, and in those with a left inguinal hernia, so exploration is often restricted to these children.

Pain after surgery usually lasts for a day or two and can easily be controlled with painkillers. The child can resume full normal activity as soon as the pain subsides.

Complications

Serious problems occur after surgery in less than 1 percent of cases. Swelling in the scrotum is common, especially when the processus vaginalis extends into the scrotum. This swelling, caused by a collection of fluid or blood at the site of the operation, is unlikely to be due to recurrence of the hernia or hydrocele. It usually disappears within a week or two without treatment.

Recurrence of a hernia after surgery occurs in about 0.1 percent of children — a much lower rate than in adults. Injury to the vas deferens or the testicular blood supply is very rare, although possible in every hernia operation in boys, because these structures adhere to the processus vaginalis. Leaving the testis in an abnormal position above the scrotum in the groin is perhaps the most common testicular complication with this type of surgery. When this occurs, a second operation is necessary to put the misplaced testis into the scrotum so that it will function normally.

Chapter 6

General Surgery Adult

Robert Stone
Professor of Surgery
University of Toronto
Surgeon-in-Chief
Toronto Western Hospital

Sari O'Sullivan
Illustrator

Before World War I there was no specialization within surgery. All surgeons treated wounds, broken bones and diseases that affected the abdominal cavity, such as appendicitis. Now that surgical specialties have emerged, general surgeons treat disorders of the digestive system, certain glands that produce hormones (such as the thyroid), and diseases of the breast.

The diseases discussed in this chapter are among the most common diagnosed and treated by a general surgeon: gallstones, groin hernia, cancer of the colon and cancer of the breast.

Gallstones

Many people in Western society develop gallstones. However, if the stones do not produce symptoms, there is often no need to treat them.

The gallbladder is a three-inch oblong sac containing one to three ounces of bile. It is loosely attached to the undersurface of the liver (Fig. 6.1). A small tube, the cystic duct, connects the gallbladder to the bile duct, which connects the liver to the upper part of the small intestine (duodenum).

The gallbladder is a storage house for

Case Study: Gallstones

Margot put it down to indigestion at first. They'd had a farewell lunch for one of her workmates, and shortly after that she'd experienced a sharp pain just below her breast-bone. Cafeteria food! she thought wryly. But she experienced the same sensation after supper at home — a meal she'd cooked herself. "Probably had too much," she thought.

For several weeks Margot went on with her usual routine: have breakfast, get the kids off to school, get herself to work, a quick lunch plus some shopping, home again for supper and whatever was planned for the evening. But gradually she began to avoid certain foods, sure that she'd have indigestion afterwards. Her husband was puzzled by her refusal of spring rolls at their favorite Chinese restaurant, since she'd always loved them.

One day the pain Margot experienced after lunch was so severe that she had to ask her supervisor if she could go home. When her husband arrived home to find her throwing up in the bathroom, he called their family doctor right away. Dr. Curtis sent Margot for ultrasound. "Sounds like a gallbladder problem to me," he told her. "The ultrasound will give us a picture of what's going on. If there are any stones, we'll be able to see them. If so, you're looking at an operation to have your gallbladder removed."

This sounded very drastic to Margot. She wanted to know why they wouldn't just remove the stones. "A gallbladder that's making stones doesn't make just one," Dr. Curtis told her. "You can have gallstones without having symptoms, but once you're having symptoms, they don't stop."

bile, a substance that breaks down and assists in the absorption of food in the intestine. Bile is produced by the liver and stored in the gallbladder. When food is eaten, the gallbladder contracts and releases bile into the intestine.

Bile contains cholesterol and other substances. If the level of cholesterol is high, or the level of some other substances is low, the cholesterol may solidify into a stone, which can grow larger over time. It is often the small stones (some no larger than a grain of sand) that cause the problems.

When the gallbladder contracts after eating, a stone may get stuck in the cystic duct, causing pain that will usually be felt somewhere between the lower part of the breastbone and the umbilicus (belly button). The pain may go right through to the back, and may be severe enough to cause nausea and vomiting. When the gallbladder relaxes, the stone may fall back into the gallbladder, and the pain will disappear almost as quickly as it began. A typical attack of such pain lasts 20 to 60 minutes and is called biliary colic.

Sometimes the stone will remain stuck in the cystic duct. In this case the pain will not disappear, but often shifts farther to the right side just under the rib cage. This condition is called acute cholecystitis, or inflammation of the gallbladder. It may cause fever and tenderness on the right side of the abdomen. Acute cholecystitis usually results in a visit to a hospital emergency department. Surgery may be necessary, but the condition will usually settle down without surgery at that time.

If the stone passes into the bile duct, three things may happen. The stone may pass into the small bowel, it may block the bile duct, or it may block the duct that drains the pancreas (pancreatic duct). If the stone is tiny, and moves into the bowel, it will be passed easily in the stool, and the pain will disappear. However, there are usually many tiny stones in the gallbladder, and similar episodes of pain are likely.

If the stone blocks the bile duct, bile

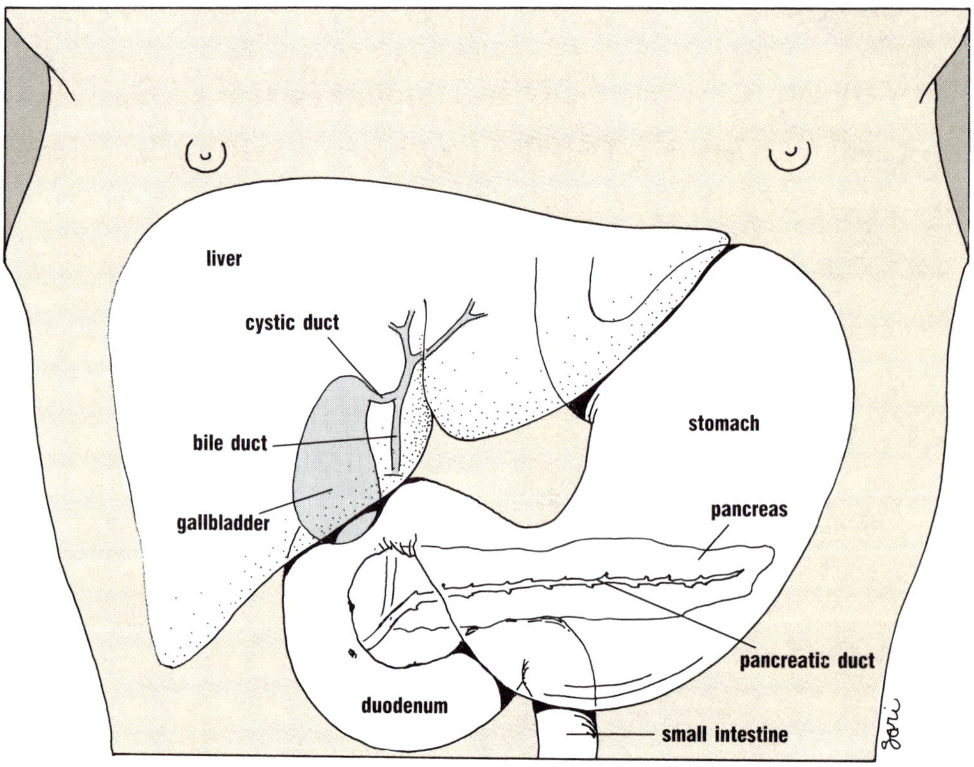

Figure 6.1
Location of gallbladder.

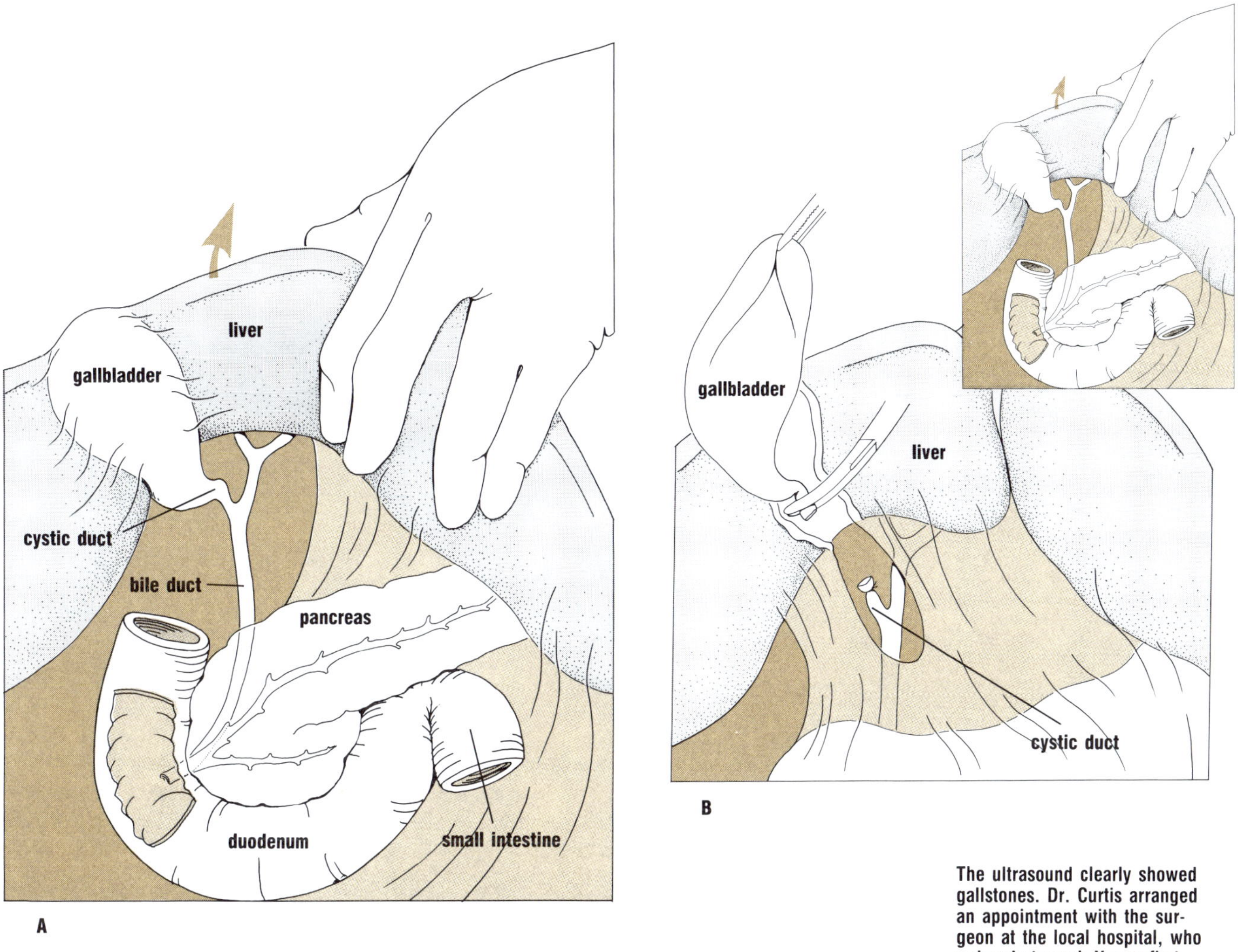

Figure 6.2
Removal of gallbladder. The gallbladder is located on the underside of the liver (A). Once the cystic duct has been tied off, the gallbladder is removed (B).

will not be able to reach the small intestine and will instead be absorbed from the bile duct into the blood. This will cause yellow discoloration of the whites of the eyes and skin (jaundice), dark-colored urine, pale-colored stools and sometimes a general itching without a rash. Bile-duct blockage is a dangerous complication of gallstones and requires immediate surgery.

If the pancreatic duct becomes blocked, the pancreas will become inflamed (pancreatitis). The pancreas produces enzymes which, along with bile, help digest and absorb food. Pancreatitis produces extreme upper abdominal pain, often with severe nausea and vomiting, and must be treated in hospital. Once the patient's symptoms have been treated with the appropriate medication, the gallstones must be surgically removed.

Frequently the symptoms of gallstones will not be clear-cut. In the early stages patients may have intolerance of fatty foods or indigestion — the uncomfortable feeling one may get after a large meal, or one that is eaten too quickly. While not serious in themselves, these symptoms are often followed by more severe

The ultrasound clearly showed gallstones. Dr. Curtis arranged an appointment with the surgeon at the local hospital, who ordered stomach X-rays first, but then agreed that the problem was gallstones. "We usually check to see that the pain isn't being caused by an ulcer," he told her. "The last episode of pain and vomiting was probably due to the stone getting stuck in the tube leading out of the gallbladder," he said. "This sometimes happens. The stone may drop back into the gallbladder again, or it may pass out through the bile duct and eventually be passed in stool. Since you're no longer in pain, one of those two things has happened. But your ultrasound showed many small stones, so it could happen again." "But until then, I don't need an operation?" Margot asked hopefully. "My advice would be to have the operation now, rather than wait until we have to bring you in as an emergency."

She decided to call Dr. Curtis again. He assured her that the operation was very common, that she'd probably be in hospital no longer than she had been with the birth of each of her children, and the symptoms would be immediately relieved, even though she'd feel sore from the operation. "How is it that I'll be able to manage without a gallbladder?" she asked. Dr. Curtis laughed. "You won't miss it," he promised. "The gallbladder is just a storage house for bile. It has no other function."

The operation seemed to be over very quickly. One minute Margot was listening to the anesthetist saying, "And now we put you to sleep," and before she knew it she was back in her room with a sore right side. That night she felt pretty groggy, and gratefully took the sleeping medication the nurse offered. But even so, she managed to get out of bed for a couple of minutes. The next day she felt "hung over," but otherwise not too bad. When the surgeon came to see her, he explained that now she was at no further risk of getting gallstones, and she was no more likley to get any other gastrointestinal problem than someone who hadn't had gallbladder surgery.

Margot returned home after four days in the hospital. By 10 days, Margot was able to be up and about. She revisited the surgeon to have the clips removed. She'd been surprised to see the wound closed with these small metal clamps, but relieved that the scar wasn't going to be too obvious once it had healed. "It's coming along nicely," the surgeon told her. "Just take it easy for a couple more weeks."

complications weeks, months or years later.

The doctor will examine the patient, ask about symptoms and do some tests to "see" the stones. The most frequently used test today is abdominal ultrasound, which will show up the stones by bouncing ultrasonic waves off them. This test is highly reliable, but X-rays can be used if there is any doubt. The patient is given pills containing a substance that is passed through the liver and becomes concentrated in the gallbladder. Any stones can then be seen in silhouette on X-ray.

Non-Surgical Treatment

There is currently no effective non-surgical treatment for gallstones. A low-fat diet may decrease the frequency of the attacks of pain, but it is no substitute for removal of the gallbladder.

Surgical Treatment

Treatment is recommended only if the stones are producing or have produced symptoms. Exceptions to this rule might include patients under age 30, diabetics and young women contemplating a pregnancy. Once the gallbladder is removed, bile continues to be supplied to the small intestine directly from the liver, via the bile duct.

The best treatment for symptom-producing gallstones is surgical removal of the gallbladder containing the stones, because stones are very likely to form again. Any stone in the bile duct or pancreatic duct should be removed as well. Most patients are admitted to hospital the day before surgery. Blood and urine samples are taken for testing, all patients have chest X-rays and patients over age 40 have an electrocardiogram (ECG) to check the heart. No food or drink is permitted within eight hours of surgery, and an intravenous drip is usually set up on the morning of the operation.

In the operating room the patient is given a general anesthetic. The surgeon then disinfects the front of the abdomen to get rid of bacteria on the skin and covers the patient with sterile towels, except over the area of the operation, which is a four- to six-inch incision in the upper part of the abdomen.

The surgeon cuts through the abdominal wall, which is one to two inches thick. The cystic duct and the artery that carries blood to the gallbladder are located and cut, and the ends are sutured. With scissors, the gallbladder is gently separated and removed from the undersurface of the liver (Fig. 4.2).

After the gallbladder has been removed, fluid will sometimes accumulate in the area of the surgery, requiring drainage. A soft plastic or rubber tube may be pushed through the abdominal wall down to the area of the operation. The tube is removed after 48 hours and the wound in the abdominal wall is then closed using both deep and superficial stitches. The deep stitches remain in place indefinitely; the stitches or clamps in the skin are removed in seven to ten days.

Recovery from the anesthetic takes up to two hours. Patients then return to their rooms. They may be given pain-killing injections, but often by the first or second day after surgery these drugs can be taken by mouth. An intravenous is left in place until normal drinking can be resumed — usually in two to three days.

Patients are encouraged to get out of bed the evening of the operation and are frequently ready to go home by the fourth day. However, patients should not resume household or child-care activities for seven to ten days.

Most patients are away from work for up to three weeks if their occupation is sedentary and six weeks if the occupation involves manual labor. It usually takes six weeks before a normal sense of well-being returns.

Complications

Complications can occur, but fortunately are uncommon. They include the complications possible from any surgical operation (see chapter 4), plus those specific to gallbladder operations. Bile duct injury is rare. To avoid this complication the surgeon must be meticulous in accurately identifying the cystic duct before it is divided. Infection occurs in the abdominal wound in up to 4 percent of cases; this can cause wound tenderness, redness and frequently fever. It is usually treated by removing one or two skin stitches and allowing the infection to drain out.

Recent Advances

Patients with gallstones are now having surgery earlier. Delay in treatment often leads to scar tissue formation around the gallbladder, which can make surgery more difficult.

During the past decade researchers have tried to learn whether gallstones can be dissolved by medicine. Although the outlook for this method is promising, it is not yet recommended treatment.

A new method using shock waves to break up stones (lithotripsy) has been very useful in treating certain types of kidney stones. Lithotripsy is now being investigated as a possible method for treating gallstones. At present, we do not know how to prevent gallstones from developing.

Groin Hernia

A hernia occurs when part of an organ or tissue protrudes through an abnormal opening. Hernias can occur in many parts of the body, but they are most often found in the groin, where the leg connects with the trunk. A groin hernia is frequently called a rupture.

There are two common types of groin hernia which occur in males — indirect inguinal and direct inguinal. Femoral hernias, which are much more rare, usually occur in women. Indirect inguinal hernias occur in babies due to an abnormality at birth (see chapter 5). Direct inguinal hernias occur later in life as a result of physical strain.

In a groin hernia, an abnormal opening occurs in the abdominal wall, which has several layers — skin, fat, muscle and inner lining (peritoneum). The muscular layers in this area are often weak, and abnormal openings can occur, causing tissue — usually the small intestine — to protrude. In the standing position, this part of the abdominal wall is subject to the greatest pressure from within the abdominal cavity. Straining, coughing, sneezing and even laughing increase intra-abdominal pressure.

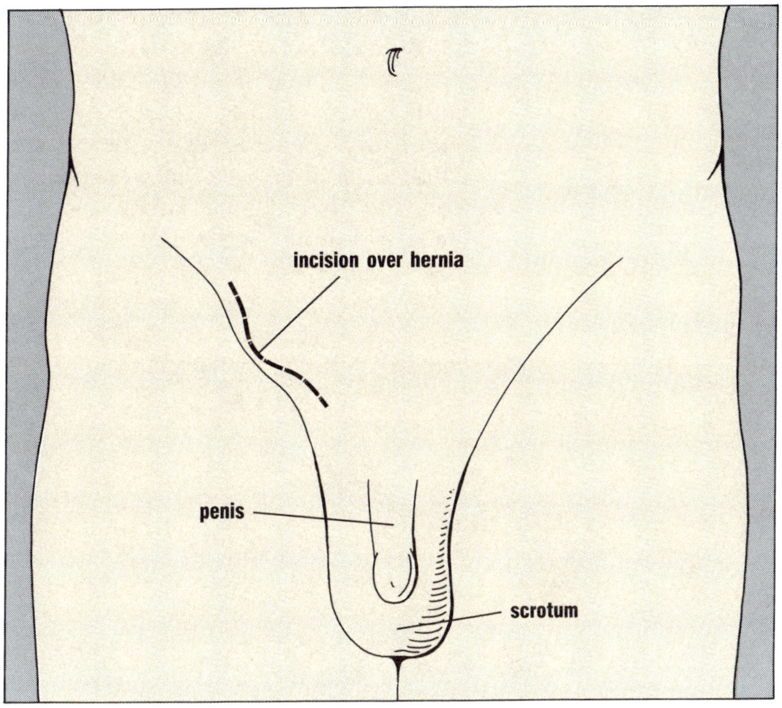

Figure 6.3
Groin hernia incision.

Diagnosis

A hernia is usually easily diagnosed on physical examination and no tests are usually required. Patients with a hernia will become aware of a lump in the groin, which may be tender at first. The lump will often appear when the patient stands; it may be ''gone'' in the morning, only to reappear by evening.

Hernias increase in size with time,

because they gradually enlarge the abnormal opening in the abdominal wall. There is a risk of a piece of bowel getting stuck in the hernia, obstructing the bowel and necessitating emergency surgery. If the contents of a hernia cannot be pushed back into the abdominal cavity, the hernia is said to be "incarcerated." When this happens, the blood supply of the bowel may be cut off, and the hernia becomes "strangulated." This also requires emergency surgery.

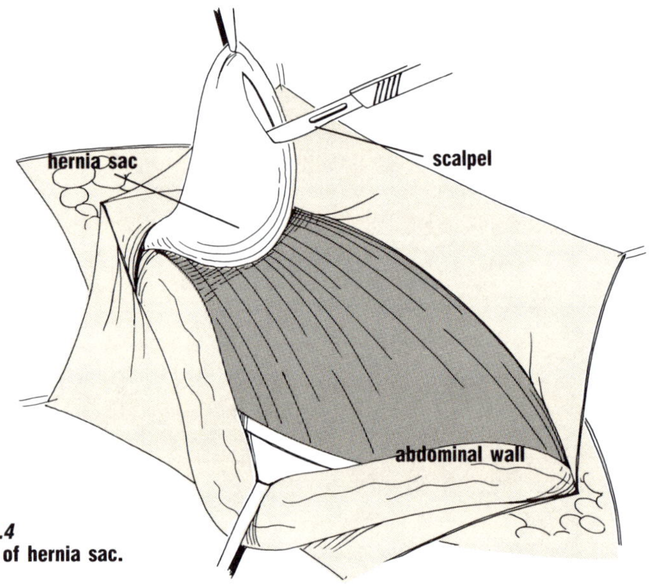

Figure 6.4
Opening of hernia sac.

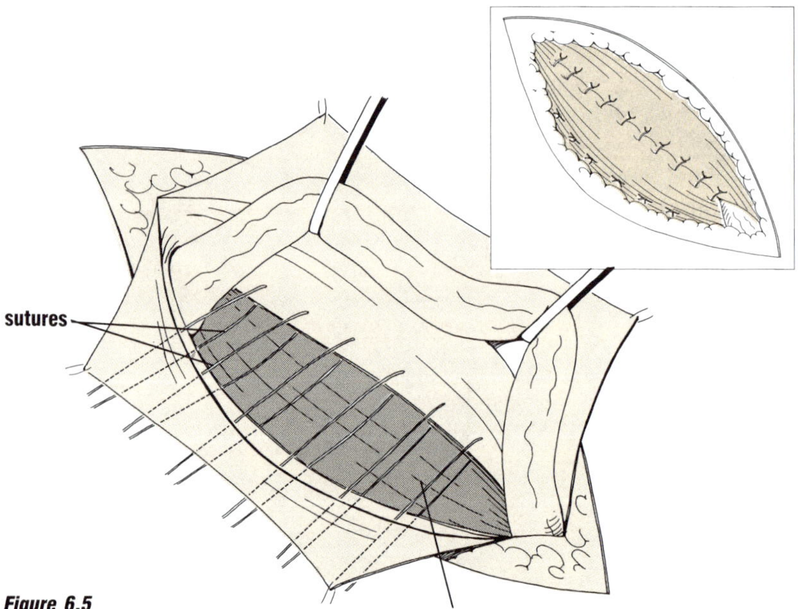

Figure 6.5
Repair of hernia.

Non-Surgical Treatment

In most circumstances a groin hernia should be treated by surgery, to push the contents back into the abdominal cavity, repair the abnormal opening and prevent a recurrence of the hernia. In patients who would not be able to withstand surgery, such as the very elderly, hernias are treated by wearing a truss, which places pressure over the abnormal opening, making it difficult for the intestine to protrude.

Surgical Treatment

If the patient is fit, surgical repair is recommended to prevent the hernia from enlarging or becoming strangulated. The larger a hernia gets, the harder it is to repair, and greater are the chances that the repair will not hold, causing the hernia to recur.

Many hernias can be repaired under local anesthetic, but surgeons tend to prefer general anesthetic, because the muscles are more relaxed. Most hernias can be repaired in 30 to 40 minutes.

Once the patient has been anesthetized, the surgeon makes an incision in the groin over the area of the abnormal opening in the abdominal wall (Fig. 6.3). The hernia sac containing the protruding intestine is then opened (Fig. 6.4). The intestines are returned to the abdominal cavity, the sac is removed, and the opening in the abdominal wall is closed.

There are several ways to strengthen this part of the abdominal wall with stitches to prevent a recurrence. The closure of the opening and the repair itself are carried out with non-absorbable stitches that remain permanently in the wound (Fig. 6.5).

The patient is usually discharged from hospital one to two days following surgery; some go home the same day. Skin stitches are removed in approximately one week. Patients are instructed to avoid heavy lifting or straining for six weeks. Most people are able to return to sedentary work within two weeks, but those doing heavy work should wait six weeks.

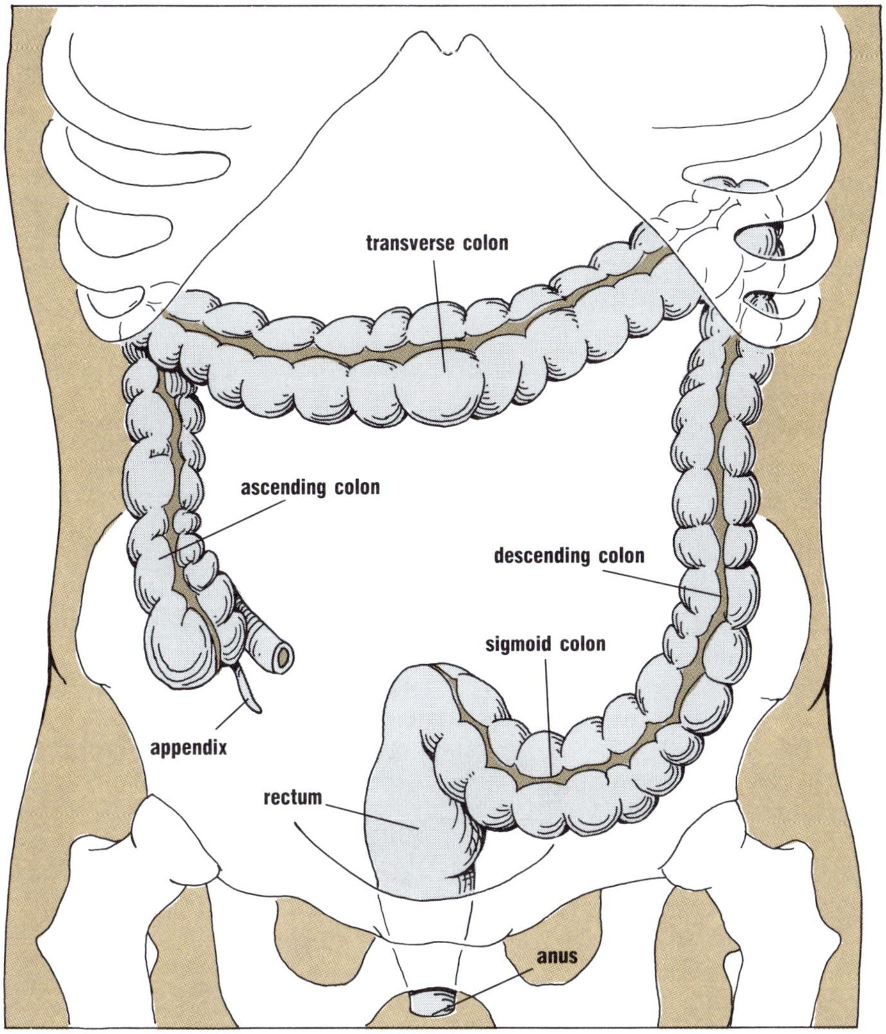

Figure 6.6
Location of colon (large intestine).

Cancer of the Colon

The colon (large intestine) extends from the end of the small intestine to the anus, and is approximately four feet long. It begins on the right lower side of the abdominal cavity, passes upward and across to the left upper part of the cavity, then down to the rectum and finally the anus (Fig. 6.6).

The colon is a storage organ. About one quart of liquid enters the colon each day; 90 percent is absorbed back into the bloodstream, and the rest is passed as stool.

Cancers of the digestive system occur most frequently in the colon. If these cancers are detected and treated early, more than half of them are completely curable. Colon cancer appears more frequently in Western civilization than in other cultures, which may be due to a lower intake of dietary fiber. Otherwise, the cause of colon cancer is unknown.

Early colon cancer usually produces no symptoms. When symptoms do occur, they may include a change in bowel habits, cramps or blood in the stool. This disease occurs most frequently in people over 40, but may occur earlier. Some patients are at high risk of developing colon cancer. Included are those with a family history of colon cancer, those who have had ulcerative colitis, and those who have had benign polyps (small tumors)

Case Study: Cancer of the Colon

Eugene had always thought of himself as the healthy type. He rarely got sick, and didn't make a big deal about it if he did. At 60, he thrived on routine, took regular walks to exercise both himself and the dog, and wasn't overweight.

His first inkling of a problem was a change in bowel habit. Always regular, he now seemed to be permanently somewhat constipated. Then he began to get abdominal cramps.

His wife, Martha, was the first one to point out how tired he seemed to be. When she suggested that he ask someone else to take over his committee work at the university, he acknowledged that he worried about being tired, because he'd always been full of energy.

When he experienced some rectal bleeding, he finally took the time to go to the university health service. The physician who saw him could find nothing wrong during the physical examination and rectal exam, but referred him to a surgeon for a sigmoidoscopy — the insertion of a rigid tube into his bowel to see if any abnormalities could be causing the bleeding.

The sigmoidoscopy was unpleasant, but mercifully over in a short time. The surgeon looked thoughtful, prompting Eugene to say, "Look, Dr. Weatherall, I hope you realize that I want to hear everything that you know about my condition."

Dr. Weatherall sat down beside Eugene. "I'll tell you what I know to date, which isn't very much. You have a growth inside your colon about the size of a raspberry." He stopped. "A growth, you said?" Eugene asked, "What kind of a growth? What do you mean?" The surgeon eyed Eugene. "I've removed a small piece of the growth. We have to examine this biopsy specimen to find out if it's malignant. If it is, we should remove it. If it isn't, we should probably remove it anyway, and keep an eye on you for a time." "You said tumor," Eugene asked, "Does that mean cancer?" "If it's malignant, yes," said Dr. Weatherall, watching Eugene closely. "When will you know?" he asked quietly. "In a couple of days — I'll call you."

Dr. Weatherall's call came through to Eugene's office a few days later. Eugene, I'm afraid the tumor is malignant. We'll have to remove it." Dr. Weatherall was very matter of fact about the future. He explained that because the tumor was relatively high in the bowel, they'd be able to cut it out and rejoin the intestine. If it had been lower, Eugene would have had to have a colostomy. He also told them that the prognosis depended on the tumor's penetration into the intestinal wall. The more superficial the tumor, the more chance they had of getting it all.

Within a week Eugene was admitted to the university hospital to begin two or three days of bowel preparation before surgery. The nurse told him that the laxatives and enemas would continue until his bowel was completely clean, to reduce the chance of infection. Looking back on it, this was the worst part of the procedure — the two-hour operation itself left him feeling sore and groggy, but otherwise reasonably comfortable.

removed from the colon in the past. High-risk patients should have periodic colon examinations, even if they have no symptoms.

Early in the disease the cancer usually remains confined to the colon. Later the cancer cells can migrate to the lymph glands around the colon (Fig. 6.7), and from here cancer cells may spread to the liver. In most cases, once the cancer cells have spread, cure is no longer possible. Even in these circumstances, however, treatment of the cancer is usually worthwhile, because the patient may live for several more years in good health.

Two basic tests are used to diagnose colon cancer: X-ray of the bowel and a direct inspection of the inside of the bowel (sigmoidoscopy or colonoscopy).

A sigmoidoscope, a rigid tube that examines the lower part of the bowel, is frequently used as the first diagnostic test. Liquid barium is put into the colon through a tube inserted into the anus. This is called a barium enema. The barium is visualized by X-ray, outlining the wall of the large bowel. In some situations this test can define the problem. In others, colonoscopy is also necessary.

The colonoscope is a flexible tube that is inserted into the anus and can be passed through the length of the colon, allowing inspection of the entire inside surface of the colon. If a suspicious area is seen, a small piece of this area can be removed through the colonoscope, to be examined under a microscope. This is called a biopsy.

Before any of these tests, the colon must be properly cleaned out. This usually involves a strong laxative by mouth the night before and a laxative suppository on the morning of the test.

If cancer of the colon is confirmed, tests may be needed to find out if the cancer has spread to the liver. This will depend on the type of symptoms, the patient's age and the type of treatment planned. These tests may include an ultrasound examination or computerized axial tomography (CAT scan).

Surgical Treatment

Most patients with cancer of the colon are best treated with surgery. The

Figure 6.7
Colon cancer.

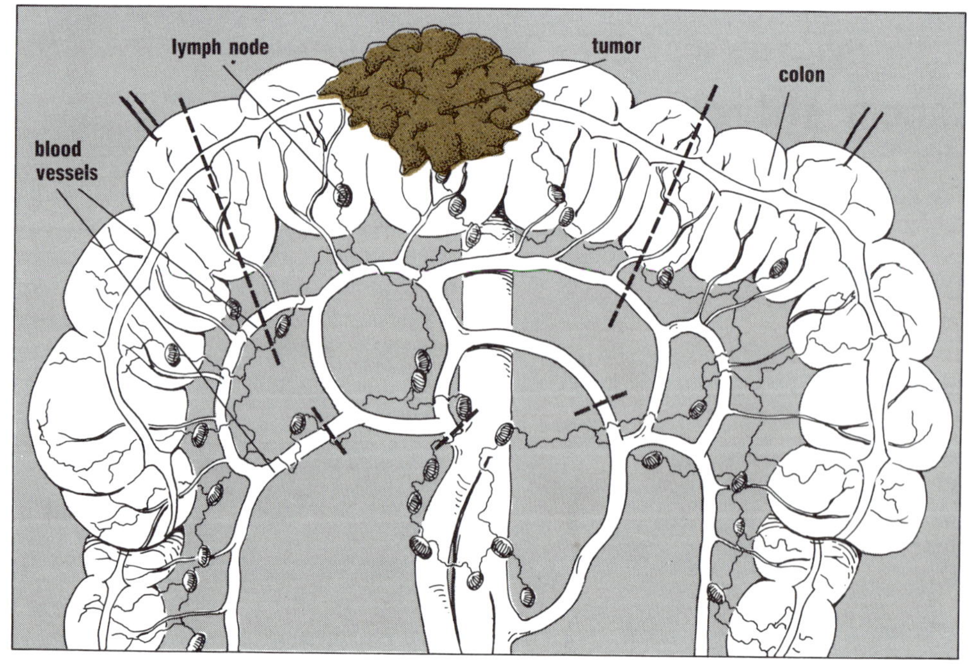

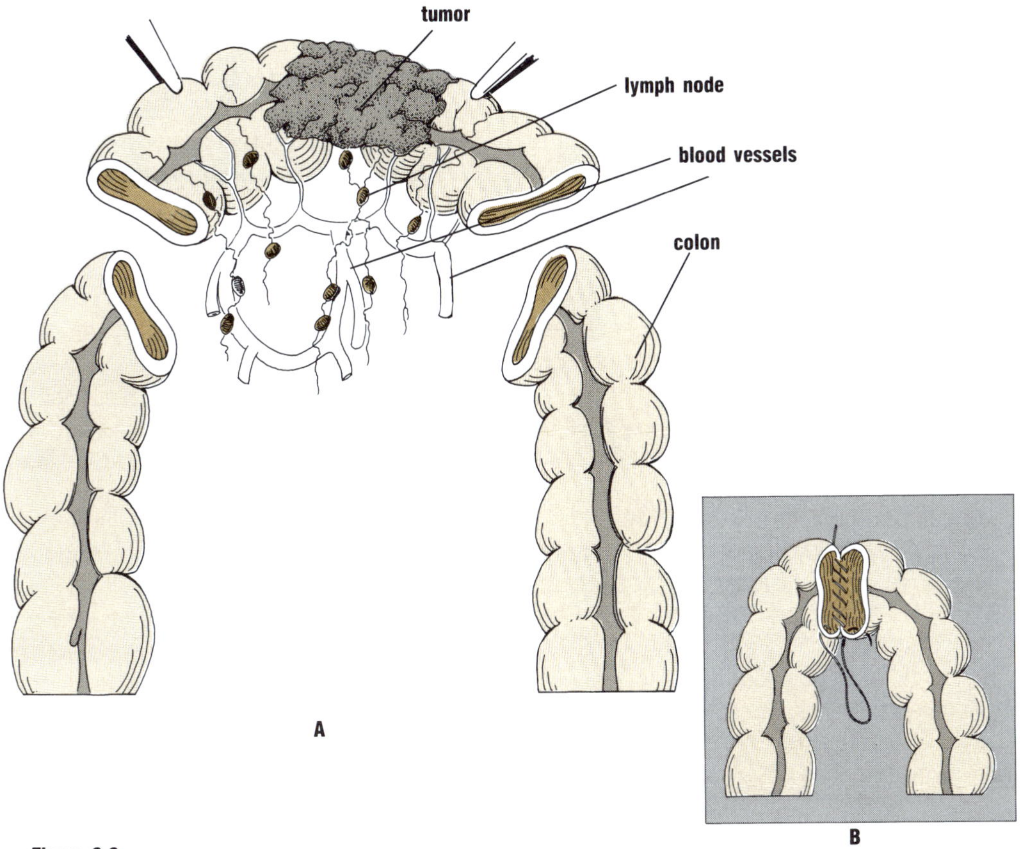

Figure 6.8
Colon surgery. The diseased portion of colon and surrounding lymph node are removed (A); then the remaining ends of colon are sewn together (B).

For the next three days Martha was constantly at Eugene's side, helping him in and out of bed, getting him to and from the bathroom. His pain medication made him somewhat drowsy, but after two days he didn't need it anymore.

The big moment came when Dr. Weatherall came with the pathologist's report. As usual, he was very matter of fact. "The tumor was reasonably superficial, so I think we got it all. From the type of tumor, I'd say that the prognosis is hopeful. Patients with this type of tumor tend to have a fairly lengthy survival time." "If the patient survives for five years with no recurrences, then we consider him cured. However, there is a statistically higher chance of getting another tumor. That is why regular checkups are necessary."

He continued to see Dr. Weatherall every six months for a checkup. Each time the surgeon said, "Nothing there," Eugene felt even more optimistic.

affected portion of bowel and the surrounding lymph glands are removed. Then the two remaining ends of bowel are sewn together (Fig. 6.8).

The patient must come to surgery with a perfectly clean bowel, which may require up to three days of preparation. Some of this can be done at home, but some is usually done in hospital. This surgery requires general anesthetic.

Some patients undergoing colon surgery will require a colostomy. A colostomy is an "artificial anus" on the front of the abdominal wall. If the lower part of the rectum must be removed, the colostomy will be permanent. In other circumstances the surgeon may find it necessary to create a temporary colostomy which may be closed in a few weeks. Most patients learn to manage a colostomy in a trouble-free fashion within a few weeks of surgery. The new appliances will allow such people to lead a normal life, including swimming.

The patient remains in hospital for seven to 14 days. It is frequently six to eight weeks before patients regain their normal sense of well being. Some help at home is advisable for the first three to four weeks.

Complications

The major complication of colon surgery is a breakdown of the joint or connection that is made in the bowel after the diseased portion has been removed. An additional complication is the development of a wound infection. Both of these complications can be minimized if the bowel is carefully prepared before surgery, and if antibiotics are used.

Case Study: Cancer of the Breast

Connie grinned as she got into the shower. With the kids at camp, having the bathroom to herself was sheer luxury! Her husband, Mike, was right. They'd have to put in an extra bathroom. After all, she thought, at age 45 she should be able to spend as long as she wanted in the shower.

It was then that she noticed the lump. It seemed like a thickened patch just underneath and a little to the left of her right nipple. She felt it as she was running the soap over her breast. Thoughtfully, she dried herself and felt again.

At breakfast, Connie told Mike what she thought she'd found. They agreed that an appointment with their family doctor should be made immediately.

Dr. Watkins knew Connie well, he'd delivered her second child and been her doctor ever since. "Connie, since we both know your mother died of breast cancer, I'm not going to wait around on this. I'd like you to have a mammogram right away. It will either put both our minds at rest or it will tell us what we have to do next."

Connie had the mammogram two days later. Connie's mother had died at age 50, and Connie remembered very well her mother's five-year battle to stay alive.

Dr. Watkins called her. The mammogram showed a lump that a surgeon should look at. He'll do a biopsy that will tell us more."

Connie thought she had never been examined quite so thoroughly as Dr. Trinkgeld examined her the next day. After checking both breasts very thoroughly, he then gave her a complete physical and ended with a needle biopsy of the lump. It was a quick and relatively painless procedure, which he said would show whether the lump was benign or malignant. "We'll make an appointment for you to come back in three days when we have the results. Then we'll discuss more fully what our options are."

Cancer of the Breast

The breast consists of 12 to 20 segments that converge at the nipple, much like the segments of a pie. On the upper, outer side of the breast, a portion of breast tissue extends up toward the armpit. Each segment of breast tissue contains clusters of cells arranged in circles, like a bunch of grapes. These clusters produce milk. Each segment is drained by a duct that leads to the nipple. There is also fat and other supporting tissues in each breast segment. The combination of fat tissue and milk glands gives the breast its finely lumpy texture.

Breast cells increase in size and number in response to certain hormones. When the hormones are withdrawn, they decrease in size and number. This accounts for the change in breast size and texture that often accompanies the monthly menstrual cycle.

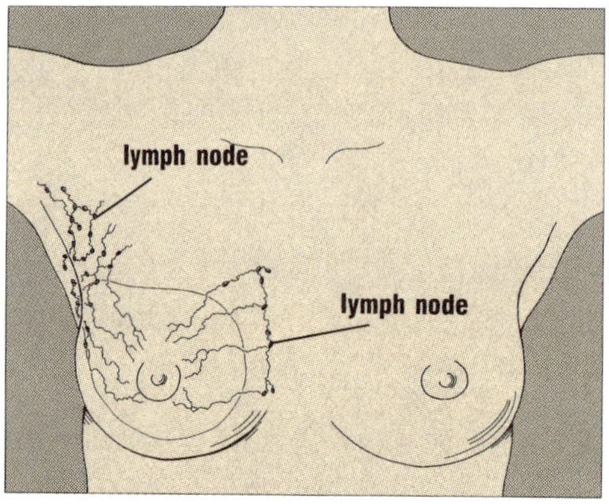

Figure 6.9
Breast tissue and lymph nodes.

Breast tissue is nourished by oxygen and nutrients that come to it in blood from arteries on the chest wall. Veins carry the blood away and back to the heart, as do other tiny tubes called lymphatics which drain toward the armpit and the chest wall, entering tiny lymph glands (Fig. 6.9). The glands collect lymph, which is then passed into the bloodstream in the lower part of the neck.

Many women develop breast lumps. Men sometimes get breast lumps, too, but much less frequently. The discovery of a breast lump should be followed by prompt medical attention. Only one lump in ten discovered by the patient is malignant. Prompt attention allays anxiety for the patient with a benign lump and provides early treatment if the lump is malignant. Early diagnosis and treatment leads to good expectation for cure in the majority of patients.

Infections, cysts, benign tumors, malignant tumors and injury may all cause breast lumps. Breast infections occur most often in women who have just had a baby or who are breastfeeding. The overlying skin may be red and hot, and the patient often has a fever. A lump due to injury may be caused by a sudden impact with the steering wheel of a car.

Cysts, benign tumors and malignant tumors may show up in a very similar way. Often a lump is noted by accident while bathing or dressing. The patient is frequently convinced that it was not there the day or week before and is therefore frightened by what appears to be rapid growth. In fact, most lumps have been present for some time before they are noticed.

A cyst is a cluster of breast cells surrounding a collection of fluid. This condition is common. The lumps are usually painless, but some tenderness may occur with pressure. They usually have a smooth surface. Benign tumors are generally of two types — fibroadenoma and fibrocystic disease (mammary dysplasia). Fibroadenomas are hard, smooth, not tender and move around within the breast. They occur most frequently in women aged 16 to 30. Fibrocystic disease may cause a breast lump which may or may not be tender, or it may cause breast pain without a demonstrative lump.

At times a lump due to fibrocystic disease or a fibroadenoma may be indistinguishable from one due to cancer, in which case a biopsy is necessary. A portion of the lump may be sucked out with a needle, or removed through a small incision in the breast. In most instances

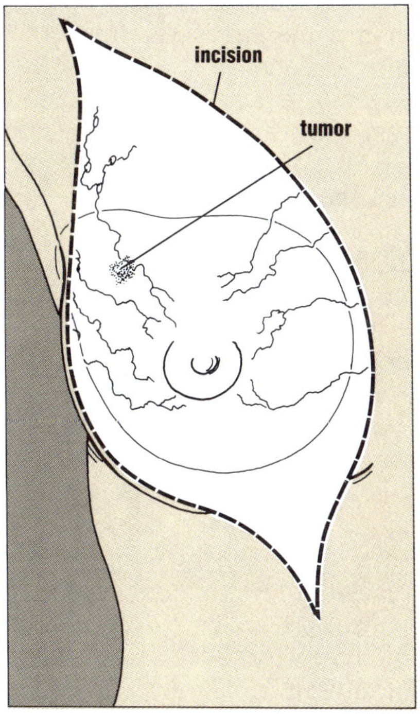

Figure 6.10
Modified radical mastectomy.

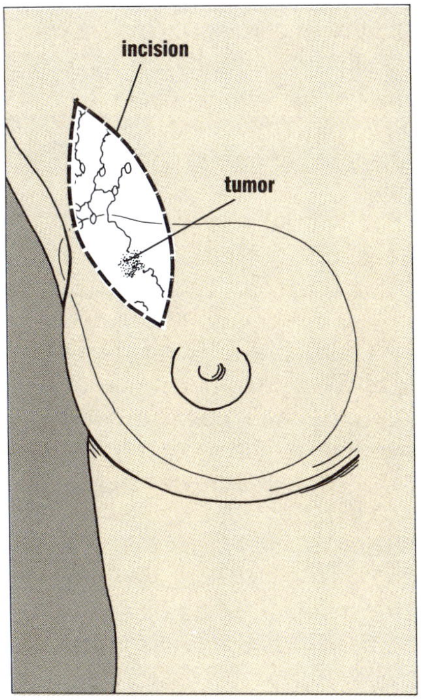

Figure 6.11
Lumpectomy.

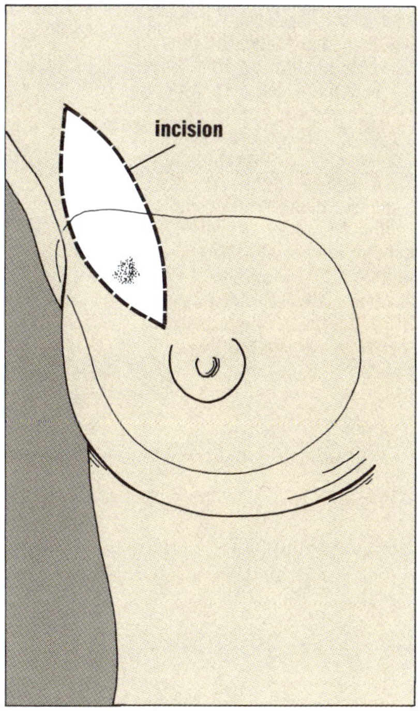

Figure 6.12
Wide local excision.

the incision method is more accurate. Local anesthetic can be used, but usually the patient is given a general anesthetic.

Malignant tumors of the breast arise either from the cell clusters or from the ducts that drain these clusters. Once a breast cancer becomes large enough to be felt as a lump, it has usually been present for about five years. It is sometimes possible to detect such a tumor using X-rays (mammography) before it becomes large enough to be felt. These tumors are usually hard, not tender and are somewhat irregular in shape.

Sometimes the surgeon will be able to make a diagnosis from the patient's history and a physical examination. Usually, however, some additional testing is required. This may include mammography and biopsy (see chapter 20, page 251).

Mammography, an X-ray of the breast, is usually not definitive, but is often helpful is deciding whether to proceed with biopsy.

There are a number of different biopsy techniques. Needle aspiration is the easiest way to make a definitive diagnosis of a breast cyst. If fluid is drawn from the lump and the lump disappears, the surgeon will likely be able to reassure the patient that the condition is benign. Open breast biopsy is the definitive test for a breast lump. This test is usually performed if there is any reasonable suspicion that the lump could be malignant.

Surgical Treatment

If a lump is diagnosed as benign, no treatment is required. However, all malignant breast lumps require more treatment than biopsy alone.

The treatment of breast cancer is controversial even among experts. This is partly due to the fact that these cancers behave differently in different women. In some women minimal treatment produces a cure, while in others even radical treatment is not enough. Generally, there are two ways to treat the local breast disease: surgery and radiation. In some circumstances both methods may be used. If some malignant cells have

The biopsy was positive. The lump was malignant. Dr. Trinkgeld explained that he was going to remove just the lump, not the whole breast, and that he would also check the lump he had found in Connie's armpit. When the pathology report on the lump was available they'd make a decision together about further treatment.

Connie had the operation the next day. Apart from nausea when she was recovering from the anesthetic, and soreness where the lumps had been removed, she felt well. A week later they were back in Dr. Trinkgeld's office. The lump and two involved lymph nodes in the armpit had been removed, with no evidence of any further spread. That was good news. It meant they had a chance to prevent recurrence or spread with treatment. Now they had to consider the options. Dr. Trinkgeld recommended radiation therapy to prevent a recurrence of the lump in the breast, and suggested this be followed by chemotherapy to lessen the possibility of the disease spreading to other sites.

The chemotherapy began a few weeks after the radiation had finished. She found she needed a couple of days off work after the injections, but otherwise the side-effects were minimal. At six months the chemotherapy was over. Dr. Trinkgeld said there was no sign of any disease, but told her he would continue to see her every three months for the next two years. Although follow-up would be life-long, it would decrease in frequency to once every six months at the end of three years.

traveled to the lymph glands under the arm or further, these cells can not usually be treated by surgery or radiation but require drug treatment (chemotherapy). In some circumstances hormone treatment might be substituted for chemotherapy.

In the 1950s, radical mastectomy was the most frequently used treatment for malignant breast lumps. This involved removal of the entire breast, the underlying muscles and all the lymph glands under the arm. This operation produced marked deformity and complications, such as swelling of the arm. By the 1960s, radical mastectomy was largely replaced by modified radical mastectomy, in which the underlying muscles are not removed (Fig 6.10). This operation provides a better cosmetic result than radical mastectomy and rarely results in arm swelling. Follow-up shows that results are just as good as with the more radical procedure. Many surgeons still recommend modified radical mastectomy for most breast cancers.

During the 1970s, a number of surgeons began doing lesser operations for many breast cancers. For many women, the lesser operations are just as good as more radical ones. These lesser procedures may include lumpectomy (Fig 6.11, simple removal of the breast lump), wide local excision (Fig 6.12, removal of the lump plus a wide margin of apparently normal tissue), and segmental resection, in which a segment of the breast containing the lump is removed. These lesser procedures are referred to as partial mastectomy. There is a risk of leaving some malignant cells in the remaining breast tissue, and therefore after partial mastectomy the breast is frequently treated by radiation.

If the tumor is small and confined to the breast, the chance of permanent cure is about 80 percent. However, if the tumor is large or has spread to the lymph nodes under the arm, the cure rate is much lower. Chemotherapy may then be added to the treatment program, which produces a cure for many women.

If the breast has been completely removed, the patient may wish to have some type of special brassiere fitting. The use of cosmetic surgery to help repair the defect may also be possible. In most cases, however, surgeons are concerned that cosmetic surgery may obscure evidence of tumor recurrence and are therefore hesitant to recommend it.

From an emotional perspective, the diagnosis of breast cancer can be devastating. It is often several months before a woman can look back on the event with any equanimity. Understanding this diagnosis takes time — it is a process rather than an event.

Complications

The major complication of surgery for breast cancer is stiffness in the shoulder, so early use of the arm and shoulder are encouraged. Sometimes physiotherapy is required. A long-term complication is swelling of the arm, which can occur following extensive removal of lymph glands under the arm. However, with more conservative surgery and early movement of the shoulder, this complication is rare.

Chapter 7

Thoracic Surgery

Robert J. Ginsberg
Professor and Chairman
Division of Thoracic Surgery
University of Toronto
Surgeon-in-Chief
Mount Sinai Hospital, Toronto

Terry Watkinson
Illustrator

Thoracic surgery involves the organs of the chest, except for the heart and large blood vessels (Fig. 7.1). The operations most frequently performed by the thoracic surgeon include tests to diagnose lung disease, such as viewing the airway (bronchoscopy), biopsying lymph glands draining the lung (mediastinoscopy), removal of lung tissue—either the whole lung (pneumonectomy) or half lung (lobectomy)—and esophageal surgery, such as hiatus hernia repair.

In Canada, cardiac and thoracic surgery are usually separate areas of specialization, but in the U.S., they may be practiced by the same surgeon.

Lungs

The nasal passages and mouth help transport oxygen to the lungs by a series of tubes — the windpipe (trachea), which branches into smaller tubes called bronchi. The oxygen reaches the lung, which acts like a sponge, and is picked up by the blood and then delivered to the rest of the body (Fig. 7.2).

To get air into the lungs through these passages, the chest wall (ribs) and diaphragm expand, producing a suction effect. Air is sucked in through the mouth

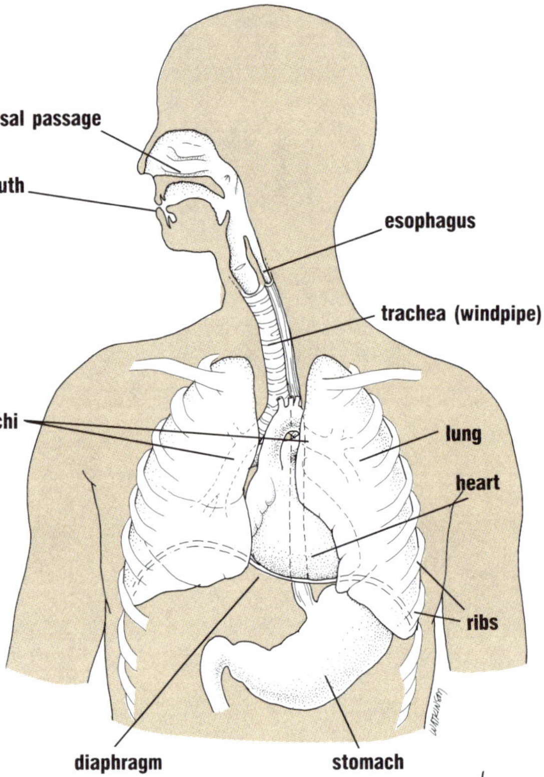

Figure 7.1
Thoracic organs

and nasal passages, through the trachea and bronchi into the lung. In the lung, oxygen is exchanged for carbon dioxide (one of the waste materials the body produces in converting oxygen to energy), and the carbon dioxide is blown out of the lungs. The average person breathes 16 times per minute, taking in about a pint of air with each breath.

Because of the high incidence of smoking, North Americans frequently get lung disease, including bronchitis (inflammation of the bronchi), emphysema (loss of elasticity in the lungs) and cancer. Lung cancer is the leading cause of death from cancer in men, and will soon overtake cancer of the breast to become the leading cause of cancer death in women. Over one million people in the world die

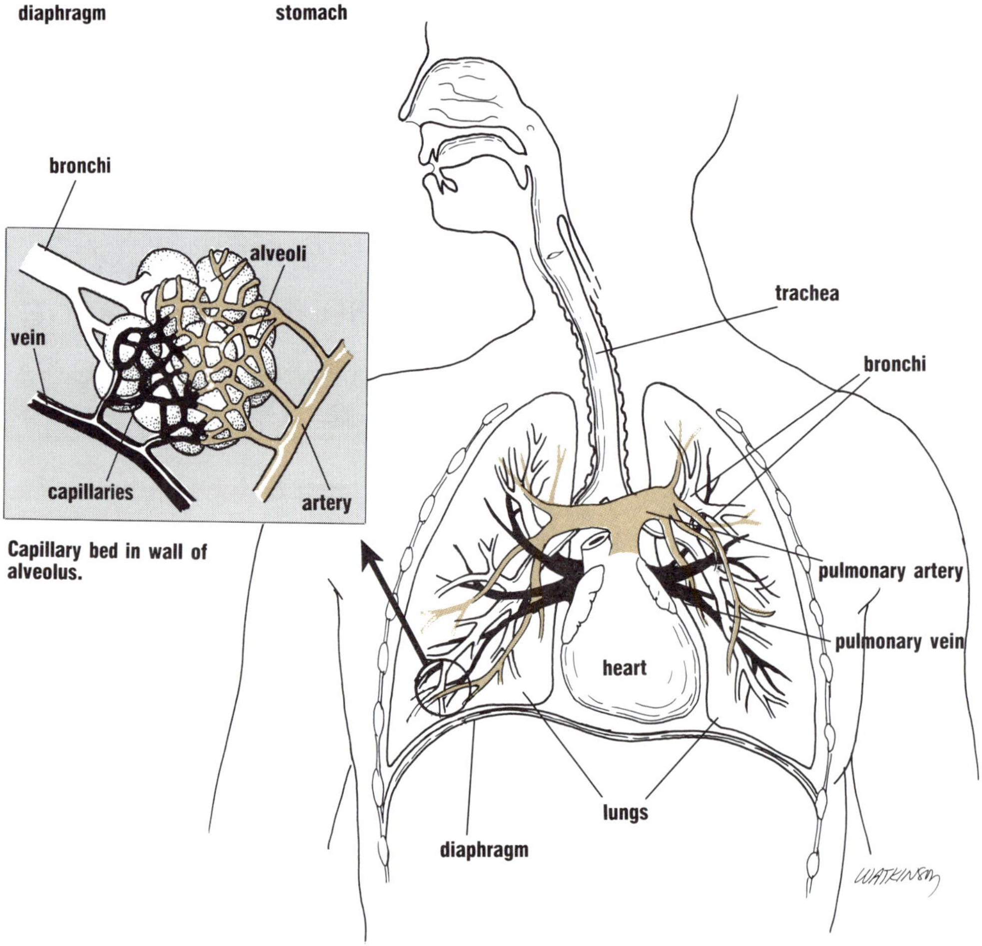

Figure 7.2
Lungs. The bronchi deliver oxygen to tiny sacs called alveoli, where it is picked up by the pulmonary capillaries (small blood vessels). The oxygenated blood is taken to the heart via the pulmonary veins. Unoxygenated blood is returned to the lungs via the pulmonary arteries.

of lung cancer each year. By the year 2000, the figure will likely be two million.

The most common reason for removing portions of lung is to treat lung cancer. In most cases surgical removal is the most effective way of curing the disease, although in only about one-third of all patients developing this highly lethal cancer is the disease caught early enough for surgery to be advised.

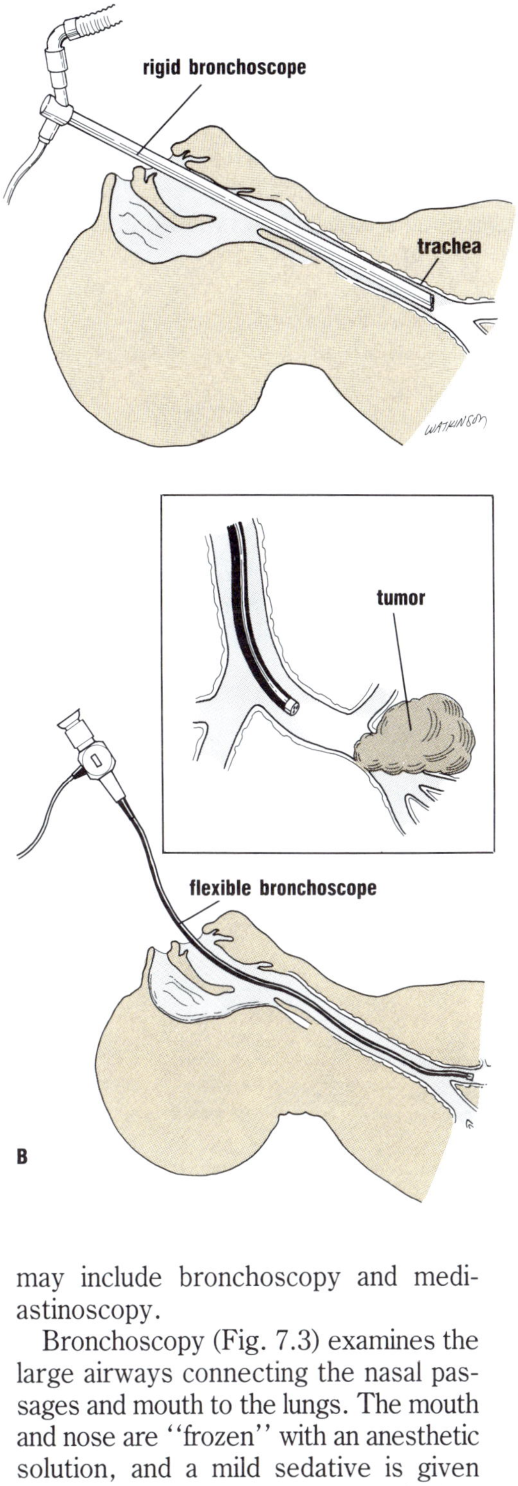

Figure 7.3
Bronchoscopy. A rigid (A) or flexible (B) bronchoscope can be passed down the trachea for the purposes of inspecting the airway or withdrawing a specimen for examination.

Lung Cancer

The chronic irritation caused by the tars in cigarette smoke produces changes in the cells lining the air tubes. These cells can eventually change into cancer cells. A tumor may develop in the smallest of the air tubes without the patient noticing any change. However, if it develops in one of the larger air tubes, it will obstruct the flow of air back and forth, causing a cough, shortness of breath, and possibly pneumonia (acute inflammation of the lungs). If the tumor grows very quickly, its growth can outstrip its blood supply, and it will start to disintegrate, causing blood flecks to appear in the sputum. If the tumor continues to enlarge, it can invade the chest wall, causing pain.

Diagnosis

Unfortunately, the best time to treat lung cancer is before it causes symptoms. Often a routine chest X-ray will pick up a shadow on the lung or a change that suggests lung cancer. If the diagnosis is made at this point, the cancer is more likely to be in a curable state. Once symptoms develop — cough, pneumonia, blood-spitting — the tumor is usually more advanced and less curable.

Frequently, the diagnosis of lung cancer is made by microscopically examining sputum samples or, when the cancer is in the outer regions of the lung, by needle biopsy (removing cells from the tumor by inserting a needle through the chest wall into the tumor). Other tests may include bronchoscopy and mediastinoscopy.

Bronchoscopy (Fig. 7.3) examines the large airways connecting the nasal passages and mouth to the lungs. The mouth and nose are "frozen" with an anesthetic solution, and a mild sedative is given intravenously. The bronchoscope is then passed through the mouth or nose into the airway. Usually a flexible bronchoscope with a fiberoptic system that contains lenses is used. Occasionally a rigid hollow metal tube is required. Any abnormalities of the airway can be inspected,

Case Study: Lung Cancer

Lily thought it was all a bit of a fuss, really, this chest X-ray every two years. She told Dr. Smith, "My parents both smoked twice as much as I do. They didn't go for chest X-rays." Since both her parents had died of heart disease, Dr. Smith wasn't too impressed with this argument. "A pack a day is a significant risk factor, Lily, and as long as you're my patient I want you to keep having the X-rays."

This time he'd called her back. "There seems to be a spot on your right lung that wasn't there two years ago. We'll wait a couple of weeks, then we'll do another X-ray, just to be sure." Lily wasn't worried. She'd had a bit of a cough lately, but she wasn't sick. After all, she was only 55.

But two weeks later the spot was still there. Dr. Smith said she'd have to see a specialist for a test called a tomography. Lily didn't like the sound of that. She told her niece about it on the phone that evening. Maureen was a nurse. She'd probably know about this tomography business. "Why don't you get an appointment on my day off, Auntie Lil? Then I can come with you to see the surgeon." "Surgeon?" yelped Lily. "Dr. Smith said a specialist." "A surgeon's a specialist, Auntie Lil. I know Dr. Minander. I've worked with him in the operating room."

Lily didn't like the sound of this at all. Dr. Smith had said it was just a test. But Maureen told her all about the CAT scan, and it really wasn't bad, just a big machine. She didn't like the waiting around, though. She kept asking Maureen why they couldn't just go home. "But, Auntie, Dr. Minander's going to tell you the results as soon as the picture's ready." "Oh, I can wait. Can't he just tell Dr. Smith?"

"The spot looks very much like a malignant tumor, Mrs. Anderson," said Dr. Minander. "We need to do another test called a bronchoscopy, and we'll do a needle biopsy at the same time." Lily glanced at Maureen and was surprised to see how pale her niece was. "Would surgery be — successful, Doctor?" her niece asked. "I don't know yet, but if there's no spread, yes, the chances are good," replied Dr. Minander. "What would I need surgery for?" asked Lily. "Do you know what malignant tumor means, Auntie?" Maureen asked. Lily didn't answer.

and specimens can be withdrawn for examination by the pathologist.

Bronchoscopy usually causes only slight discomfort. The patient will frequently experience coughing during the examination, but very little else. The patient receives enough oxygen and sedation to make him or her as comfortable as possible.

If a rigid tube is to be used, general anesthetic is usually preferred. After this procedure, the patient may have a sore throat, but very little other discomfort.

Non-Surgical Treatment

Once the diagnosis of lung cancer is made, the doctor will order other tests, such as isotope scans, computerized axial tomography (CAT scan) or ultrasound examination, to see whether the cancer has spread. If it has, surgery is unlikely to remove the disease and is usually not recommended.

Non-surgical treatments may include chemotherapy (drugs that kill cancer cells) and/or radiation. These treatments can shrink the tumor, and may even cause it to disappear. However, on the whole, this type of treatment relieves only the symptoms of the disease by shrinking the tumor; eventually, the cancer will likely recur.

Surgical Treatment

When surgery is being considered for lung cancer, biopsy of the lymph glands draining the lung (mediastinoscopy) is frequently necessary to evaluate infections and types of cancer. If the cancer has spread to the lymph glands around the windpipe, the tumor has usually spread beyond the stage which can be cured by surgery (Fig. 7.4). Since mediastinoscopy is a fairly minor procedure, many surgeons perform this operation first, to avoid subjecting patients who cannot be cured to major surgery.

Mediastinoscopy is done through a small cut in the neck, just above the breast bone. The cut extends down to the area of the windpipe, and the biopsies are taken through an instrument inserted in the front of the trachea into the area between the breastbone and lungs (mediastinum).

The operation is simple and safe, and is performed under general anesthetic. Usually the only problem after the operation is mild pain related to the incision.

Before major surgery is considered, the patient will be advised to stop smoking and will be taught breathing exercises, as well as exercises to regain activity of the shoulder. Because large muscles of the chest and shoulder are divided and then sewn up again, movement of the shoulder can become restricted after the operation unless exercises are done every day to mobilize it. Breathing exercises are important to prevent pneumonia from developing after the operation.

If the lung cancer can be cured by removing a portion of the lung, the operation will be performed in three stages. First, the muscles of the chest in front of the ribs will be cut, and the chest

Figure 7.4
Lung tumor.

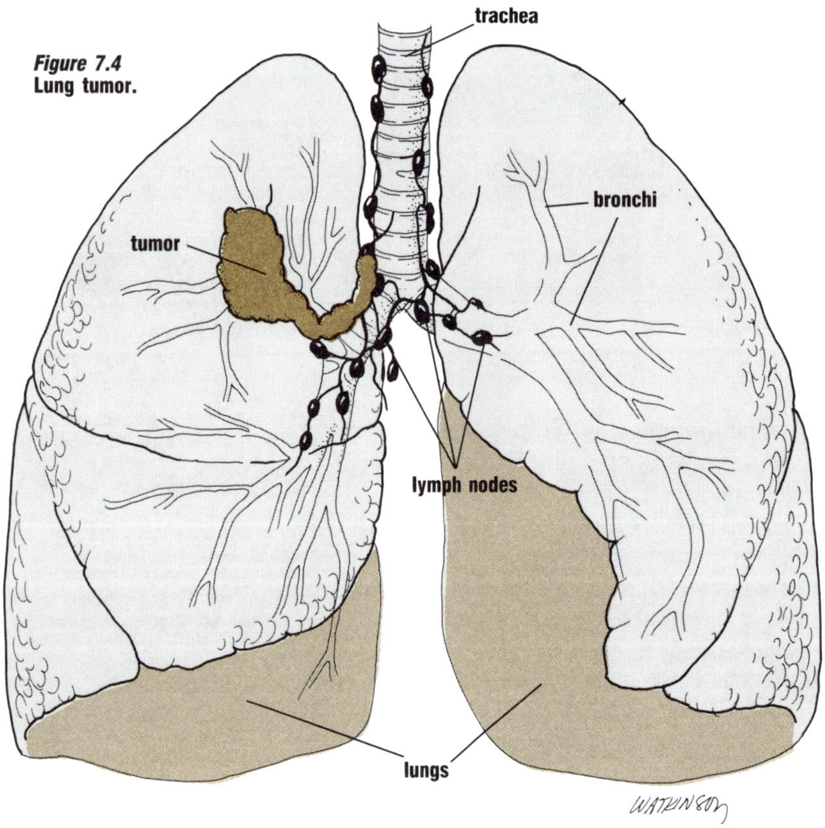

cavity will be entered either between ribs or by removing a rib (Fig. 7.5). Then the airway and the blood vessels supplying the affected part of the lung are divided and closed off, and the diseased portion of the lung is removed. The final step includes closing the incisions in the ribs, muscles and skin.

To remove the cancer, the surgeon may remove the whole lung (pneumonectomy), half the lung (lobectomy), or sometimes even less than half a lung (segmentectomy or wedge resection). The operation that removes the least amount of lung necessary will be chosen.

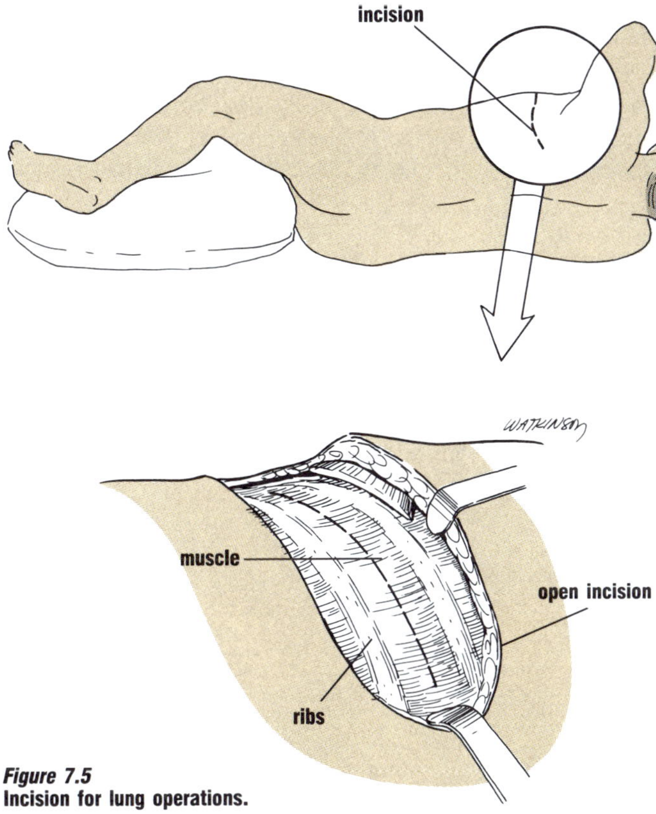

Figure 7.5
Incision for lung operations.

Complications

About 1 percent of all patients under 60 will succumb to complications arising from the operation. This figure rises to 4 percent for those aged 60 to 70, and to 6 to 7 percent for those over age 70. Complications after this surgery are infrequent but if they do occur are usually not life-threatening. Because most patients with cancer are elderly, problems related to the heart and lungs are the most common. The surgeon will monitor heart and lung function continuously for a few days after the surgery, often in an intensive care unit.

One or two tubes will usually be left in the chest after the operation to drain the chest of air and fluid leaking from the remaining portion of the lung until spontaneous healing occurs (Fig. 7.6). Once air and fluids stop leaking from the lung, the chest tubes will be removed. This normally occurs within a few days of surgery. Once all tubes are removed, recovery is quite speedy.

Since the surgeon either spreads the ribs or removes a rib to get at the lung, the patient will experience pain when coughing or moving for a few days after the operation. Pain-relieving drugs are given to control the pain.

The patient remains in hospital for about seven to ten days. After this, the patient is quite mobile and self-sufficient, but needs further convalescence at home to regain strength. Few patients will require nursing care at home. The family can usually provide the little assistance that is needed. Most patients can return to work four to six weeks after the operation.

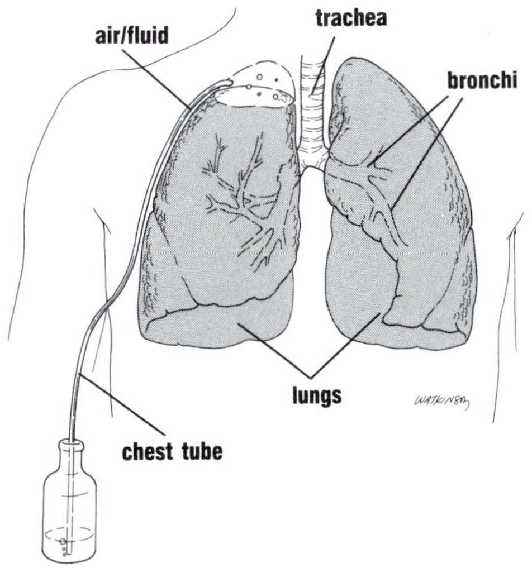

Figure 7.6
Chest tube.

Dr. Minander said she'd have a local anesthetic for the bronchoscopy. Afterwards, she didn't feel too bad — a bit groggy, a sore throat, but nothing to it, really. Her sister was coming to take her home at the end of the day. She hoped that would be the end to it, but Maureen seemed to think she'd be back in the hospital in a couple of weeks, and had told her to get the time off work. Her boss had asked if it was serious. Lily had said it wasn't, but Maureen had got really annoyed with her, and said she was to ask for six weeks off. Six weeks! She'd never been off work that long in her life.

Both her sister and Maureen were there when Dr. Minander came back to see her. "The pathologist's report shows a malignant tumor at the base of your right lung. It doesn't look as though there's any spread, although we'll check for that. I recommend surgery, to remove that portion of your lung." This time, they didn't have to tell her. Lily knew they were talking about cancer.

Lily didn't really have much time to brood on it. There always seemed to be some test or other in the two weeks before she had surgery.

Maureen had assured her that she had a good chance of being cured, but Lily didn't feel so optimistic. It seemed she was to have something called mediastinoscopy before the operation to take out part of her lung.

"The mediastinoscopy is a kind of biopsy that tells the surgeon if the cancer has spread to your lymph glands," one of the nurses explained.

She hadn't expected to feel so much pain after the operation. The incision was very sore, which Maureen said was because they'd had to pull her ribs apart to get at her lung. But Dr. Minander's news was good. "We found no spread, and we got out all the tumor, so the outlook is good. We'll have to see how things progress over the next few months." He was pleased to see that she'd stopped smoking. She didn't tell him she'd given it up mostly because the pain was so bad when she coughed.

It was a week before Lily left the hospital. She still felt a lot of pain around the incision, but Dr. Minander had said he could give her something for the pain if it seemed too bad. Although it took a few months, the discomfort did eventually disappear.

She saw Dr. Minander every three months at first. Each time he gave her a good report, she felt on top of the world. When she went to see Dr. Smith again she told him, "Those chest X-rays of yours weren't a waste of time, after all." After 18 months, she was down to two visits a year to Dr. Minander. Maureen had told her that was a good sign, and that at the end of five years she'd only have to see him once a year. Lily never did start to smoke again. Suddenly it didn't seem like there was all the time in the world to quit, after all.

Removing small portions of a lung has minimal effect on breathing. If a whole lung is removed, the patient likely will no longer be able to participate in strenuous activities such as running or tennis. However, the routine activities of daily living and less active sports, such as golf and swimming, can easily be undertaken.

The cure rate from lung cancer depends entirely on the stage of the disease at surgery. As a general rule, if the cancer is totally removed, there is a good chance of cure. Very early cancer (without spread to the lymph glands) can be cured in about 80 percent of cases. The cure rate lessens with spread to the lymph glands.

Recent Advances

Forty years ago all lung cancers were treated by removal of the whole lung. In the last 30 years, removal of half a lung has been done wherever possible and, recently, removal of only a portion has been found to be just as effective in curing certain types of lung cancer.

Recent research has combined chemotherapy, radiotherapy and surgery in the hope that more patients will be cured. We do not yet know the results of this type of treatment.

Esophagus

The esophagus, or gullet, is a hollow muscular tube connecting the throat to the stomach. It propels swallowed food into the stomach to be digested. The esophagus itself does not digest food. It is simply a means of transportation.

Once food enters the upper esophagus, the muscular valve between the lower esophagus and stomach opens up to allow easy passage of food into the stomach (Fig. 7.7). When one is not eating, this valve is usually closed to prevent food or stomach juices from traveling back into the esophagus, where the acid and digestive enzymes could "burn" the inner lining of the esophagus, producing an uncomfortable heartburn sensation. On the other hand, this intricate valve must allow belching and, in certain circumstances, vomiting.

The valve is located just below the diaphragm within the abdominal cavity. Because of the weight of all the abdominal organs, this cavity exerts a pressure that helps keep the valve closed. There is another upper muscular valve between the throat and esophagus. If food does happen to get back into the esophagus, this valve can prevent it from returning to the mouth, where it may "go down the wrong way" into the lung.

Reflux Disease and Hiatus Hernia

Diagnosis

Because of the higher pressure in the abdominal cavity compared to the pressure in the chest cavity, the upper part of the stomach is sometimes pushed into the chest through the opening in the diaphragm that allows the esophagus to pass through to the stomach (Fig. 7.8). This results in a hiatus hernia, which may weaken the lower valve mechanism. If the valve is not weakened, few problems occur. Only about 5 percent of patients with hiatus hernia experience any significant symptoms.

A weakened valve allows food and stomach juices to "reflux" back into the esophagus, burning the esophagus lining because of the acid nature of the stomach contents. Eventually ulceration can occur. The ulcers will heal, but the resulting scar tissue can narrow the lower end of the esophagus and interfere with food traveling into the stomach. During all of this, the patient may experience reflux symptoms such as heartburn or spontaneous regurgitation of food or acid to the back of the throat.

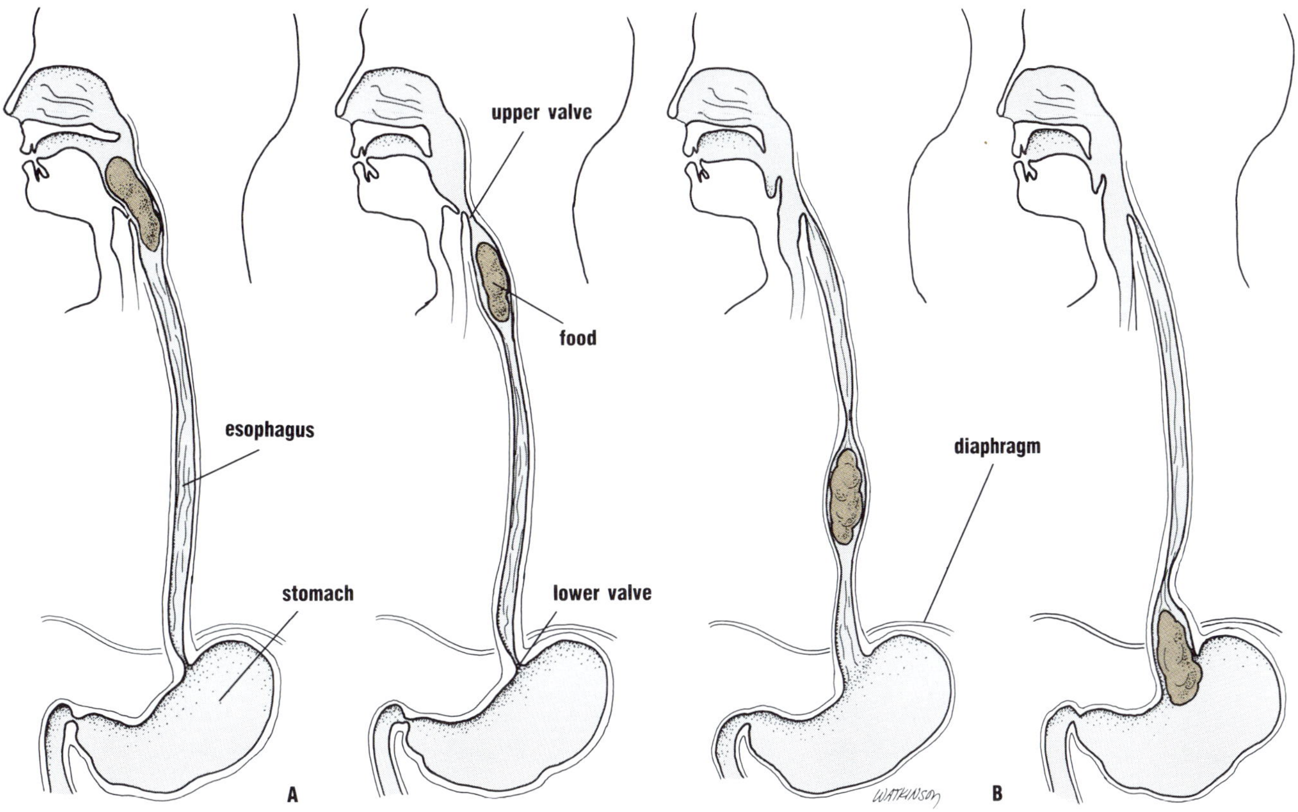

Figure 7.7
Esophagus. Food is swallowed (A) and transported down the esophagus to the stomach. A lower muscular valve closes to prevent food from passing back into the esophagus (B).

Acid regurgitation can cause choking, especially if the patient is lying flat. Occasionally, the acid simply irritates the esophagus, causing spasm of the esophageal muscle which can result in chest pain, either spontaneously or when eating.

With increasing abdominal pressure (obesity, pregnancy, etc.) or simply with time, further herniation of the stomach into the chest may occur. A large hernia (Fig. 7.9) can produce a heavy feeling in the lower chest, or even significant pain. Extreme herniations can interfere with heart and lung function. In the worst instance, the whole stomach herniates into the chest, and may completely twist, cutting off the blood supply and causing gangrene. This is very rare, but it can occur.

Non-Surgical Treatment

Most patients with a hiatus hernia require no treatment, since there are no symptoms. However, if the symptoms of reflux do occur, especially heartburn, the patient will often seek help. In most

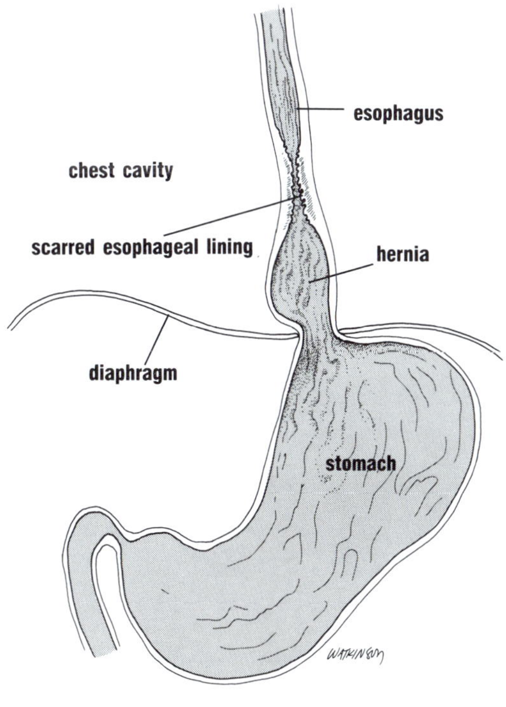

Figure 7.8
Hiatus hernia. Scarring can be caused by acids that are regurgitated back into the lower esophagus.

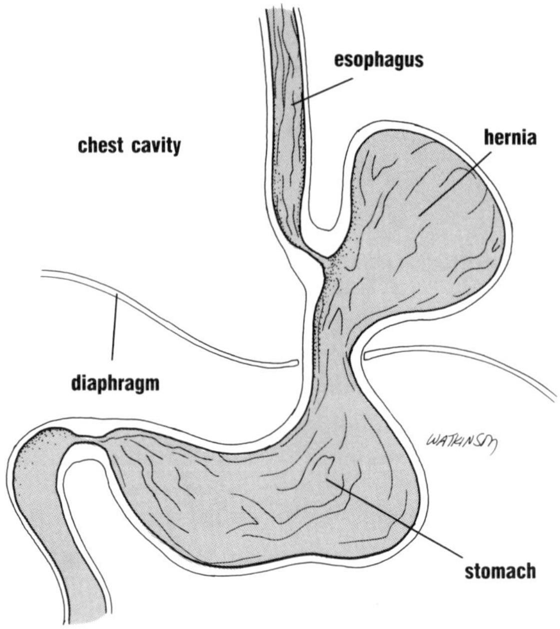

Figure 7.9
Advanced hiatus hernia.

instances a barium X-ray examination of the esophagus and stomach will reveal the diagnosis. With mild symptoms, no further tests are required. The treatment may include avoiding smoking and fatty foods (both of which weaken the valve), elevation of the upper body in bed to prevent liquid from refluxing (Fig. 7.10) and avoiding foods that aggravate the heartburn, especially alcohol and acid foods such as juices. Antacids or drugs to reduce acid production are frequently prescribed to counteract the acid in the stomach.

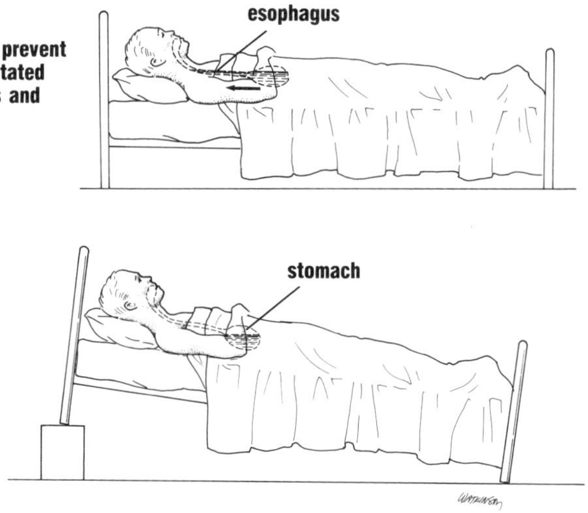

Figure 7.10
Elevating upper body to prevent acids from being regurgitated back into the esophagus and throat.

Very frequently, this treatment will control the symptoms. Since the symptoms of reflux occur only periodically, treatment may be necessary for a few months and then only intermittently. If symptoms persist, however, or it is suspected that the esophagus has been damaged, further tests and possibly surgical treatment may be required.

The most common test other than a barium X-ray is esophagoscopy. After the throat has been frozen, a flexible esophagoscope — a relatively thin, movable fiberoptic tube — is passed through the mouth and into the esophagus (Fig. 7.11), so that the whole of the esophagus, valve area, stomach and duodenum (upper part of the small intestine) can be inspected. If the esophagus is abnormal, tissue specimens can be taken for examination by the pathologist.

Although rare, a "rigid" esophagoscopy, using a hollow metal tube, may be necessary. This is almost always done under general anesthetic, and is done only when there is extreme narrowing of the esophagus, or when a piece of food is stuck in the esophagus and has to be removed.

Other tests include special fine probes passed through the mouth into the esophagus and stomach to test the amount of acid that is regurgitating into the esophagus over a fixed period of time (pH test), or to determine the muscular function of the esophagus (esophageal manometry). Isotope tests can also be used to evaluate the function of the esophagus, the abnormal valve and the stomach. This requires swallowing small amounts of radioactive material, which can then be followed through the esophagus and stomach by the use of a "gamma camera," much like a geiger counter. The amount of radioactive material used in this examination is minimal and noninjurious.

Surgical Treatment

Surgical correction of hiatus hernia or the symptoms of reflux disease can be done

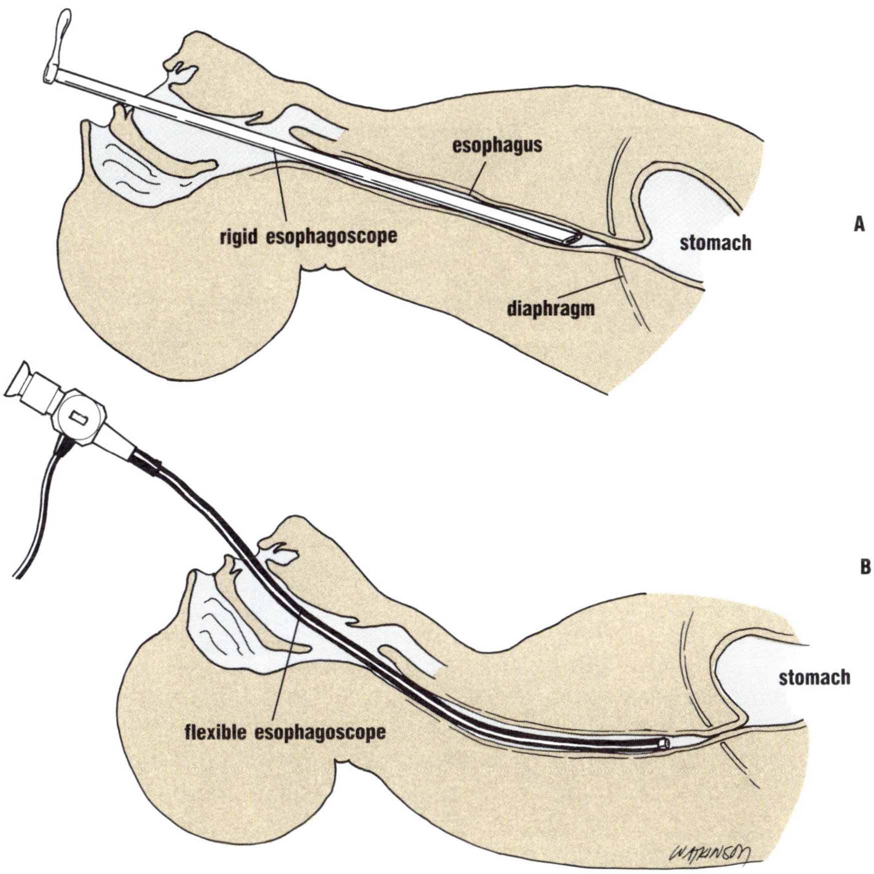

Figure 7.11
Esophagoscopy. A rigid (A) or flexible (B) esophagoscope can be used to examine the esophagus and stomach.

in a number of ways, and the surgeon may choose to approach the problem through a chest incision or abdominal incision. First, the stomach and the lower end of the esophagus have to be brought down into the abdominal cavity to allow the valve to function again. In addition, various techniques are used to reinforce the valve and stop the stomach from pushing back up through the diaphragm (Fig. 7.12). If, for example, the esophagus has been seriously damaged and scarring has occurred, the surgeon may have to reconstruct the esophagus using a portion of the stomach (Fig. 7.13).

In general, convalescence from hiatus hernia surgery is smooth. Patients should be eating within a few days of surgery and should leave the hospital in seven to ten days. After surgery, food may stick at the lower end of the esophagus due to swelling, so the patient should avoid

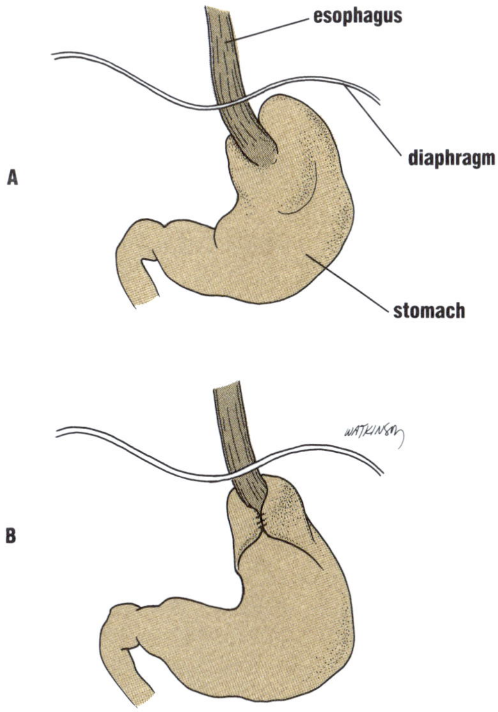

Figure 7.12

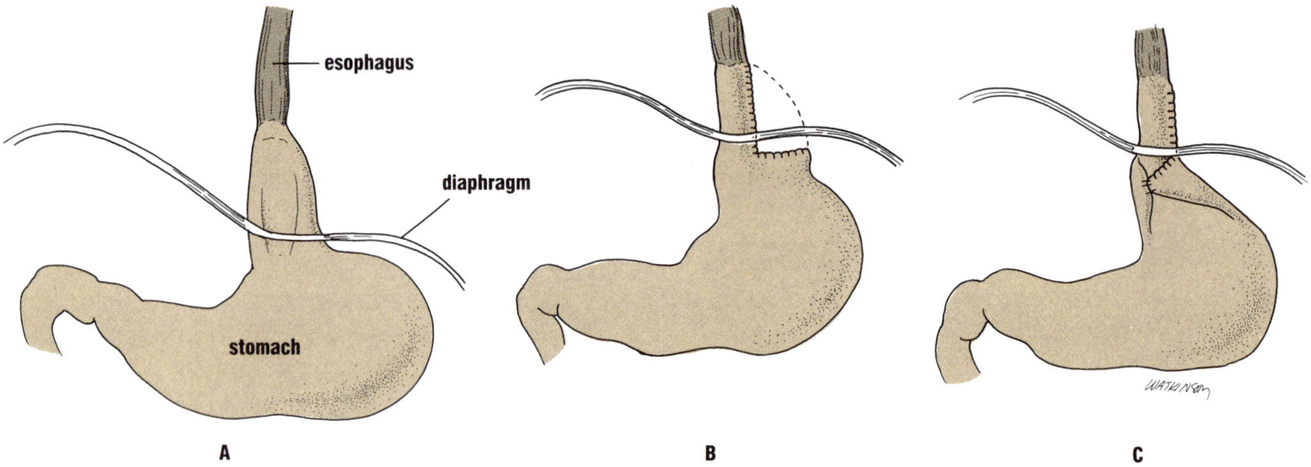

Figure 7.13
Hiatus hernia repair. In some cases, the bulging hernia (A) may be corrected by surgically lengthening the esophagus using a portion of the stomach (B and C).

bulky foods for the first few weeks. If the incision is made through the abdomen, there is often less postoperative pain, but a longer convalescence is required before normal eating can begin. If the incision is made through the chest, there is usually more pain, but return to normal eating occurs more quickly.

Complications

Unfortunately, the valve mechanism is a delicate one and perfect reconstruction can be difficult. The operation is designed to allow food to pass easily through the valve, prevent food and acid from regurgitating, but allow the patient to belch and/or vomit when necessary. If the valve is reconstructed too tightly, the patient will not be able to belch or vomit normally.

Over several years, about 10 to 15 percent of patients will develop recurrent symptoms. On the whole, however, if the operation is expertly done, the symptoms will be much less severe than the original ones.

The real problem for the surgeon in this illness is the careful selection of patients for whom surgery should be advised. Many patients with reflux and hiatus hernia symptoms have unrelated symptoms such as nausea, chest pain, headaches, back or arm pain, which may not be relieved by the operation.

A few decades ago, it was not uncommon for this operation to fail. However, with more advanced surgical techniques, and with careful selection of the appropriate patient, anti-reflux surgery can now be advised if non-surgical treatment fails to control the problem.

Recent Advances

A recently popularized technique of surgically treating hiatus hernia involves wrapping a plastic collar around the lower end of the esophagus to mimic the function of the valve that has been damaged. Although these plastic collars have been used for the past eight to ten years, they are associated with a high incidence of complications due to the plastic dislodging. Most surgeons are wary about recommending this approach.

Chapter 8

Obstetrics and Gynecology

Obstetrics and gynecology is the specialty of medicine concerned with women's reproductive health and disease. It encompasses pregnancy and childbirth, infertility, menstrual abnormalities, pelvic infections, cancer of the female reproductive organs and problems with pelvic support.

Walter J. Hannah
Professor and Chairman
Department of Obstetrics
and Gynecology
University of Toronto
Obstetrician and Gynecologist
Women's College Hospital, Toronto

Sari O'Sullivan
Illustrator

Uterus

The uterus (Figs. 8.1 and 8.2) is a hollow, pear-shaped structure that lies in the pelvis between the bladder in front, and the rectum and large intestine behind. The inner lining of the uterus is called endometrium. This lining is shed every month as menstruation, and is the place where the fertilized egg implants itself if a woman becomes pregnant. During pregnancy, the primary function of the uterus is to provide a home for the developing fetus, allowing it to grow, providing its nourishment, and finally expelling it when it is ready to be born. The lower portion of the uterus (neck or cervix) is attached to the upper end of the vagina and protrudes into it for a short distance. The physician can feel or see the cervix during a pelvic examination. During labor, the cervix must widen to allow the fetus to pass out of the uterus and into the vagina.

The uterus or "womb" is the vital organ in the reproductive process. Even

Figure 8.1
Posterior view of female pelvis.

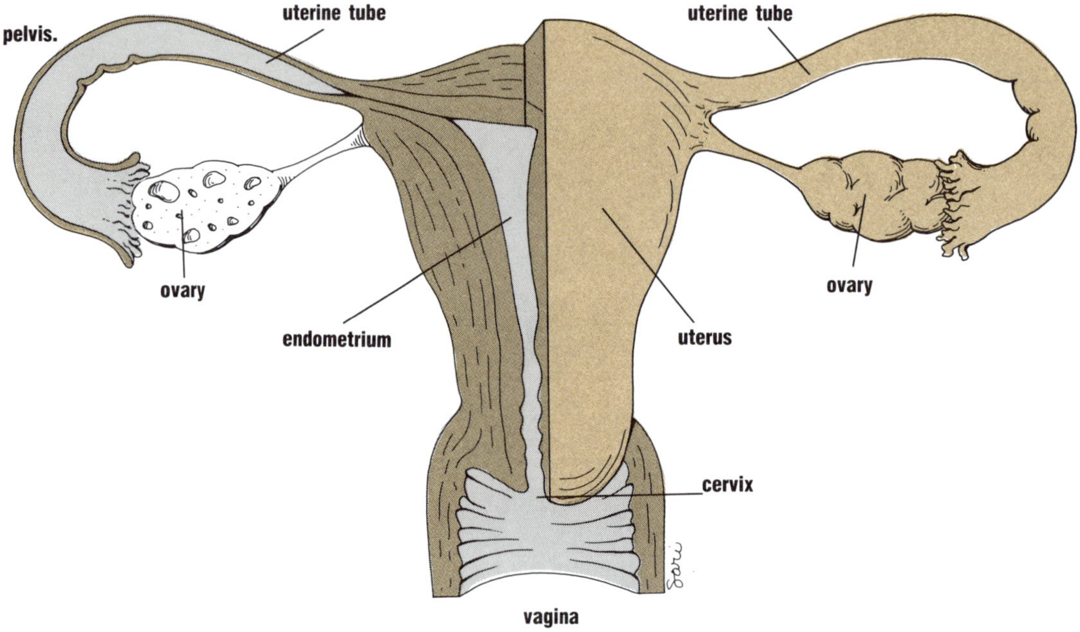

though babies can now be conceived outside the uterus, it is not possible for a pregnancy to be completed successfully outside the uterus.

Surgery on the uterus may consist of removal of fibroid tumors (myomectomy), correction of congenital abnormalities to facilitate childbearing (metroplasty), cesarean section in childbirth (hysterotomy), and total removal of the uterus (hysterectomy). Hysterectomy is most often performed because of a disabling disturbance in menstrual function, or failure of supporting ligaments to maintain the uterus in its proper position.

Figure 8.2
Side view of female pelvis.

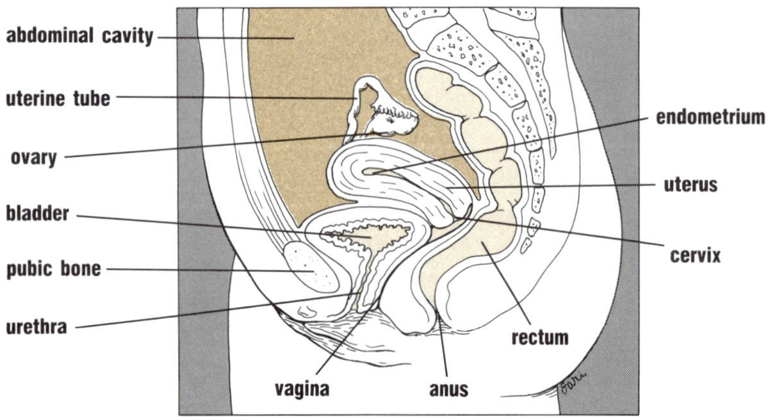

Dysfunctional Menorrhagia

Under ordinary circumstances, menstrual flow is not excessive. Occasionally, however, menstruation becomes excessive and/or prolonged for no apparent reason, especially in the later reproductive years. In most cases there is no uterine abnormality. This condition is called dysfunctional menorrhagia, and is the reason for most of the hysterectomies performed in North America.

The typical menorrhagia patient is in her late thirties or forties. Her periods were previously normal but are now much heavier and/or prolonged. She may pass clots of blood, indicating that a large amount of bleeding is taking place. She may have endured the embarrassment of a social accident. In many instances, she feels dragged out by the end of the period because of the excessive blood loss. It is often a very disabling condition, detracting significantly from her enjoyment of life and her ability to meet the demands of her day-to-day schedule.

The cause of this problem is still unknown. Recent research suggests that a group of substances called prostaglandins, which are contained in uterine mus-

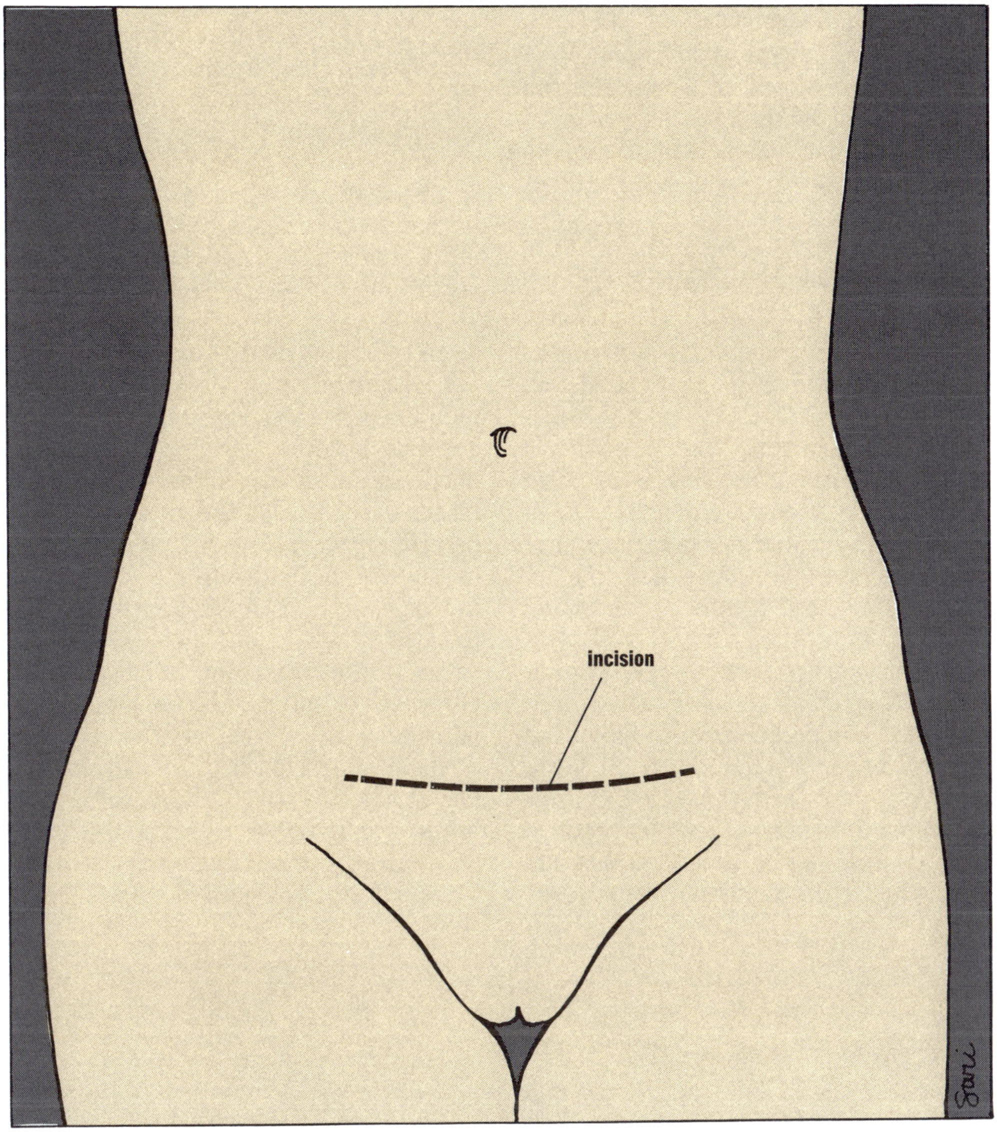

Figure 8.3
"Bikini" Incision used for most gynecologic surgical operations.

Case Study:
Dysfunctional Menorrhagia

As a career person, Carol found taking a day off work every month because of her period out of the question. For about three months now, her periods had been really heavy — and they'd been longer than usual, too. It seemed as though one had only just finished when the next one started. She had thought that as you got older your periods got lighter, not heavier, until they gradually stopped altogether. Today she was flooding. She'd been up an hour and had already changed her pad and her underwear three times. At this rate, she was afraid to go anywhere. She decided to see her gynecologist for an examination.

Dr. Laxner did a pelvic exam, but everything looked just fine. She recommended that Carol have a dilatation and curettage — a D and C. "It's not a remedy; it's to let us know what's going on in your uterus. Once we know that, we'll be able to decide on a course of treatment."

cle, may affect the blood clotting mechanism and the uterine blood vessels' ability to contract. Reduction in both of these actions will increase bleeding. In many cases, menorrhagia may be associated with menstrual cycles in which ovulation does not take place, as is often the case in women in their forties. Absence of the hormone progesterone leaves the endometrium stimulated by estrogen only. The resultant shedding of the endometrium is irregular, leading to periods of up to 14 days or even longer.

Occasionally the bleeding is so heavy that urgent treatment is required. More often the problem is chronic, with month after month of heavy disabling periods.

The diagnosis of dysfunctional menorrhagia is not difficult. It is based on the history of the menstrual periods along with the finding, on pelvic examination, of normal pelvic structures. The hemoglobin is measured to see how much blood has been lost.

Dilatation and curettage (D and C) done in the premenstrual phase of the

Carol managed to have the D and C fairly quickly. Dr. Laxner had stressed that it must be in the second half of her cycle, so they could find out if she was ovulating. Dr. Laxner had also given her iron pills to take, and they did seem to make her feel less tired. Who knew, maybe this was just a temporary thing. Her first period after the D and C was certainly nothing like the 10 to 12 days she'd been getting used to.

Her second period coincided with her postop checkup. "Dr. Laxner, it's back. I was almost afraid to leave the house today, I was flooding so much." "Well, Carol, you're still ovulating, so hormone treatments aren't going to help. I think we're looking at a hysterectomy if you really want to get rid of this."

Carol was shocked. She thought that a hysterectomy was something you had when you had cancer — and then not until you were well into your fifties. "Dr. Laxner, I'm only 44. It isn't . . .?" "Cancer? Extremely unlikely. If you didn't smoke, I'd recommend trying the birth control pill, because it often corrects this situation, but you'd likely be taking it until the menopause."

The doctor made Carol feel much better. "The most common reason for doing a hysterectomy is heavy menstrual bleeding, and we usually find nothing else wrong in a woman of your age." They talked about family size. Carol was adamant that at age 44 she didn't want any more children, which Dr. Laxner said was the only final thing about having a hysterectomy. "It *is* major surgery and I don't want to minimize that, but women with your condition usually find that after the healing period they feel much better than they did when they were having such debilitating periods."

cycle will rule out any abnormality in the endometrium, and tells the physician whether ovulation has taken place. In a D and C the cervix is dilated and the uterus is scraped. In 25 to 30 percent of women, the procedure alone improves the situation for varying periods of time.

Non-Surgical Treatment

The only effective non-surgical methods of treating this problem are hormones. The choice of hormones depends on whether ovulation is occurring. If ovulation is not occurring, progesterone is lacking, so oral progesterone is given during the last ten days of the cycle. If ovulation is occurring, a combination of synthetic estrogen-progestin (birth control pill) often produces dramatic improvement. Since patients with dysfunctional menorrhagia are often in their forties, they are at increased risk of cardiovascular complications such as stroke or thrombophebitis if they are smokers. If they are not, and if no other contraindication to the use of the birth control pill exists, it can be an acceptable and very satisfactory method of treatment.

Surgical Treatment

If neither D and C nor hormones resolve the problem, then hysterectomy is considered. The operation may be performed through the abdomen or the vagina. When the uterus has fallen down (prolapsed), the vaginal route is chosen so that a vaginal repair can be carried out at the same time. The abdominal route is most often chosen under other circumstances.

An incision is usually made just at the pubic hairline (Fig. 8.3). While the abdomen is open, the surgeon will check to see that no other disease exists. The uterus is removed by cutting the attached blood vessels and ligaments, which must be properly tied (Fig. 8.4). Finally, the cervix is detached from the top end of the vagina, which is then sewn together to close or narrow the opening. In most cases, the skin incision is closed with absorbable sutures which do not need to be removed.

The ovaries and fallopian tubes may or may not be removed. Removal of the tubes and ovaries forestalls the very small possibility of developing an ovarian tumor or malignancy at some time in

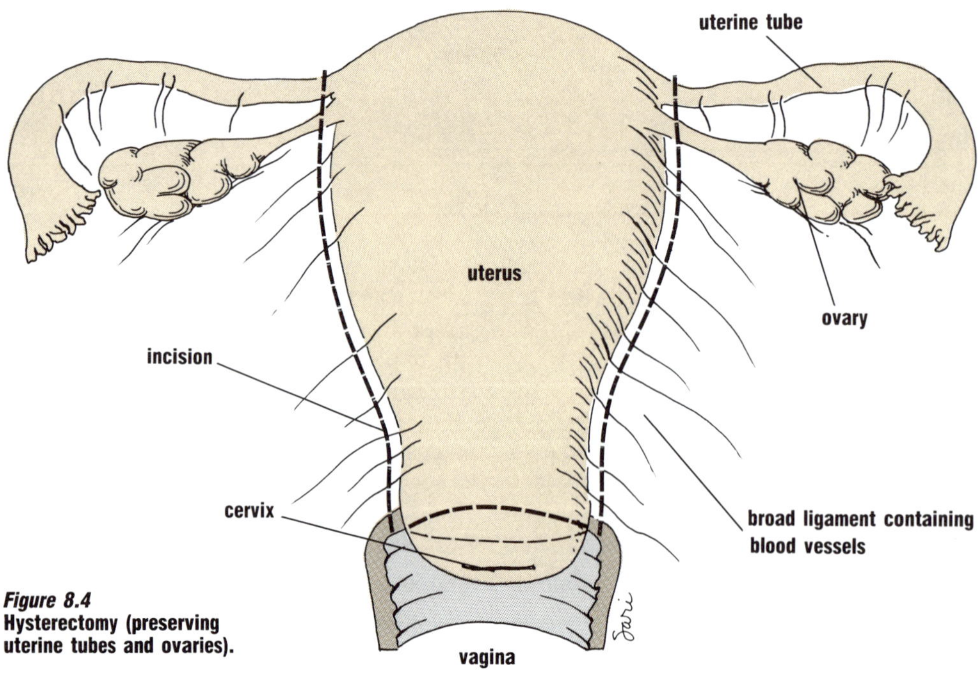

Figure 8.4
Hysterectomy (preserving uterine tubes and ovaries).

the future. Ovarian cancer is a serious disease because it tends to become extensive before it is discovered.

However, the ovaries are the source of estrogen. Their removal causes an acute menopause, with hot flushes, which will begin within a few days of the operation. Many women in their late forties choose to have the tubes and ovaries removed because ovarian function usually ceases around age fifty. Removal of the ovaries does not extend the scope of the operation.

For the first 12 to 24 hours, the most common symptoms are nausea from the anesthetic and pain-relieving drugs, and pain around the incision. Medication is usually given for both symptoms. Intravenous fluids are given for 24 hours to ensure that the patient is getting enough liquid.

By the second day, the patient will usually notice "gas pains" as the digestive tract returns to normal. Within the next 24 hours, this intestinal gas is passed and the cramps are dramatically relieved.

The patient is encouraged to get up and walk soon after the operation to prevent blood clots forming in the legs, and to maintain muscle strength.

Patients usually stay in hospital for five to seven days after an uncomplicated abdominal hysterectomy. Convalescence at home ranges from four to six weeks. As the top end of the vagina heals, the patient usually experiences a vaginal discharge — at first red, then yellowish. The most common complaint of patients during the convalescent period is that they tire easily. This is temporary, and is best handled by a nap in the afternoon and an earlier bedtime. At the same time, physical activity should be increased each day.

Complications

Complications following hysterectomy are relatively uncommon. The most frequent problem is an infection at the top end of the vagina (vaginal vault), which cannot be rendered bacteria-free before the operation. When the vaginal vault is opened, these bacteria can gain entrance to the pelvic floor, where the raw area from the recent surgery provides a nourishing medium for them.

Infection is minimized by ensuring that all bleeding in the operative site has been controlled. A small opening is often left at the vaginal vault to ensure adequate drainage of any blood. If the vault does become infected, antibiotics are used.

Occasionally the return of normal gastrointestinal function is delayed (paralytic ileus, see page 40). The symptoms are bloating of the abdomen, nausea, vomiting and no bowel activity. This rare complication is managed by intravenous fluids and decompression of the stomach by a thin tube attached to a suction apparatus (nasogastric tube).

Very occasionally, bright-red vaginal bleeding may occur after the patient returns home. This is due to erosion of a blood vessel during the healing process. Usually one or two stitches are applied around the bleeding vessel, but sometimes the vagina is packed to stop the bleeding.

If both ovaries have been removed, almost all patients will begin to have hot flushes shortly after the operation, often while still in hospital. This "surgical menopause" is treated with estrogen.

Recent Advances

Surgical technique for abdominal hysterectomy has been modified over the last 10 years to achieve better drainage. Combined with improved anesthesia, this has reduced complications and shortened the hospital stay.

Research is aimed at finding the cause of dysfunctional menorrhagia, so that an effective non-surgical treatment can be found.

Ablation or destruction of the endometrium by laser is being undertaken in a few centers, but it is too early to make judgements about its place in the treatment of this problem.

One of Carol's fears had been how Ted, her husband, would feel towards her after the operation. "Why don't you bring him to your next appointment?" Dr. Laxner suggested. She gave Carol some pamphlets about "dysfunctional uterine bleeding" and suggested that she think it over for one more cycle. Then she and Ted should come to see her.

Dr. Laxner put Ted at ease right away. "Why don't we talk about best hopes and worst fears? And don't be embarrassed to ask questions. Most people don't know a lot about how their bodies work, until something goes wrong." Ted was very frank, which helped Carol, because she suspected that he was worried about "how things would be afterwards," but hadn't said anything, focusing only on her health. Aside from a six-week healing period, when sex wasn't advisable because the top end of the vagina would still be sore, Dr. Laxner said that most couples found their sex lives improved.

At the end of the appointment Carol and Ted looked at one another. Then Carol said to Dr. Laxner, "When can I have it done?"

The worst thing about the operation, Carol decided, was that she could not expect to be out of the hospital in under five days.

The operation hadn't felt much worse than her appendectomy at age 17. She'd been admitted the afternoon before surgery, had had the routine blood tests, and had been given a mild sedative before going down to the operating room in the morning. Her next memory was of the recovery room ceiling, and of wondering what she'd done to feel so sore. At that point a nurse came over to give her something. The next time she woke up she was back in her room, feeling a bit woozy and still sore, but otherwise not too bad.

Case Study: Sterilization

Emily and Alan weren't sure before the baby was born whether this would be their last. They had a beautiful little girl already. Neither of them really cared whether the second baby was a girl or boy, but until it was born they really couldn't think of anything else.

A boy! Caitlin was delighted with her little brother, although her enthusiasm had to be restrained some of the time. Patrick thrived, however, and Emily found that six months had gone by before she even noticed the passage of time.

When she asked her family doctor about sterilization, he said she should be absolutely sure she didn't want any more children. Two children were about as much as she could manage, she thought.

Alan found the idea of not having any more children a lot easier to accept than the idea of surgery. "Can't we just go on as we are?" Emily had been using an IUD since Patrick's birth, but wasn't totally comfortable with it. She'd had some cramping, but worse, a close friend had just become pregnant — and she had been using an IUD. Emily wasn't crazy about the idea of surgery, either, but she decided to get more information from their family doctor. She wanted to know what was involved — and whether vasectomy was preferable to tubal ligation.

"Well, Emily, I guess it comes down to a question of who's most determined to go through with it," Dr. Pinner told her. "There's no doubt that vasectomy is a much simpler procedure. The important thing is to be sure that you don't want any more children, and to decide which one of you wants to be sterilized. The effectiveness is about the same for both operations." He mentioned that his gynecologist consultant did most tubal sterilizations by laparoscopy and coagulation, which meant you could leave the hospital the same day, after an operation that lasted only 30 minutes.

Fallopian Tubes

The Fallopian or uterine tubes (Figs. 8.1 and 8.2) are thin-walled, hollow tubes that extend four to five inches from the upper corners of the uterus out to the ovaries. The ovarian end of the tube is tulip-shaped; at ovulation it wraps itself around the ovary to catch the egg and transport it to the uterus.

If fertilization takes place, it does so in the outer end of the tube. Muscular contractions of the tubal wall then propel the fertilized egg along the tube, helped by the beating action of fine hairs (cilia). If the tube has been damaged by infection, fertilization may not be possible, or the fertilized egg may not be able to migrate to the uterus, and a tubal pregnancy may result.

Surgery is performed on the tube for sterilization. The tube may also be attended to surgically when a tubal pregnancy occurs. And in those situations where conception is impossible because of obstruction of the tube, some form of plastic or reparative surgery may restore continuity. Tubal damage arising from sexually transmitted pelvic infections, along with requests for reversal of surgical sterilization, has dramatically increased the number of fallopian tube operations in the last decade.

Sterilization

Surgical sterilization is by far the most common operation on the fallopian tubes today. However, any woman contemplating this procedure should be very certain that she wishes no more pregnancies. Although reversal of tubal sterilization is possible, and the results are quite good, successful reversal cannot be guaranteed.

Abdominal Tubal Ligation

Over 90 percent of surgical sterilization is done by either abdominal tubal ligation, or laparoscopic tubal ligation.

An abdominal tubal ligation is performed through a short lower abdominal incision (Fig. 8.3). Part of the tube is then removed and the remaining ends are closed. Several different methods are used. The outer end of the tube may be removed (fimbriectomy), the mid-portion may be removed (Pomeroy method), or the mid-portion may be removed and the remaining inner end may be buried in a small tunnel created in the corner of the uterus (Irving method). This last technique reduces the possibility of failure to as close to zero as possible.

The incision is small and the complication rate is very low. However, there is the usual pain and gas cramps following any abdominal incision. The average hospital stay is two to three days.

Laparoscopic Sterilization

The laparoscope is an instrument like a small telescope with a powerful light source and a sophisticated lens system. It is introduced into the abdomen through a small incision at the navel, usually under general anesthetic. A second smaller incision is made at the pubic hairline (Fig. 8.5). Looking through the laparoscope,

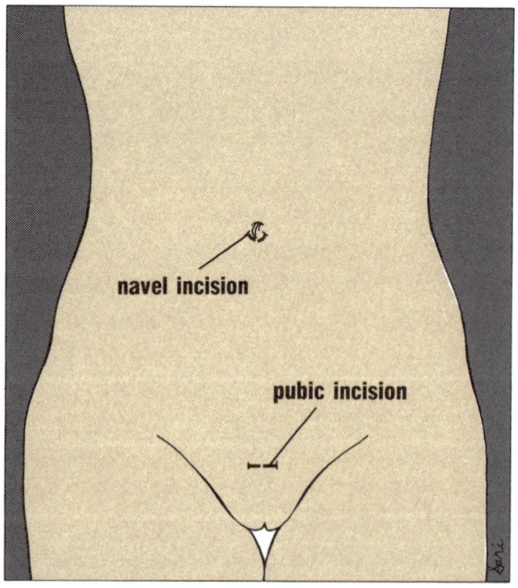

Figure 8.5
Incisions for laparoscopic sterilization.

the gynecologist can introduce a thin pair of forceps through the pubic incision and pick up the part of the tube closest to the uterus. An electric current is passed through the tube to burn or coagulate it, so that conception becomes virtually impossible.

An alternative to coagulation is the application of a small plastic clip or ring around the tube. This reduces the amount of tubal damage and increases the chances of successfully reversing the procedure in the future.

Laparoscopy is done with tiny incisions and less surgical dissection than abdominal tubal ligation. Patients can therefore return home on the same day and are often able to resume normal activities the following day. The only disadvantage is that the laparoscope is introduced into the abdomen blindly. In rare instances the bowel can be injured, especially if it adheres to the abdominal wall because of previous abdominal surgery. Many gynecologists are hesitant to recommend laparoscopy for patients who have had previous abdominal operations.

Tubal Pregnancy

The number of tubal pregnancies has increased in the past ten years, mainly due to an increase in sexually transmitted pelvic infections. Despite the availability of antibiotic therapy, tubal damage occurs but may not be severe enough to block the tube and produce infertility. In these circumstances, the fertilized ovum may be impeded in its travel down the tube and may implant in the tubal wall. As the pregnancy grows, the tube becomes distended, creating pain, until ultimately it ruptures, leading to the possibility of serious intra-abdominal bleeding. The rupture causes diffuse abdominal pain, pallor and faintness.

A tubal pregnancy can now be diagnosed at an earlier stage, thanks to two diagnostic tools: a very sensitive blood test that will diagnose pregnancy within two weeks of conception, and ultrasound — reflections of high-frequency sound waves bounced off body structures.

Once a tubal pregnancy has been diagnosed, surgery must be performed immediately, before the tube can rupture.

The standard treatment for a tubal pregnancy used to be removal of the entire tube via an abdominal incision. Now that damaged tubes can be reconstructed, the area of the tube containing the pregnancy may be cut out, and the two cut ends left open to be rejoined at a later date if necessary. This is not usually required as the other, healthy tube will allow for future pregnancies.

The postoperative course is similar to that of all other lower abdominal operations. Incision pain is present for the first few days, and gas pains are common until gas has been passed through the rectum, usually by the third day.

Surgical Reconstruction of Tubes

By injecting a dye through the cervix into the uterus and out through the fallopian tubes, X-ray or laparoscopic examination will show whether the tubes are blocked, thereby causing infertility. Reconstruction can sometimes clear the blockage or reverse a previous sterilization. The success rate for the reversal of sterilization is much higher than for clearing blocked tubes, since the tube remaining after sterilization is usually healthy.

In this type of plastic surgery, the ends of normal healthy tubes (or as much healthy tube as is available) are joined, using a microscope, delicate instruments and the finest suture material to minimize damage to the important tubal lining.

Many gynecologists will prescribe antibiotics after the operation to reduce the risks of infection. A saline solution is sometimes injected through the cervix/uterus and out into the tubes to ensure that they remain open.

Dr. Pinner gave them the name of his gynecologist consultant and told them to call when they were ready. Alan was still a little uneasy, but Emily called for an appointment the very next day. The gynecologist advised her to be sure that she wanted no more children, because although reversals were reasonably successful, nothing could be guaranteed. Emily assured him that her mind was made up. She was booked for the operation in three weeks' time.

Emily worried about the general anesthetic. She'd far rather have an epidural, as she'd had when Caitlin was born, but the gynecologist had explained that breathing would be difficult during the operation, and the anesthetists preferred to have the patient under general anesthetic so that they could assist her breathing if necessary.

Emily was well aware of everything as she was wheeled into the operating room, so her first sensation of regaining consciousness was one of surprise at having been asleep. The recovery room seemed noisy. She was glad when she was taken back to her room. Aside from a couple of visits from nurses to take her temperature and blood pressure, she really wasn't aware of much.

Suddenly it was 4 p.m., and a nurse was telling her that her husband had called to find out when he could take her home. All she could think of was sleeping, but it would be nice to do that in her own bed.

Caitlin and Patrick were a bit puzzled by their sleepy mother, and couldn't understand why she didn't want them to curl up in her lap for a couple of days. In retrospect, she thought that was the hardest part of the experience. The two small incisions weren't that painful, but they were in vulnerable places, and Patrick loved to kick as she balanced him on her lap.

Otherwise, she found recovery to be rapid and easy once the effects of the anesthetic had worn off. There were no stitches to be taken out, so she didn't see the gynecologist again until four weeks later. When he asked her how she felt, she suddenly realized with relief that she would never to have to worry about being pregnant again.

Recent Advances

In some centers the laparoscope is being used to manage the unruptured tubal pregnancy, in place of the standard open abdominal operation.

When tubal damage is too great for surgical reconstruction, *in vitro* fertilization (IVF) allows some women to bear children. In this situation, three or more eggs are retrieved from the ovary at the time of ovulation, formerly through the laparoscope, but now through needle puncture through the vagina under ultrasound guidance. They are fertilized with sperm and incubated in a suitable culture medium. At an appropriate time, the fertilized eggs are introduced into the woman's uterus, in the hope that the pregnancy will continue.

Although there is a high success rate for egg retrieval and fertilization, no more than 20 percent of women in whom IVF is attempted become pregnant and carry to term. The reasons for this are not entirely clear, and research is aimed at finding out what the problems are and how they might be corrected.

Cryopreservation (freezing) of embryos reduces the number of treatment cycles that are required to achieve a successful pregnancy, and may improve the success rate.

Ovaries

The ovaries (Figs. 8.1 and 8.2) lie on either side of the pelvis, attached to the uterus by ligaments. During the reproductive years, the ovaries are slightly smaller than a chestnut.

The ovaries produce the cells that develop into ova, one of which is usually released from an ovary each month during the reproductive years. The ovaries also produce two hormones — estrogen and progesterone. Estrogen is responsible for the changes in a woman's body beginning at puberty — breast development, widening of the hips and genital enlargement. Estrogen also stimulates the uterine lining (endometrium) to prepare for possible implantation of the fertilized egg. Once ovulation takes place, a structure called the corpus luteum ("yellow body") is formed in the ovary. The corpus luteum continues to produce estrogen but also produces progesterone, which also prepares the endometrium for implantation and helps support the pregnancy in the early weeks until the placenta can produce enough progesterone to take over this function.

During the menstrual cycle, the level of estrogen and progesterone produced by the ovary rises steadily until one or two days before menstruation, when hormone production drops precipitously. Without the continued support of the ovarian hormones, the endometrium is shed as menstruation.

Occasionally, ovulation does not take place. This is especially true during the first couple of menstrual years, and during the forties. When this happens a corpus luteum is not formed, no progesterone is produced, and the resultant period may be heavy and/or prolonged.

The ovaries may become infected as a result of sexually transmitted diseases, but this is usually because the fallopian tube is infected, and ovarian function is seldom affected. The conditions that most often afflict the ovaries are cysts or tumors.

Most ovarian cysts occurring during a woman's menstrual years simply result from periodic overstimulation from the hormones of the pituitary gland (located at the base of the brain), which controls ovarian function among other things. These are called physiologic cysts, and they will almost always disappear spontaneously. Not so very long ago healthy ovaries were often removed because of the presence of a physiologic cyst which would likely have disappeared on its own, given a little more time.

Benign Ovarian Cysts or Tumors

A cyst is a fluid-filled sac, lined by one of the cells contained within the ovary. Unlike the common physiologic cysts described previously, a true ovarian cyst does not disappear spontaneously. In fact, this cyst usually grows steadily and, in neglected cases, can attain a remarkable size. There have been reports in medical literature of cysts weighing over 200 pounds.

In addition to cysts, which contain fluid, another type of growth may arise from the ovary. It is often called a solid ovarian tumor to distinguish it from a cyst, but this distinction is sometimes confusing. Many gynecologists prefer to call all abnormal growths of the ovary (whether true cysts or ovarian tumors) "neoplasms." Most ovarian growths are benign; a minority are malignant. Sometimes the differentiation between a benign and malignant growth can be made before surgery, but very often the diagnosis must be confirmed at the operating table or under a microscope in the pathology laboratory.

Diagnosis

Many benign ovarian growths produce no symptoms and do not betray their presence until they have grown sufficiently to produce abdominal enlargement or lower abdominal pain from hemorrhage, twisting or rupture.

The diagnosis is made by pelvic examination. The gynecologist can feel the enlarged ovary through the vagina and the lower abdomen. The gynecologist can determine size of the growth, its consistency, location and mobility. If the patient is obese or if the physician is uncertain of the findings, an ultrasound examination may be performed, but this is often not necessary.

Non-Surgical Treatment

There is no non-surgical treatment for true ovarian growths. They must be removed, for two main reasons. First, they may hemorrhage, rupture or twist, all of which may require emergency surgery with removal of the entire ovary, rather than just the growth itself. Second, the growth may be malignant, and that diagnosis can often not be made until the tumor is examined under the microscope.

However, true ovarian growths must be distinguished from the previously described common physiologic cysts which require no surgery. Small growths (less than two inches in diameter) can be observed for four to six weeks. At the end of that time, common physiologic cysts will have shrunk or disappeared altogether. True cysts or tumors will remain unchanged or have grown larger. If the mass is larger than two and one-half inches in diameter, it is unlikely to be physiologic and will require operation.

Surgical Treatment

With the patient under general anesthetic, an abdominal incision is made (Fig. 8.3). The ovarian growth is examined carefully and removed, followed by careful examination of the other ovary. The pelvis and abdomen are usually washed with a saline solution, which is then collected and sent to the laboratory. Should the growth prove malignant, microscopic examination of the solution will determine whether cancer cells have spread beyond the tumor itself. The entire pelvis and abdomen are explored to determine if there is any evidence of malignancy elsewhere.

If the growth is benign, only the cyst or tumor is removed, preserving as much ovarian tissue as possible during a woman's reproductive years. In a postmenopausal patient, the ovary itself is usually removed as well, since it no longer has any function.

If removal of the growth alone is feasible, an incision is made at the base and the growth is cut out and removed (Fig. 8.6). The ovary is then closed with absorbable sutures. No matter how little ovary remains, it will continue to

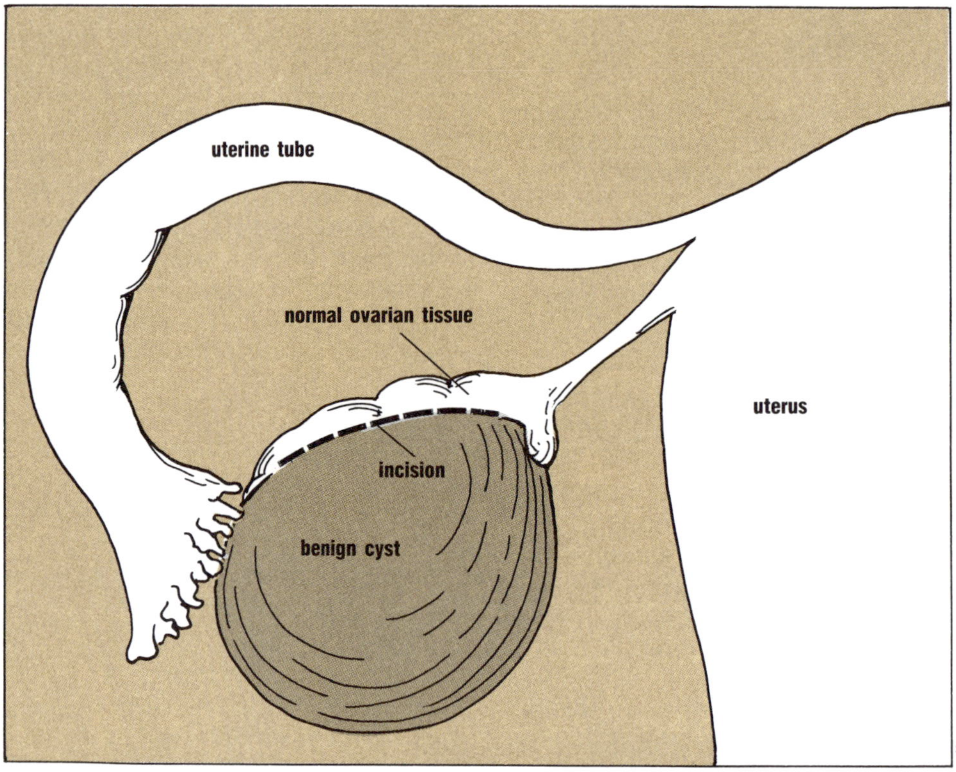

Figure 8.6
Operation for removal of benign ovarian cyst, preserving normal ovarian tissue.

produce ova and hormones until the menopause.

If there is any doubt whether the growth is benign or malignant, it can be examined under a microscope in the operating room to confirm the diagnosis.

Malignant Ovarian Tumors

Although ovarian cancer occurs less frequently than uterine and cervical cancer, it kills more frequently, because it doesn't produce symptoms until it has become extensive. Also, it has the entire abdomen in which to spread and it does so, often with frightening efficiency.

Diagnosis

The first symptom patients may notice is enlargement of the abdomen. Pain is not a frequent problem until the disease is well advanced. Gastrointestinal symptoms such as nausea, vomiting or diarrhea may occur if the bowel becomes involved, as it often does. Swelling of one or both legs occurs late in this condition.

If an ovarian tumor is extensive and immobile, chances of it being malignant are greater. Abdominal fluid and firm nodules in the tumor mass also increase the probability of it being cancerous.

Surgical Treatment

The management of ovarian cancer is primarily surgical, although there is often additional treatment with radiation or chemotherapy.

Every effort is made to remove as much of the tumor as possible, because the response to chemotherapy or radiation is greatly improved if as little tumor as possible is left behind after the operation. For this reason, and because of the technical difficulties often encountered at operation, there has been a concerted effort recently to concentrate the treatment of advanced ovarian cancer patients in university centers under a multidisciplinary group of gynecologic cancer specialists, who can coordinate the services of experts in radiation therapy and chemotherapy. In many instances even advanced ovarian cancer can be cured by aggressive surgery supplemented by chemotherapy or radiation therapy.

The basic treatment for cancer of the ovary is total abdominal hysterectomy, removal of both tubes and ovaries, including as much of the ovarian tumor as possible, together with removal of the apron of fatty tissue covering most of the abdominal contents (omentum), which is a favorite site for spread of the disease. It may be necessary to remove portions of the bowel or bladder as well, to remove as much tumor as possible.

The recovery period for ovarian cancer surgery is similar to that for abdominal hysterectomy. If the bowel is involved, the return to normal eating habits may be delayed, increasing the hospital stay to 10 to 12 days.

When the patient has recovered from the operation, the treatment team decides on the need for chemotherapy and/or radiation.

Recent Advances

A major necessity in ovarian cancer is a means of earlier detection. No satisfactory screening method has yet been devised, but researchers are trying to identify a common substance in the blood of patients with this disease. This line of research is very promising and could have a profound effect on survival rates.

As well, research is continuing in the search for more effective chemotherapeutic agents with an enhanced ability to destroy cancer cells together with a reduced effect on normal cells.

Researchers are currently working on the relationship between the body's immune system and ovarian cancer. The immune system mobilizes the body's defenses against "foreign agents," which include bacteria, viruses and tumor cells. The means may be found to encourage the body's own defense mechanisms to attack this particular form of cancer and other malignancies as well. This is one of the most promising avenues in cancer research.

Genital Prolapse

The pelvic structures — bladder, uterus and rectum — are held in place by two main sources of support.

The first is a broad platform of muscle called the pelvic diaphragm. This muscle is like a sling that holds the pelvic organs. There are perforations in the pelvic diaphragm through which the vagina, rectum and urethra pass. When these perforations widen, for example as a result of childbearing, there is less support for the structures that pass through them.

The second major source of pelvic support is the endopelvic fascia — a layer of strong connective tissue that lines the floor of the pelvis. Ligaments in this tissue are the major source of support for the uterus.

Weakened, stretched pelvic ligaments can allow the uterus to descend or prolapse from its normal position (Fig. 8.7). If the endopelvic fascia lying between the bladder and the front wall of the vagina becomes thinned or weakened, the bladder is no longer supported, and it bulges into the front wall of the vagina (cystocele) (Fig. 8.8). Similarly, if the endopelvic fascia between the rectum and the back wall of the vagina is weakened, a rectal bulge occurs (rectocele) (Fig. 8.9). Occasionally, the small intestine may bulge higher up along the back wall of the vagina (enterocele).

Some women will remember hearing the phrase "fallen womb" from their mothers or grandmothers. This descriptive term is exactly what is meant by prolapse of the uterus. In this situation,

Figure 8.7
Prolapsed uterus, viewed from below (A) and from the side (B).

A

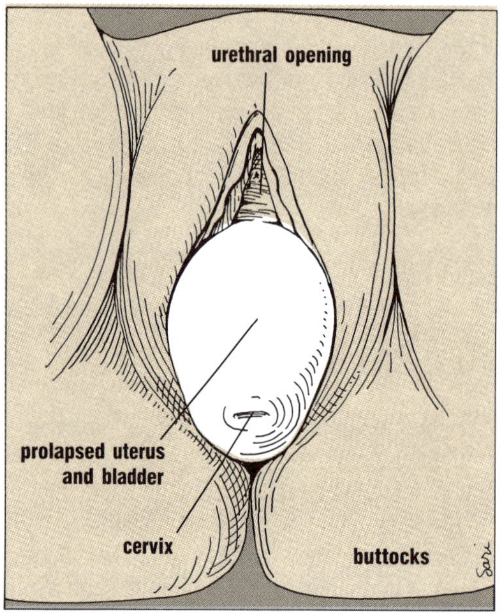

B

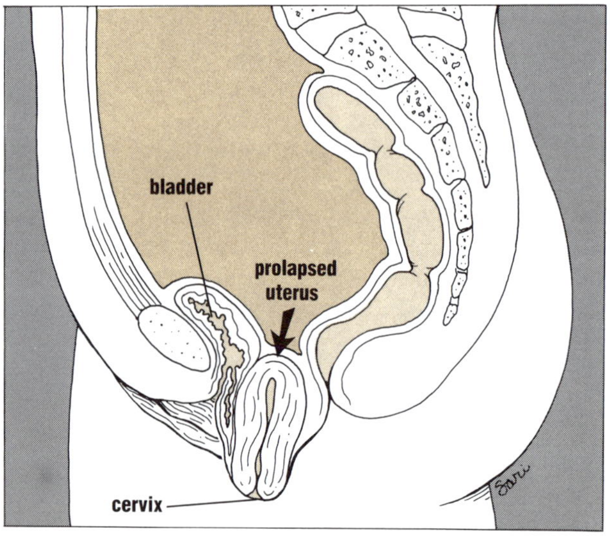

the uterus descends through the vagina from its normal position in the pelvis, until, in its most advanced state, it lies entirely outside the vagina.

Genital prolapse may occur in the reproductive years, but is more common in post-menopausal women. Contributing factors are childbirth, loss of estrogen stimulation to the genital tract and, in some cases, a predisposition to genital tract weakness.

Now that women have smaller families, better nutrition and less manual labor than their grandmothers did, genital prolapse is not as common. Nevertheless, when it does occur it can be a source of discomfort and disability, particularly for physically active women.

Diagnosis

Not all women who have genital prolapse suffer from it or are even aware of it. There are varying degrees of relaxation of the supporting tissues, and symptoms often don't occur until the disorder has become quite advanced.

The characteristic symptom common to all forms of prolapse is the presence of a bulge into the vaginal opening which may be felt and/or seen. This may be associated with a feeling of pelvic discomfort, pressure or backache.

A cystocele may be large enough to cause some difficulty in urinating, and recurrent urinary infections may occur owing to difficulty in emptying the bladder completely. Rectocele can cause difficulty in defecation. Stool may fill the bulge and women may have to insert their fingers into the vagina and press on the back wall to redirect the rectal contents.

Non-Surgical Treatment

Except in the mildest cases, there is no non-surgical treatment for this problem. Voluntary contraction of the pelvic muscles can strengthen the pelvic diaphragm, but in almost all cases with symptoms, the problem is too far advanced to respond to anything but surgical repair. The use of a pessary or ring is reserved only for elderly or frail women who are poor surgical risks.

Surgical Treatment

Genital prolapse that causes no significant discomfort requires no treatment. The problem does not always worsen, and many women with some genital relaxation have no interference with the enjoyment of their daily lives, including sexual activity. When a woman's discom-

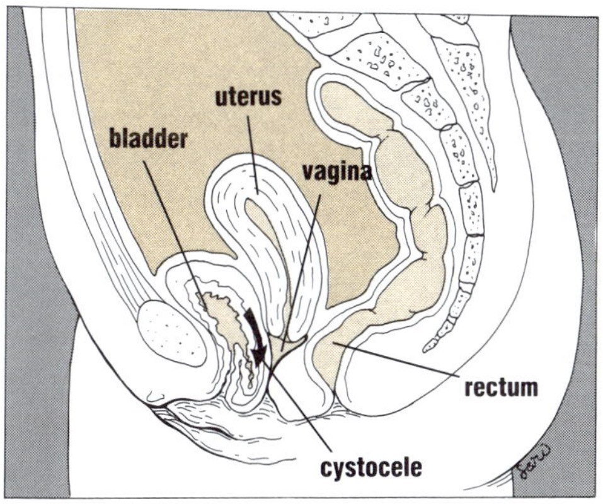

Figure 8.8
Cystocele.

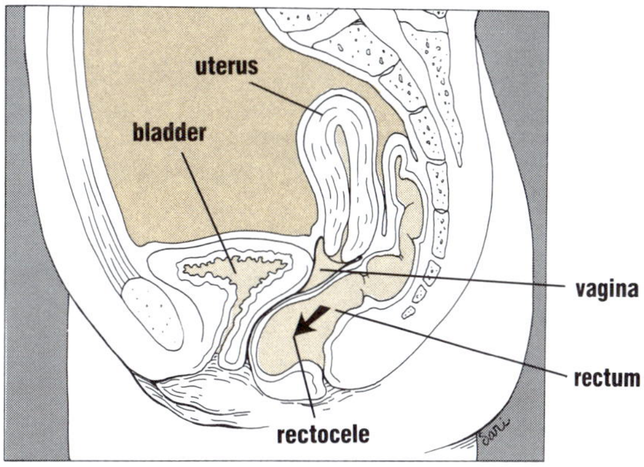

Figure 8.9
Rectocele.

fort is sufficient to require treatment, surgical repair is usually necessary.

If there is a major prolapse of the uterus, the uterus must be removed, and the ligaments that support it must be shortened to help support the upper end of the vagina, which will also prolapse without such support.

For bladder prolapse, the connective tissue between the bladder and front wall of the vagina is strengthened by "imbrication" — a series of tucks that reinforce the tissue by folding it back on itself. Recently, synthetic material has been used as an implant to further strengthen this tissue.

In a rectal prolapse, the muscles of the pelvic diaphragm are brought together to reduce the size of the defect through which the vagina and rectum normally pass, thus providing firm muscular support for the vaginal walls, both front and back.

The surgical procedure which is most often employed to deal with all components of genital prolapse is known as "vaginal hysterectomy with anterior and posterior repair." This operation is usually performed under general anesthetic and is done entirely through the vagina. An incision is made around the cervix (Fig. 8.10), and into the abdominal cavity in front and behind the uterus. The uterus is removed, and the ligaments that attach the uterus to the sidewall of the pelvis are shortened to provide support for the vaginal vault. The incision at the vaginal vault is closed.

The cystocele is repaired by opening the skin of the front vaginal wall (vaginal mucosa) and separating the bladder from the mucosa. Then follows the imbrication, with or without the synthetic implant previously described. The excess vaginal mucosa is then cut away and the front wall closed.

The rectocele is repaired by making an incision into the back wall of the vagina up to the vault and separating the rectum from this mucosa. The muscles of the pelvic diaphragm are then brought together by two or three separate stitches, forming a firm support for the rectal bulge. Once again, excess mucosa is cut away and the vaginal incision is closed.

The convalescence following this operation is similar to that for abdominal hysterectomy. It differs, however, in two important aspects. First, because the operation is performed entirely through the vagina, which contains a number of bacteria that cannot be adequately eradicated by the usual antiseptic measures, postoperative infections are more common. Most gynecologists therefore inject an antibiotic shortly before the operation, with one or two additional injections in the first 24 hours after the operation. This has dramatically reduced the infection rate.

Second, repair of the cystocele tem-

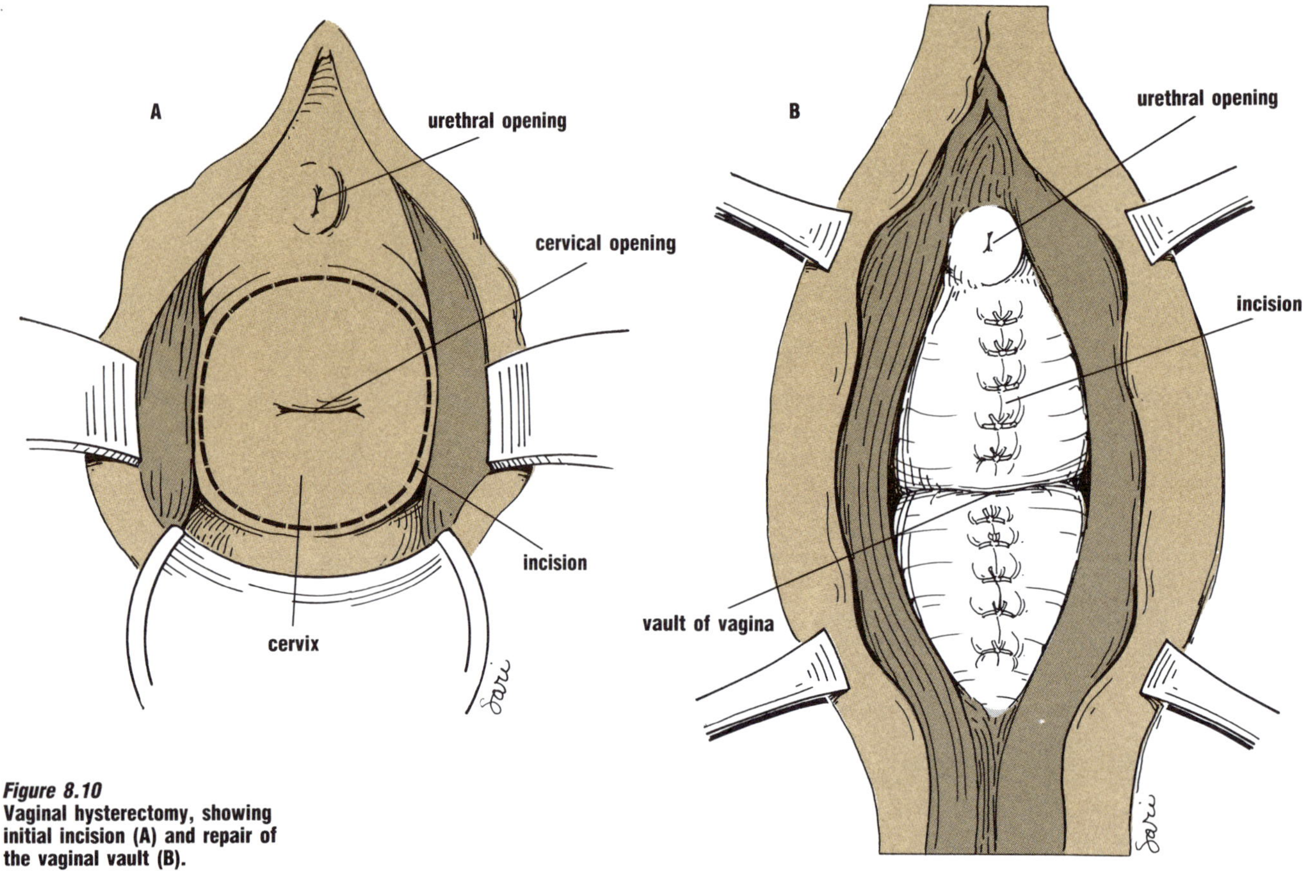

Figure 8.10
Vaginal hysterectomy, showing initial incision (A) and repair of the vaginal vault (B).

porarily produces some obstruction of the normal urinary flow from the bladder, owing to swelling around the urethra. For this reason, a catheter or rubber drainage tube is inserted into the bladder through a small incision just above the pubic hairline before the operation actually begins, but after the anesthetic is induced. This will drain the bladder until the tissue swelling is reduced. After about the fourth or fifth day, the catheter is clamped for successively longer periods of time, allowing voiding to occur in the normal way. When the normal voiding pattern has been restored, the catheter is removed.

The usual hospital stay after this operation is eight to ten days. During the next two to three months, full activity is encouraged, apart from heavy lifting or straining.

A successful operation allows a woman suffering from genital prolapse to resume full physical activities. Her sexual activity is not jeopardized in any way, even though the internal dimensions of the vagina may have been reduced by the repair (Fig. 8.10).

Urinary Incontinence

The bladder's ability to empty itself is controlled by the contraction of the detrusor muscle, which lines the bladder wall. Under ordinary circumstances, when the bladder becomes full, a signal is sent through the spinal cord to the brain.

If the detrusor muscle is functioning abnormally, the signal to void is given when there is only a small amount of urine in the bladder, so that the desire to void occurs more frequently. In this condition, the detrusor muscle also contracts with great strength and to some extent not entirely under voluntary control. Therefore, voiding may occur involuntarily, creating considerable embarrassment.

This form of incontinence related to abnormal detrusor function is called "urgency incontinence."

Under ordinary circumstances, an elaborate sphincter mechanism ensures continence when the pressure inside the abdomen is increased, as in coughing or sneezing. This sphincter is located at the junction of bladder and urethra, and can descend or become damaged from childbirth and/or tissue weakness. This can allow the increased intra-abdominal and bladder pressure to be transmitted directly to the urethra, resulting in an unchecked spurt of urine. Many women who have borne children, and a few who have not, have had the experience of losing a small amount of urine when the intra-abdominal pressure is increased, perhaps during sports, running, coughing, laughing or sneezing. This is called "stress incontinence," and it may be first noticed during a pregnancy, between pregnancies or after the childbearing years are over.

Diagnosis

The two types of urinary incontinence must be distinguished since the treatment is entirely different. Unfortunately, both conditions can exist at the same time, creating a "mixed" problem of incontinence.

The diagnosis of pure stress incontinence is easily made by a history of urinary loss on running, coughing, laughing or sneezing. On pelvic examination with a full bladder, a characteristic spurt of urine may be found with coughing. Usually, but not always, there is some sag or relaxation of the front wall of the vagina.

The diagnosis of abnormal detrusor muscle function is suggested by a history of urinary frequency with an intense desire to urinate, and not always reaching the bathroom on time. There may or may not be a history of urinary infections. There are usually no characteristic findings on routine pelvic examination.

Because these conditions may coexist in the same individual, and the treatment is so different, a series of special tests is often recommended to determine which condition is the major cause of the incontinence. These tests are carried out in specialized centers and on an outpatient basis. They measure pressures within the bladder and urethra, and determine the amount of fluid the bladder can hold before the desire to void becomes intolerable.

Non-Surgical Treatment

Abnormal detrusor function is not treated surgically, but major stress incontinence is. Medication is usually prescribed for a malfunctioning bladder muscle. Drugs are now available that relax the bladder muscle, allow it to hold more urine before stimulating the desire to void, and restore the element of voluntary control to the voiding process. The results of this treatment are remarkably successful.

Very mild cases of stress incontinence may respond to pelvic exercises, in which the muscles surrounding the vagina are strengthened by frequent voluntary contractions of these muscles over an extended period of time. Most troublesome problems of stress incontinence, however, require surgical correction.

Surgical Treatment

Since the underlying problem with stress incontinence is usually the descent of the bladder neck from its normal position, treatment is aimed at restoring the bladder neck to its original position. The operation is known as a retropubic urethropexy. There are a few variations of the basic procedure, but the principle is the same.

Following a low abdominal incision, the space between the bladder and the pu-

Figure 8.11
Retropubic urethropexy. The neck of the bladder is attached with sutures to the pubic bones or cartilage.

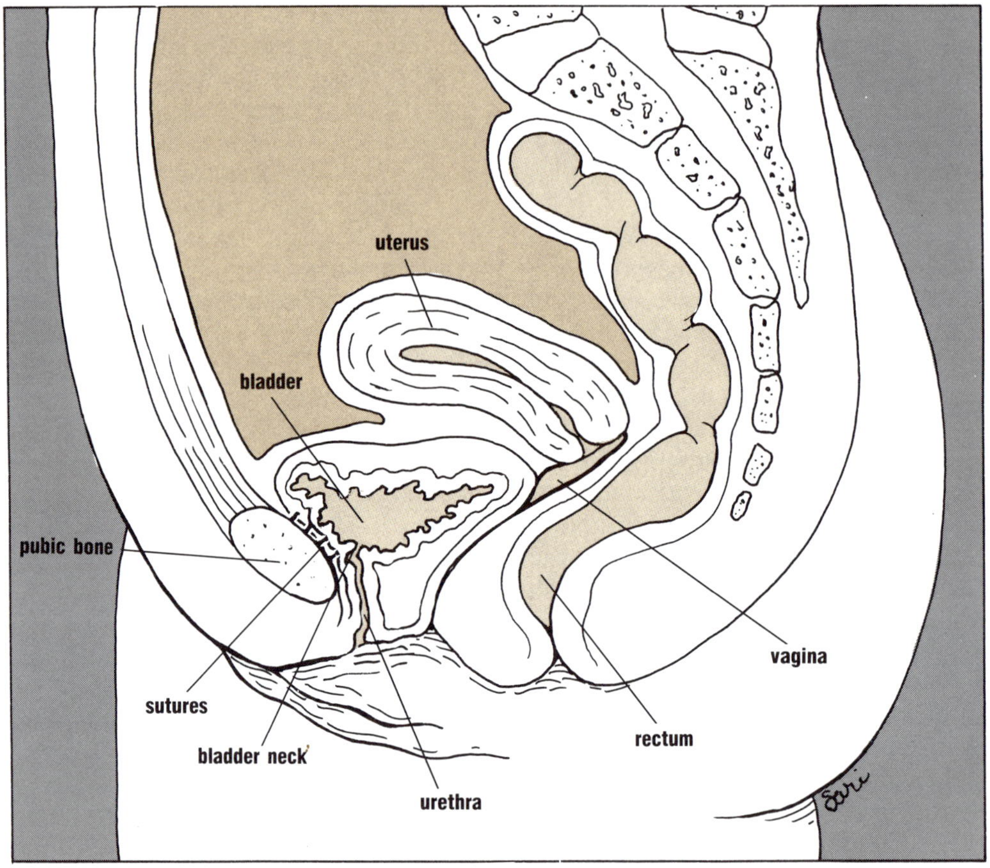

bic bone is entered (Fig. 8.11). The bladder neck and a small part of the urethra are freed from the structures to which they are attached. The bladder neck is elevated to its original position behind the pubic bones and attached with sutures either to the cartilage between the bones or to ligaments attached to the bones.

Because the abdominal cavity is not entered, recovery from this operation is usually quick. Normal voiding usually resumes quickly and many patients are ready to be discharged within five to seven days. After discharge, patients are encouraged to avoid heavy lifting or straining for six to eight weeks until healing is secure.

Although the cure rate following this operation is high, there can never be an absolute guarantee of success, especially in the long-term, because the problem can recur. Correct diagnosis is very important. If abnormal detrusor function and stress incontinence coexist (as they often do), the detrusor abnormality must be dealt with first. Surgery is reserved only for pure stress incontinence.

Chapter 9

Urology

The urologic surgeon treats urinary problems in men and women, as well as conditions related to male sex organs. Urological problems tend to be more common in the male, particularly older men with prostate problems. However, urinary infections are among the most common illnesses of females in all age groups.

Grant Angus Farrow
Assistant Professor of Surgery
University of Toronto
Urologic Surgeon
Toronto General Hospital

Margot Mackay
Illustrator
Associate Professor
Department of Art as Applied to Medicine
University of Toronto

Few problems can be more troublesome than those that affect the ability to pass urine. While some of these problems can be life-threatening, such as kidney failure or a tumor, many are minor — yet they can have a major effect on one's life.

Kidneys and Ureters

The kidneys are located on either side of the body, below the ribs in the small of the back. They have many functions, the main one being the removal of waste products from the body. Blood is filtered through the kidneys, and waste products are passed into the urine, which is collected into a series of funnels (calyces) (Fig. 9.1). These drain into the renal pelvis, a large funnel that in turn empties into the ureter.

The ureter is a long muscular tube that propels the urine from the kidney to the bladder by muscle contraction. The bladder stores urine until voluntary voiding

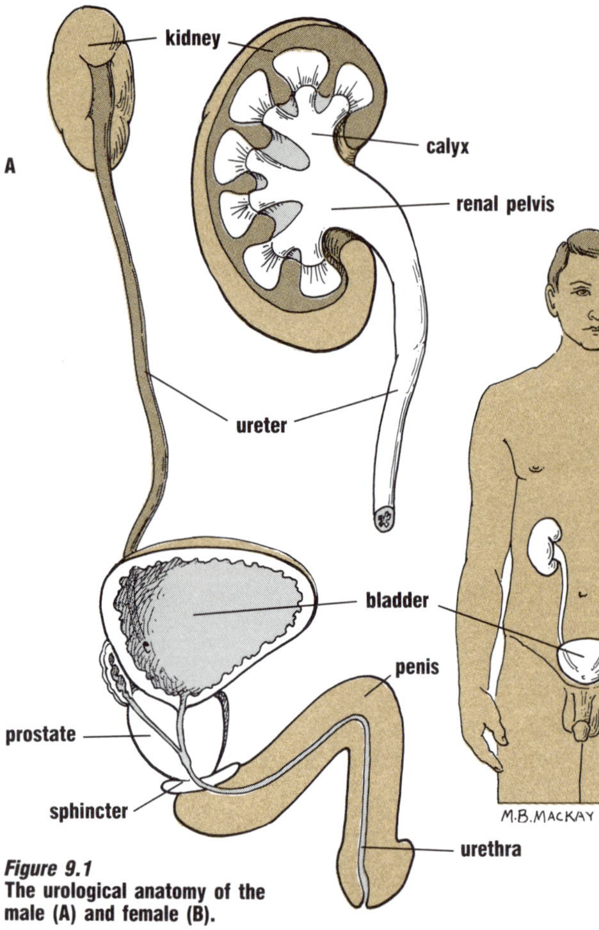

Figure 9.1
The urological anatomy of the male (A) and female (B).

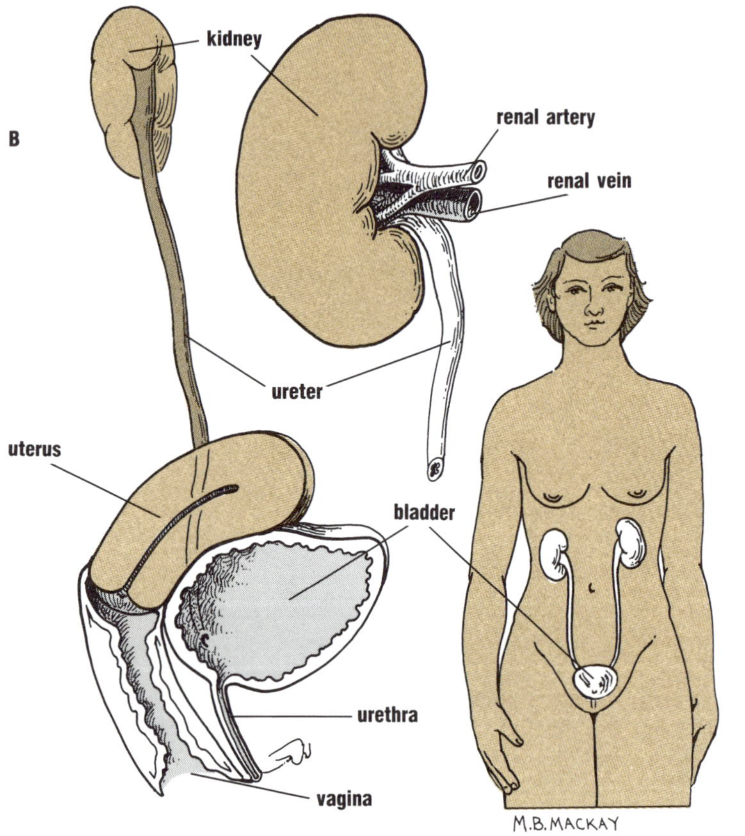

occurs, at which time the sphincter muscle relaxes and the bladder muscle contracts, forcing urine along the urethra and out of the body. At all other times the normal sphincter remains tightly closed.

The kidney also controls blood pressure and stimulates the production of red blood cells.

The development of the artificial kidney (renal dialysis) has dramatically changed the outlook for patients with kidney failure. Kidney transplantation has become a life-saving operation. (See chapter 19.)

The understanding that high blood pressure may be caused by partial obstruction of the artery to the kidney (renal artery stenosis) has provided a surgical cure for one form of hypertension. In a technique called percutaneous transluminal angioplasty, a small catheter with a dilating balloon is inserted through a tiny skin incision into the major artery in the groin and up to the kidney to dilate the blocked or narrowed renal artery.

Kidney Stones

Waste products are concentrated in the urine. If the concentration becomes too high, some waste products such as calcium, phosphate, uric acid, oxalate and cystine may crystallize and eventually form a stone. If small stones pass into the ureter, they can produce severe pain and may partially or completely obstruct the kidney. Larger stones may remain in the kidney and eventually fill the entire renal pelvis. Stones lodged in the kidney or ureter may produce bleeding, infection, obstruction and loss of kidney function.

Diagnosis

The pain of kidney stone (renal colic) can be the most severe pain experienced in the body. Felt first in the flank (the side area between the ribs and the hip bone), then the lower abdomen and groin, it gradually increases in intensity to unbearable severity and then spontaneously subsides over a 30-minute cycle. The sufferer is often nauseated and vomits with the pain.

Calcium-containing stones can be seen on X-ray, but uric acid and cystine stones cannot. Instead, an intravenous pyelogram is required — a dye is injected into a vein, causing the stone to show up on X-ray. The dye may also be injected directly into the ureter and kidney. Ultrasound can be used to diagnose larger stones or an enlarged urinary tract, but may not detect small stones. Computerized axial tomography (CAT scan) — a computerized X-ray technique that provides sectional views of the body — will also demonstrate stones.

Non-Surgical Treatment

The ideal treatment for kidney stones is prevention. Avoidance of excessive calcium inhibits the development of calcium stones. High-calcium foods include dairy products (milk, cheese and butter) as well as multiple vitamins with calcium supplement. Uric acid stones will dissolve in alkaline urine and are therefore often treated with bicarbonate to alkalinize the urine and a drug called allopurinal to decrease uric acid production. Increasing fluid intake is important in treating and preventing all urinary stones.

Surgical Treatment

Stones may be removed from the kidney in three ways: open surgery, percutaneous surgery or lithotripsy.

Although now used much less frequently, open surgery is still required for particularly large stones or stones that do not respond to other treatment. A general anesthetic is required. The surgeon makes an incision in the flank and extracts the stone from the kidney through the renal pelvis, which is then repaired (Fig. 9.2). Recovery is prompt, and there is generally no damage to the kidney.

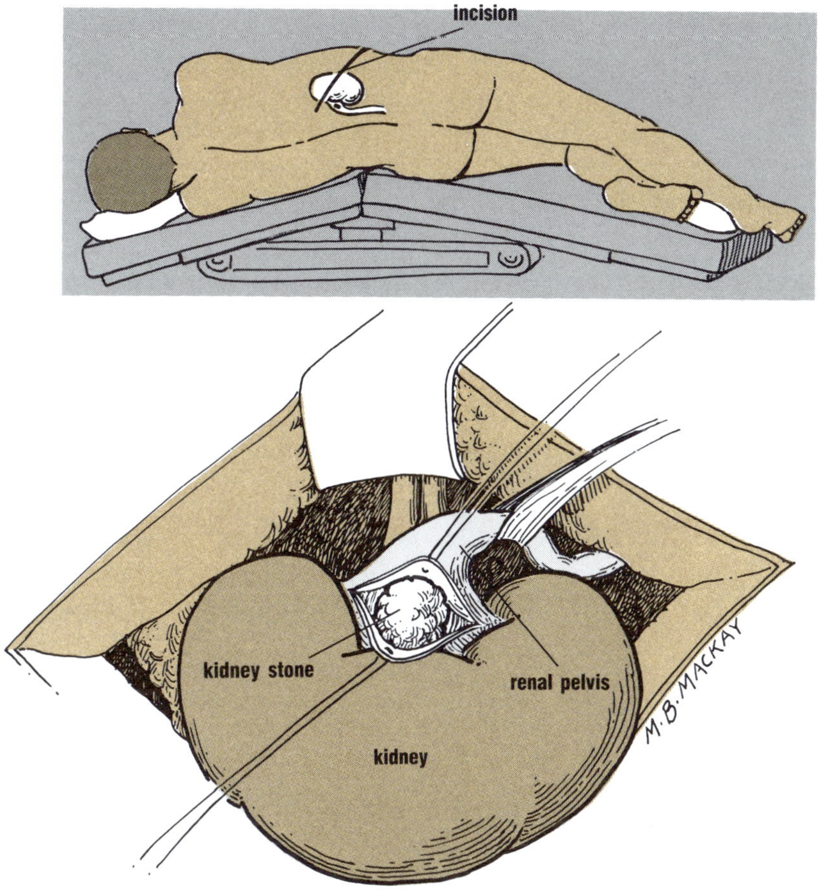

Figure 9.2
Open surgical removal of kidney stone from renal pelvis.

Large stones filling the renal pelvis and calyces may require an incision in the kidney itself to remove all fragments of the stone. During this operation, the blood supply to the kidney is temporarily clamped to prevent blood loss, and the kidney is cooled to preserve function. A tube is inserted into the kidney and brought out through the skin to maintain drainage and prevent pressure build-up after surgery.

The patient can get out of bed the next day and is usually discharged within one week. Normal activities about the house may begin after one week, with the patient usually returning to non-physical work after three to four weeks. However, heavy lifting and strenuous exercise should be avoided for six weeks.

Infection is a common complication after removal of kidney stones, so patients usually take antibiotics for two weeks. Some urine drainage from the incision for several days is common. Discomfort around the incision may continue for many months after surgery because small skin nerves have been cut. Recovery is usually prompt, however, and little postoperative care is required.

In percutaneous surgery, kidney stones are removed with an instrument called a nephroscope, which is inserted into the kidney through the skin (Fig. 9.3). A general anesthetic is required. The surgeon introduces a guide wire into the renal pelvis. Progressively larger dilating tubes are passed over the guide wire until a telescope can be passed into the kidney. Looking directly into the kidney through the nephroscope, the surgeon guides the instrument to small stones, which are then removed. Larger stones may be broken up by employing an ultrasonic or hydroelectric probe, and removed in pieces. A large drainage tube is placed temporarily in the channel made by the nephroscope, since the technique may need to be repeated if small fragments become lodged in the kidney or if undue bleeding is encountered as the channel is being enlarged through the kidney.

Figure 9.3
Percutaneous removal of kidney stone.

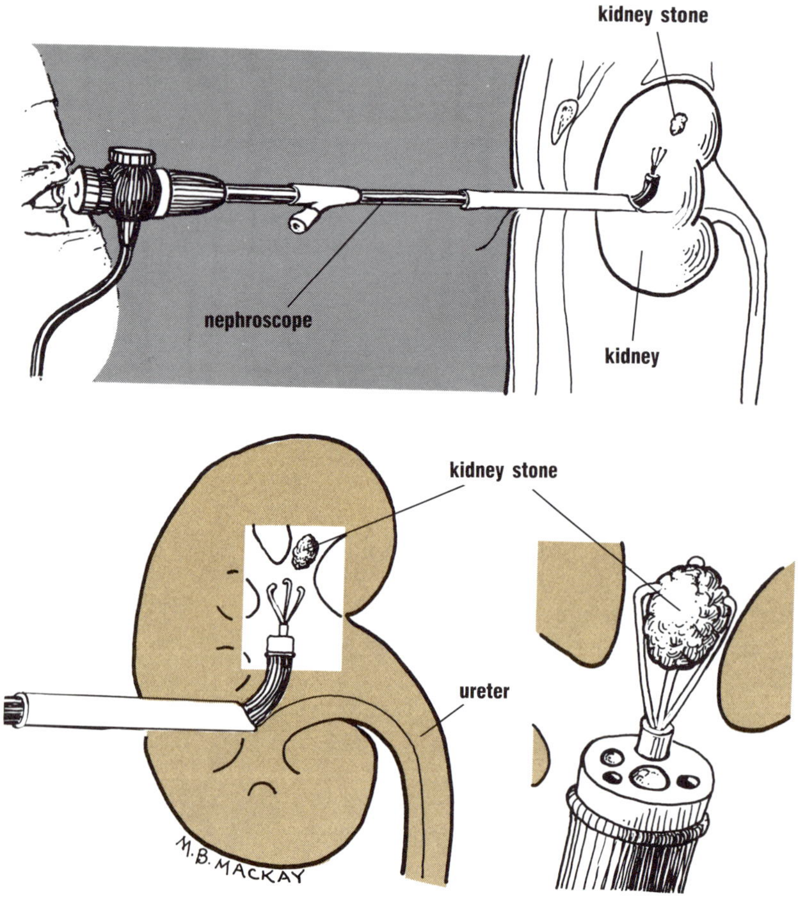

The advantages of percutaneous surgery are that no significant incision is required, recovery is prompt, and the hospital stay is short. Open surgical removal may be necessary if undue bleeding occurs, if all fragments cannot be removed, or if the other side of the kidney is perforated.

Most patients can be discharged within two or three days. There is little discomfort, and normal activity may be resumed after 10 days. The hospital stay may be prolonged if postoperative bleeding or infection occurs. The patient usually takes antibiotics for 10 days to decrease the chance of infection.

Over 90 percent of kidney stones may now be treated by lithotripsy, a technique that focuses a shock wave generated outside the body on the stone, causing it to disintegrate. The shock wave is focused by X-ray control and transmitted to the body in a water bath. Several hundred impulses are required until the stone is eventually pulverized. The patient then passes the small fragments in the urine. About 20 percent of patients experience significant pain passing the fragments and need pain medication, although most patients can be discharged from hospital the following day. Although complications are infrequent, careful monitoring of the equipment, the patient and the kidney is essential. Large stones may not be completely removed at one time, and follow-up treatments may be required.

In the past, lithotripsy patients required a general anesthetic, but with newer equipment an anesthetic is not required.

Ureteric Stones

Stones in the ureter may be removed in three ways: open surgery, endourology or lithotripsy. Small stones usually pass spontaneously. Open surgery is rarely used now, because most stones can be removed by endourology or lithotripsy.

In endourology, an instrument (cystoscope) is passed through the urethra into the bladder. The cystoscope consists of a light, observing lens and various attachments for grasping, removing, cutting and cauterizing.

A ureteroscope is a similar long, thin instrument which may be inserted through the cystoscope directly into the ureter. The ureter is dilated, allowing the ureteroscope to be passed to the level of the stone. Looking through the cystoscope, the surgeon is able to guide the ureteroscope to grasp and remove small stones (Fig. 9.4).

Larger stones may be broken up with an ultrasonic probe inserted via the ureteroscope. Stones in the upper portion of the ureter may be pushed back into the kidney and removed percutaneously, as previously described. A general anesthetic is required.

After the operation, patients may experience pain for 24 to 48 hours, passing small blood clots or small fragments of stone. Most patients may be discharged the following day, resuming full activity, including strenuous activity, within two to three days.

Stones often recur. It is therefore essential to detect any abnormality that may have caused a stone and prevent recurrence. This is done by testing calcium, phosphorous and uric acid metabolism. A rare cause of stones is a tumor of the parathyroid, an endocrine gland in the neck that regulates calcium metabolism.

Recent Advances

Lithotripsy has been the major advance in the treatment of kidney stones. Newer technology has eliminated the need for the water bath and simplified the apparatus.

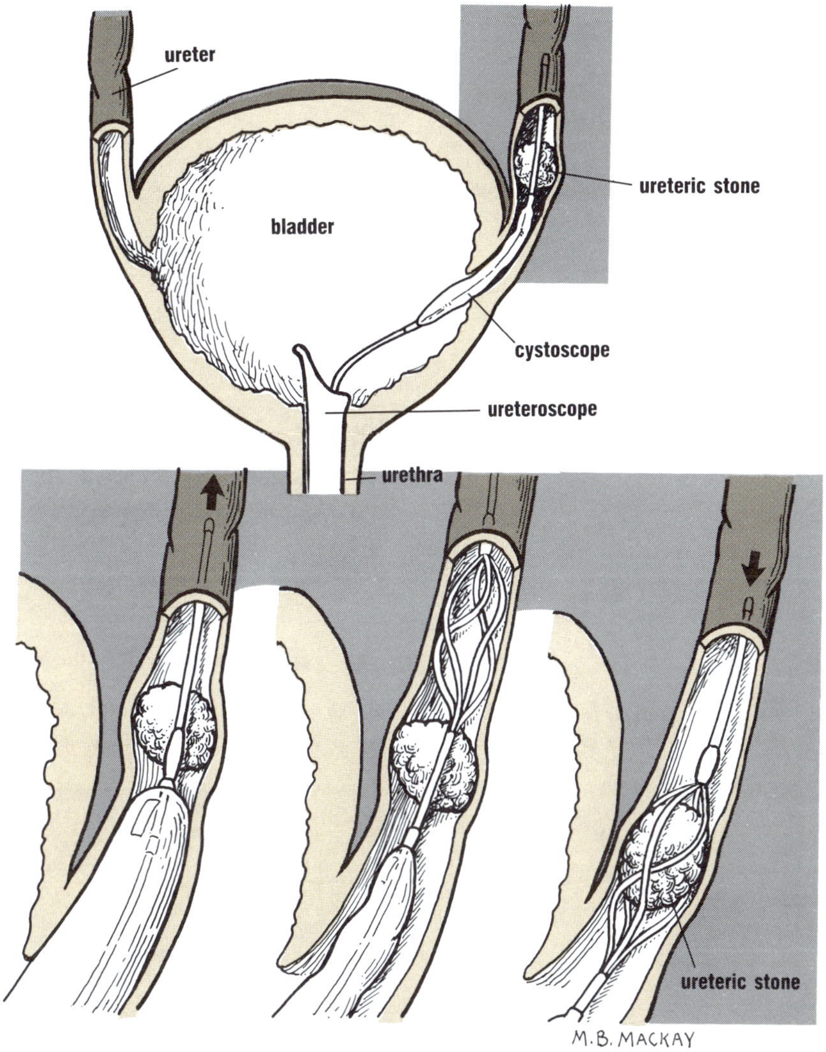

Figure 9.4
Removal of ureteric stone.

Kidney Tumors

Malignant tumors may develop in either the kidney tissue (renal cell carcinoma) or the renal pelvis (transitional cell carcinoma). With both kinds of tumor, the affected kidney must be surgically removed. One kidney can be removed and the second kidney will maintain satisfactory function. In fact, the remaining kidney grows (hypertrophies) over the next six months, so that it can take over approximately 70 percent of the original function of both kidneys.

The usual first symptom of a kidney tumor is blood in the urine. Pain and a palpable lump are late signs. Kidney X-ray, ultrasound, and CAT scan will usually reveal the presence of a tumor. An angiogram — dye injected into the renal artery via a catheter in the femoral artery of the leg — will outline the tumor and its blood supply so that the surgeon can see the extent of the problem before surgery.

Non-Surgical Treatment

Kidney tumors generally do not respond well to radiation and chemotherapy, which are reserved for palliative care when surgery is not an option.

Surgical Treatment

Removal of a kidney is called radical nephrectomy. A large incision is made in the chest and abdominal cavities to allow removal of the kidney, its surrounding envelope of fatty tissue and the adjacent adrenal gland (Fig. 9.5).

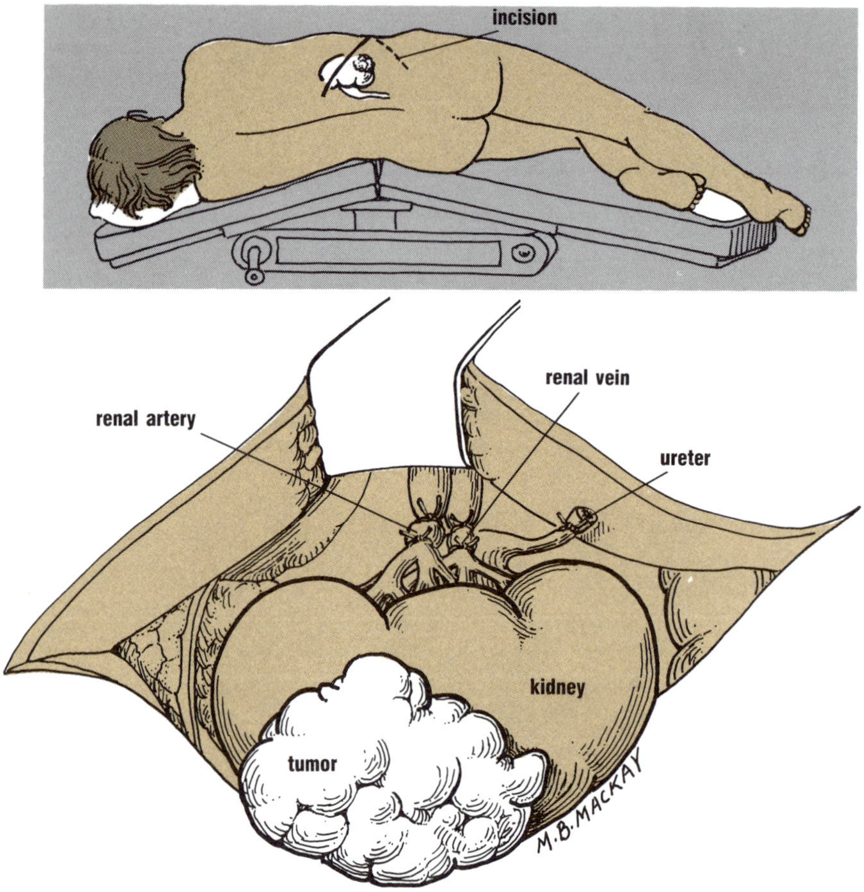

Figure 9.5
Radical nephrectomy (removal of kidney) for kidney tumor.

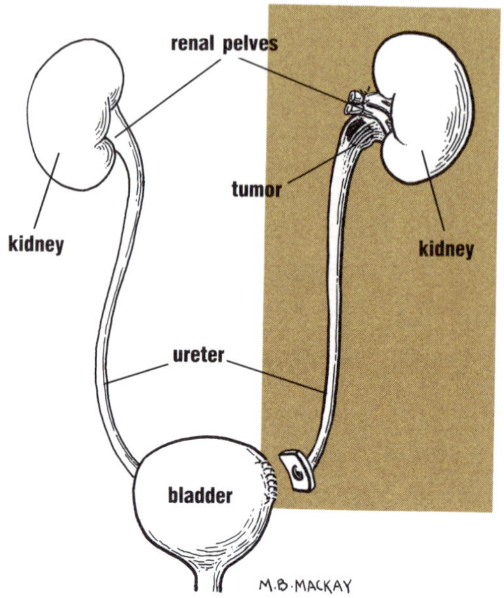

Figure 9.6
Nephroureterectomy (removal of kidney and ureter) for tumors of renal pelvis or ureter.

Tumors of the renal pelvis are treated by removing the entire ureter and its junction with the bladder, as well as the kidney (Fig. 9.6). Tumors of the ureter are usually treated similarly to renal pelvic tumors, with removal of the entire ureter and associated kidney. Small ureteric tumors may be treated by cutting out the affected segment of the ureter, rejoining it, and preserving the kidney. Very low-grade tumors have an excellent chance of cure when treated this way. However, because the ureteric wall is thin, tumors of the ureter can invade adjacent structures early.

Because one normal kidney remains, the patient is left with no disability, and recovery from surgery is usually prompt. The usual hospital stay following radical nephrectomy is seven to 10 days. Normal physical activities may be resumed in two to three weeks, and strenuous activity in six weeks. Complications are rare, and usually relate to wound infection.

Renal cell carcinoma has a reasonably good prognosis; if the tumor is confined to the kidney, the chances of 10-year survival are excellent.

Because renal pelvic tumors (transitional cell carcinoma) have a 20 percent chance of developing in the bladder at a later date, these patients must have regular follow-up cystoscopic examinations — insertion of a special viewing telescope into the bladder via the urethra, under local or general anesthetic.

Recent Advances

Endourological techniques are developing to a point where a ureteroscope may be passed via the urethra through the bladder, along the ureter and into the renal pelvis, where biopsy and even removal of small superficial tumors can be performed.

Large kidney tumors can sometimes be treated by injecting solid material or alcohol directly into the arteries supplying the tumor. This can be helpful in controlling hemorrhage and may reduce the size of large tumors, but it will not cure the tumor.

Bladder

The bladder acts as a reservoir for urine delivered from the kidneys via the ureters (Fig. 9.7). The bladder is made of interlacing bundles of muscle with a lining. It can expand to hold about three cups when full and contract to a capacity of less than two tablespoons following voiding. The two ureters enter, and the urethra leaves the bladder at a small fixed triangle called the trigone.

Diseases of the bladder may originate in the bladder itself, or be caused by disease of the prostate or urethra. Primary bladder infection (cystitis) is the most common bladder problem; in women, it is simply treated with antibiotics. Bladder infections in the male or recurrent infections in the female may be caused by outlet obstruction and require further investigation. Bladder stones and diverticuli (out-pouchings of the bladder wall) are also usually caused by obstructions in the prostate and urethra. Cancer of the bladder is a malignancy found in both sexes.

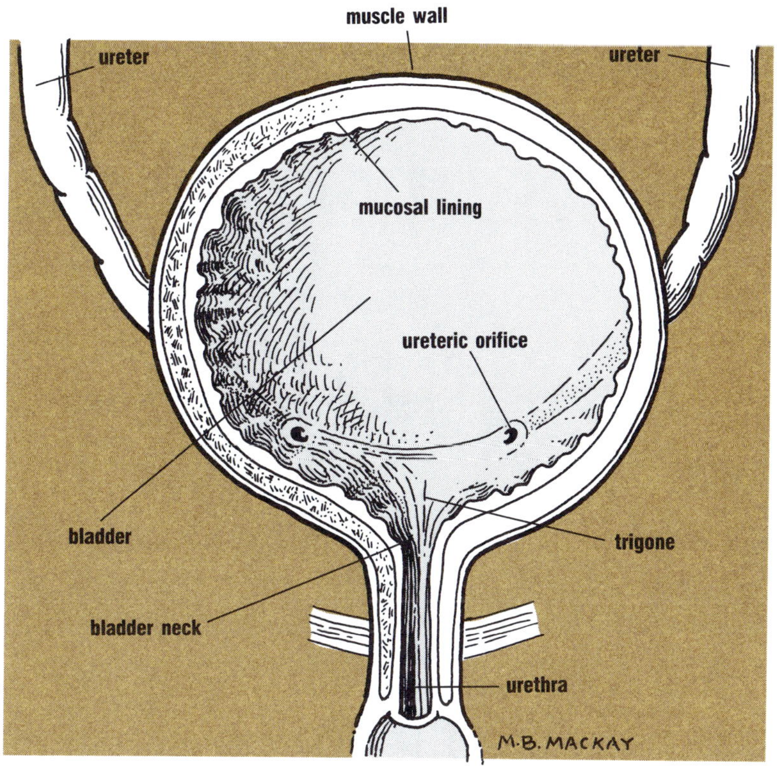

Figure 9.7
Bladder

Bladder Tumors

Cancer of the bladder develops in the bladder lining. It is believed to be caused by a carcinogenic substance in the urine, but aside from rare specific chemicals, few such substances have been identified. However, if a tumor develops anywhere in the surface lining (transitional epithelium) of the collecting system (i.e., in the kidney, ureter or bladder), there is a 20 to 30 percent chance of developing other tumors of the transitional epithelium. This supports the belief that a substance in the urine causes the tumors.

Because they originate in the lining surface, bladder tumors tend to be superficial and multiple. As tumors increase in size they grow into the bladder cavity. They may also infiltrate the bladder wall, involving the deeper muscle layer, and may eventually extend through the wall (Fig. 9.8). They vary widely in their degree of malignancy, from benign to very malignant.

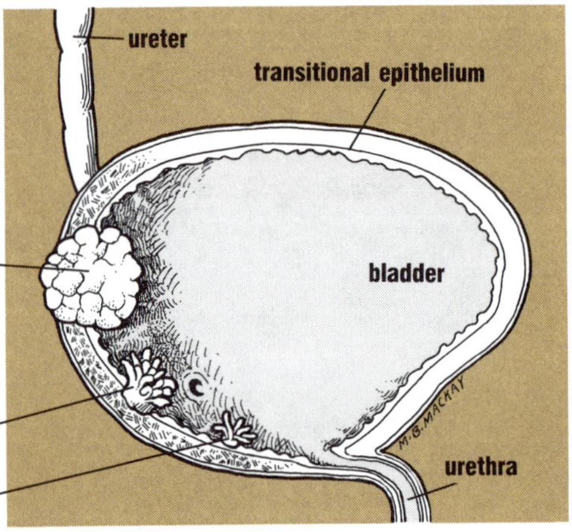

Figure 9.8
Bladder tumors.

Diagnosis

The first noticeable symptom of bladder tumors is blood in the urine, which may be obvious, or evident only under a microscope.

The bladder can be inspected by cystoscopy. The cystoscope is inserted into the bladder via the urethra, the bladder is filled with water, illuminated with a light source, and observed through a telescope. The surgeon can biopsy tumors (remove a piece for examination under a microscope) via the cystoscope. X-ray, ultrasound and CAT scan may show larger tumors, but may not detect small growths.

Non-Surgical Treatment

Surgery is the initial treatment in virtually all cases. Non-surgical treatment is used as an adjunct to surgery, or for palliative treatment. (See Recent Advances.)

Surgical Treatment

In transurethral resection (Fig. 9.9) an operating instrument (resectoscope) is passed into the bladder via the urethra. Using a high-frequency electrical current, the tumor is removed in small fragments, which are washed out of the bladder with water. This allows the removal of single and multiple tumors situated in the bladder lining or infiltrating the superficial muscle. Tumors extending into the deep layer of the muscle are not suitable for this technique, which might perforate the bladder wall. However, the extent of deeply infiltrating tumors can be seen by cystoscopy, and a biopsy performed. These deep tumors must then be treated with open surgery, radiation or chemotherapy.

Following transurethral resection of a bladder tumor, there is a 20 to 30 percent chance of another tumor developing elsewhere in the bladder. These patients must therefore undergo cystoscopic examination at regular intervals several times a year to detect early recurrence before invasion occurs. Cells found in the urine are microscopically examined at this time as well. X-ray examination (intravenous pyelogram) is performed at less frequent intervals.

The most common site for malignancy of the bladder is at the base of the bladder (trigone), next to the bladder neck and openings of the ureters. Infiltrating malignant tumors in this area require removal of the entire bladder and creation of a new bladder to provide drainage from the kidneys. Because the prostate and seminal tract in the male are very close by, they must also be removed in this operation, which is called cystectomy.

The most common bladder replacement is an ileal-conduit urinary diversion (Fig. 9.10). In this operation a loop of small intestine (ileum) is isolated with the blood supply intact. The intestine is then reconnected so that normal bowel function is preserved. One end of the isolated loop of small intestine is closed and the other end is brought out to the skin of

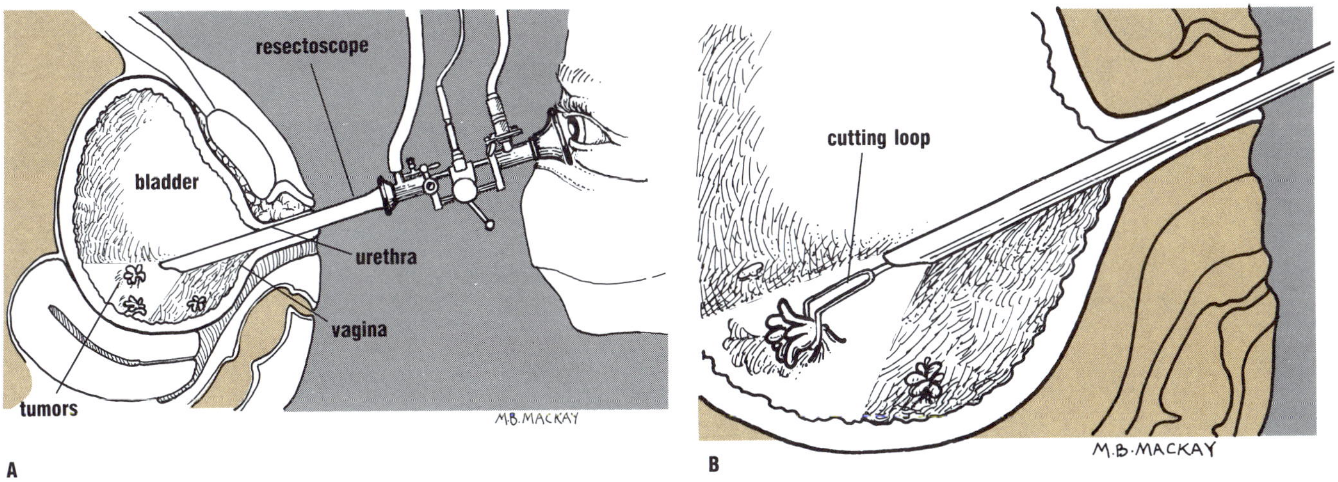

Figure 9.9
Transurethral resection of bladder tumors.

the abdomen through an opening called an ileostomy stoma. The ureters are attached to the small bowel so that the urine flows through it and out through the stoma. Discharge of urine through the stoma is continuous, because there is no reservoir for it to collect in. The urine drains into an ileostomy appliance or bag attached with adhesive to the skin.

In rare cases the bowel loop may be attached to the urethra, to preserve normal voiding. However, it is not often possible to use this technique because it does not permit complete removal of the cancer.

Occasionally tumors arise on the expandable dome of the bladder. These tumors can often be treated by removing that part of the bladder only (partial cystectomy), preserving bladder function.

With modern ileostomy appliances and the support of skilled therapists, patients with an ileal conduit are able to resume a normal, active life with no restrictions of diet, activity or travel.

Because the bowel is involved in the operation, temporary delay in small intestine function occurs following surgery. This requires suction drainage from the stomach by a tube through the nose for several days. The hospital stay is 10 to 14 days; during the last few days the patient is taught to manage the skin stoma and change the collecting bag. Temporary leakage of urine from the anastomosis sites is common and usually subsides within one or two weeks. Strenuous physical activity should be avoided for two months. Superficial bladder tumors that do not invade the underlying muscle have a 90 percent chance of cure, but tumors invading the muscle have a much poorer prognosis.

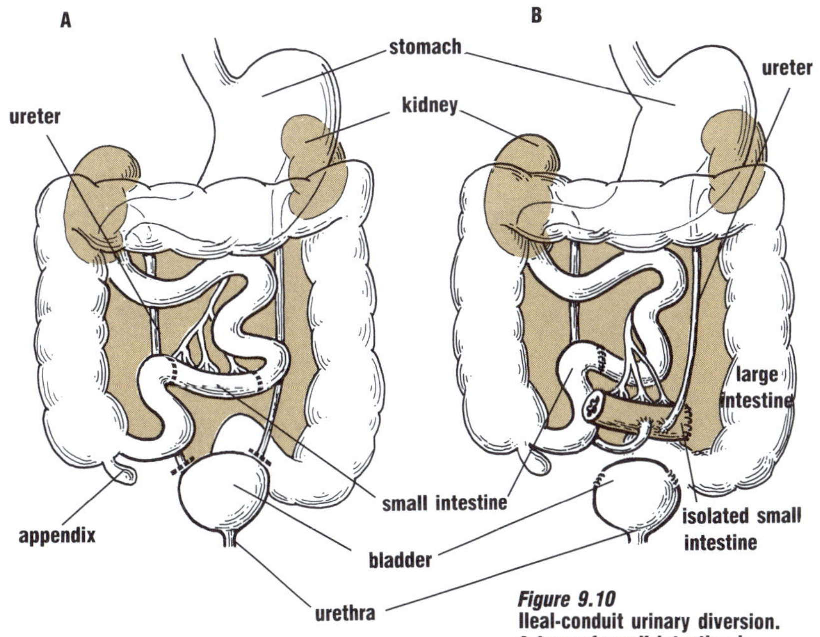

Figure 9.10
Ileal-conduit urinary diversion. A loop of small intestine is isolated (A) and the ureters are attached to it. The small intestine is then repaired (B).

Recent Advances

A transurethral instrument employing a laser is now available for treating bladder tumors, but as yet the technique is not precise and does not allow accurate microscopic assessment.

Chemotherapy can control superficial bladder tumors, and when used at weekly or monthly intervals following transurethral resection, may prevent the recurrence of tumors as well. Patients receiving this treatment must be closely observed, because the drugs are very toxic and cause complications; also, many bladder tumors do not respond to chemotherapy.

Bladder cancer often responds to radiation therapy, which may be used for patients whose general health makes them unsuited for major surgery, or may be used as a treatment before surgery. Unfortunately, infiltrating tumors at the base of the bladder still require surgical urinary diversion, and because of the high dose of radiation required to be effective, complications are frequent. Radiation to the bladder may damage adjacent structures. As a result, radiation to the bowel may produce diarrhea, bleeding and even perforation, with bowel leakage into the bladder. Scarring and obstruction of the urethra may also occur. There can be severe bladder irritation, with bleeding and loss of bladder control. Radiation can result in a small contracted bladder, causing frequent urination and incontinence.

Bladder Stones

Stones develop in the bladder because of sedimentation of waste products due to obstruction of the urethra, which is most frequently caused by an enlarged prostate gland. Stones may also form around an indwelling bladder catheter. Treatment of the stones must therefore include treatment of the primary condition. Bladder stones are usually multiple and are often associated with bladder infection. The patient may experience pain, burning on urination and bleeding.

Non-Surgical Treatment

Stones may be prevented by early treatment of the outlet obstruction. Stones associated with a catheter are prevented by high fluid intake, bladder irrigation and frequent change of catheter.

Surgical Treatment

Bladder stones can usually be removed via the cystoscope. Smaller stones are extracted intact; larger stones may be crushed or fragmented by an ultrasonic probe. However, multiple large stones must be removed by open surgery. Small stones may be removed under local anesthetic as an outpatient, but larger stones require the patient to have a general anesthetic. The patient usually leaves the hospital the day after surgery.

The obstructive condition (most commonly prostate enlargement, see page 103) must be corrected to prevent stones from recurring. The main complication is infection, which is readily controlled with antibiotics when the stone and obstruction have been removed.

Prostate

The prostate is an internal male sex organ. It sits like a donut at the base of the bladder, and the urethra passes through it, draining the bladder (Fig. 9.11). The vas deferens, carrying sperm from the testes, enters the urethra through the prostate. The prostate is made up of many small glands embedded in muscle, which contract and empty on ejaculation. The gland produces a gelatinous fluid, which acts as a nutrient and vehicle for the sperm.

Because of its location at the base of the bladder, diseases of the prostate may cause urinary voiding symptoms, either

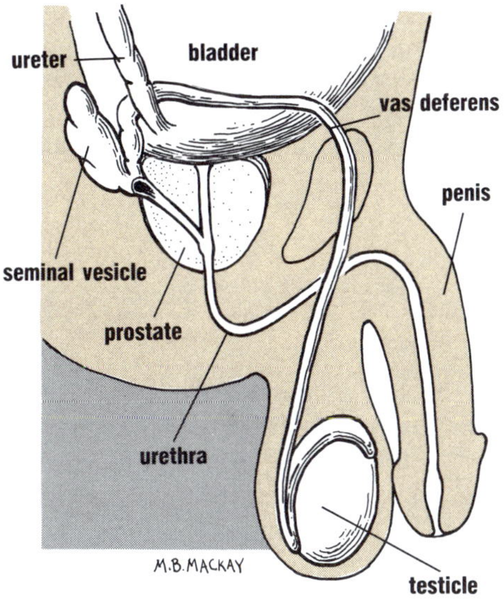

Figure 9.11
Bladder and male genitalia.

irritative or obstructive. The prostate is examined by digital rectal palpation and direct observation by cystoscope through the urethra.

Diseases of the prostate are probably the most common urological problems in men. Prostate problems that may require surgery include prostatic hypertrophy and cancer of the prostate.

Benign Prostatic Hypertrophy

Benign prostatic hypertrophy (enlargement of the prostate) usually begins to develop around age 50, obstructing the bladder outlet (Fig. 9.12). However, like graying hair, it begins and progresses at varying times and rates. A small enlargement developing near the urethra often causes more symptoms than a bigger enlargement away from the urethra. The bladder muscle compensates by becoming stronger, which delays the onset of symptoms. Resulting changes in the bladder can include bladder stones, outpouchings in the bladder, and infection. Advanced cases may produce enlarged ureters and kidneys, with eventual kidney failure.

Benign prostatic hypertrophy causes the prostate gland to enlarge, encroaching on and obstructing the urethra, causing poor urinary stream and poor bladder emptying, forcing the patient to make frequent trips to the bathroom, even at night.

Diagnosis

The enlarged prostate can be felt by rectal examination. The diagnosis is confirmed by cystoscopy (see page 100) where the surgeon can observe the enlarged prostate and detect changes in the bladder. Because this condition occurs in most males to some degree, the decision to operate is only made when symptoms interfere with normal activities, and obstructive changes in the bladder are seen on cystoscopy and X-ray.

Non-Surgical Treatment

There is no drug treatment for benign prostatic hypertrophy. However, in the early stages of the condition, the symptoms may be helped by careful bladder emptying, not allowing the bladder to become overfilled, and avoiding excessive tea, coffee and alcohol.

Case Study: Benign Prostatic Hypertrophy

Giles was concerned about the number of times he found he had to relieve himself over the course of a day. It was becoming a bit of a headache at work, and since the condition persisted, Giles made an appointment with his physician.

Tests were scheduled and done, and at his follow-up appointment his doctor came straight to the point. "Tell me, Giles, have you been having any problems voiding lately?" "If you mean do I pee a lot, the answer's yes. But so what? That happens to all of us as we get older, doesn't it?"

His doctor asked him further questions about whether his bladder still felt full after voiding, or if he had trouble getting the urine to flow when he got to the bathroom. Finally he recommended a consultation with a urologist.

Giles didn't like the rectal examination, and liked all the probing tubes even less. But at the end of the investigations, the urologist was reassuring. "First of all, I expect you're wondering if there's a serious problem." Giles, who didn't like to mince words, growled, "By that I take it you mean cancer." "That's one serious problem."

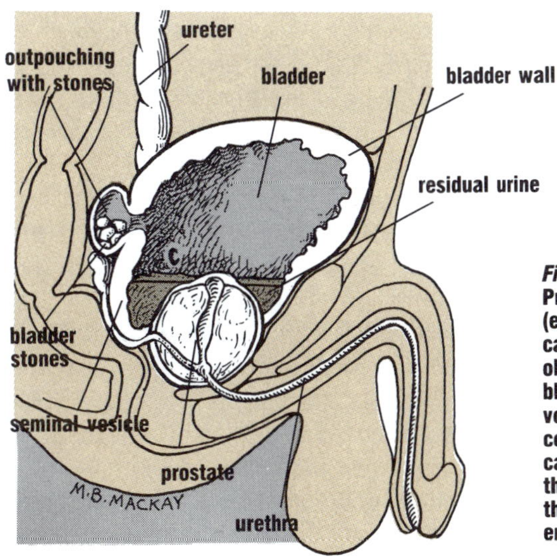

Figure 9.12
Prostatic hypertrophy (enlargement of the prostate), causing bladder outlet obstruction. The wall of the bladder is thickened after voiding and the bladder contains residual urine. Stones can occur in outpouchings in the bladder. In advanced cases, the ureters can become enlarged.

Dr. Webster did not take offence. He'd dealt with many worried men who weren't sure what was wrong with them, and didn't like other people probing them to find out. "But we can tell from your X-rays and the other tests we've done that you simply have an enlarged prostate gland, which is making it difficult for you to empty your bladder properly. Because it never really empties, it fills up again very quickly — and you end up running to the john every half hour."

"So I just have to put up with it?" Giles wasn't keen for further probing. "Not at all," replied Dr. Webster. "But since this condition tends to get worse, to a point where the bladder is really obstructed, we also have an operation to remove the enlargement. We don't believe in subjecting people to unnecessary surgery, so we don't operate unless we see the obstruction getting worse, or until the patient feels really hampered by the condition."

Dr. Webster explained in detail what would be done, and what effects Giles could expect. He was careful to emphasize that recovery wouldn't be instantaneous. It was important for Giles to do nothing that might cause bleeding in the first month after surgery. The operation itself seemed surprisingly simple. There was no incision. The enlargement in Giles' prostate was scraped out by an instrument inserted through the penis. Afterwards Giles was sore, and he had to have a catheter for a few days, but otherwise he felt fine. When the catheter was taken out, Giles was a little disappointed that he still had to go to the bathroom as often, but Dr. Webster had prepared him for the sight of blood in his urine. That disappeared by the time he went back to work 10 days later.

At his three-month check-up Dr. Webster was encouraging — the prostate had healed well — but he warned Gilles not to tax his health too soon after surgery. He also reminded him that regular checkups were important. Serious problems could often be prevented or held in check if they were caught early.

Surgical Treatment

The aim of surgery is to remove the enlargement of the prostate that is causing the urethra to narrow. The obstructive portion of the prostate may be removed through an abdominal incision (retropubic or suprapubic prostatectomy) or through insertion of an instrument into the urethra (transurethral resection of the prostate). Both techniques remove the same tissue and are equally effective. The transurethral resection without an incision is easier for the patient, has a more rapid recovery, and is therefore much more common. The open incision is generally used when the prostate has become very large.

After the core of the prostate is removed, a raw surface similar to a burn is left, so a catheter is used for several days to continuously drain the bladder.

After the catheter is removed, there is usually blood in the urine for several days; red blood cells will be seen on microscopic examination of the urine for three months until the lining of the urethra is restored. Strenuous activity such as lifting, exercising, straining for bowel movement, and sexual activity may cause bleeding and should be avoided for one month after surgery.

Frequency and urgency often persist for several days or weeks. However, normal urinary function and control are usually rapidly restored. Slight loss of urine with straining may be experienced. Sexual function is generally restored to pre-surgery level, although some patients do experience retrograde ejaculation into the bladder, making it difficult to effect a pregnancy. Treatment may be less effective in older patients with larger glands and with more obstructive changes before surgery.

Because the cavity caused by removal of the prostate core is large, regrowth of the prostate usually does not cause obstruction. Less than 10 percent of patients need repeat surgery.

Scarring in the urethra or bladder outlet occurs in 10 to 15 percent of cases, requiring subsequent treatment. The presence of benign hypertrophy has no effect on later development of cancer of the prostate. However, the patient should have regular follow-up visits, including regular rectal examinations.

Cancer of the Prostate

Cancer of the prostate is one of the most common cancers in men, especially older men. Although 30 percent of males over age 75 have a microscopic malignant tumor of the prostate, the majority will be unaware of their tumor and will require no treatment. Cancer in the younger patient, and large malignant tumors in any patient, can behave in a more aggressive fashion and do require treatment.

Diagnosis

Patients with prostatic cancer may have urinary symptoms such as urinary obstruction and frequency, although small tumors cause no symptoms and are usually discovered on routine rectal examination. The tumor feels like a hard lump in the normally rubbery gland. Cancer is sometimes discovered during surgery for benign prostatic hypertrophy.

Ultrasound may also pick up a tumor in the prostate. A blood test for an enzyme, prostatic phosphatase, is usually elevated if the tumor has spread beyond the prostate, but this is not an effective screening test for early tumors.

Cancer of the prostate spreads very quickly to the bones of the spine and pelvis, because veins link them directly. The cancer stimulates the bone to grow, causing a dense appearance on X-ray.

Non-Surgical Treatment

Stopping testicular function will control 85 percent of prostate tumors to some degree, whether the tumor is in the prostate or has spread beyond it. Testicular function may be stopped either by surgical removal of the testicles, or by taking stilbesterol, a female hormone, which causes the testicles to atrophy. Tumors in men over age 70 or tumors that have spread beyond the prostate in younger men can be treated with hormones. (Once the tumor has spread, surgery is no longer an effective treatment.) Hormone treatment will not eradicate cancer of the prostate, but it will often control further spread for five to 10 years. For this reason, patients over age 70 are not subjected to radical surgery.

Radiation has been used to treat localized tumors, but long-term results show marginal benefit over hormone therapy. Complications are frequent following radiation therapy, and include radiation damage to the bowel, bladder and urethra, bowel and bladder irritability, and bleeding. Serious late complications include obstruction and breakdown of the bowel and bladder with leakage of bowel contents or urine. Because radiation damage can take a long time to show up, these changes may continue over five to 25 years.

Hormone treatment with female hormones or the removal of the testicles always stops normal erections. Approximately 50 percent of patients treated with radiation lose sexual function as well.

Surgical Treatment

Tumors confined to the prostate gland in men under age 70 may be cured by surgical removal. Bone, liver, lung and CAT scans must confirm that there is no demonstrable tumor beyond the gland.

Surgery requires removal of the entire prostate (radical prostatectomy) (Fig. 9.13). The bladder is then reattached to the urethra, preserving the muscle of control. The initial part of the procedure includes exploration and lymph node biopsy, to be sure the tumor has not spread beyond the prostate. If it has, removal of the gland would not be curative, so the operation would be terminated and hormone therapy would be instituted instead.

A catheter is left in place until the reattachments begin to heal, at which time the patient must relearn normal voiding and urinary control. The major complications of radical prostatectomy are incontinence (loss of urinary control) and impotence (inability to have an erection). Stress incontinence (losing a small

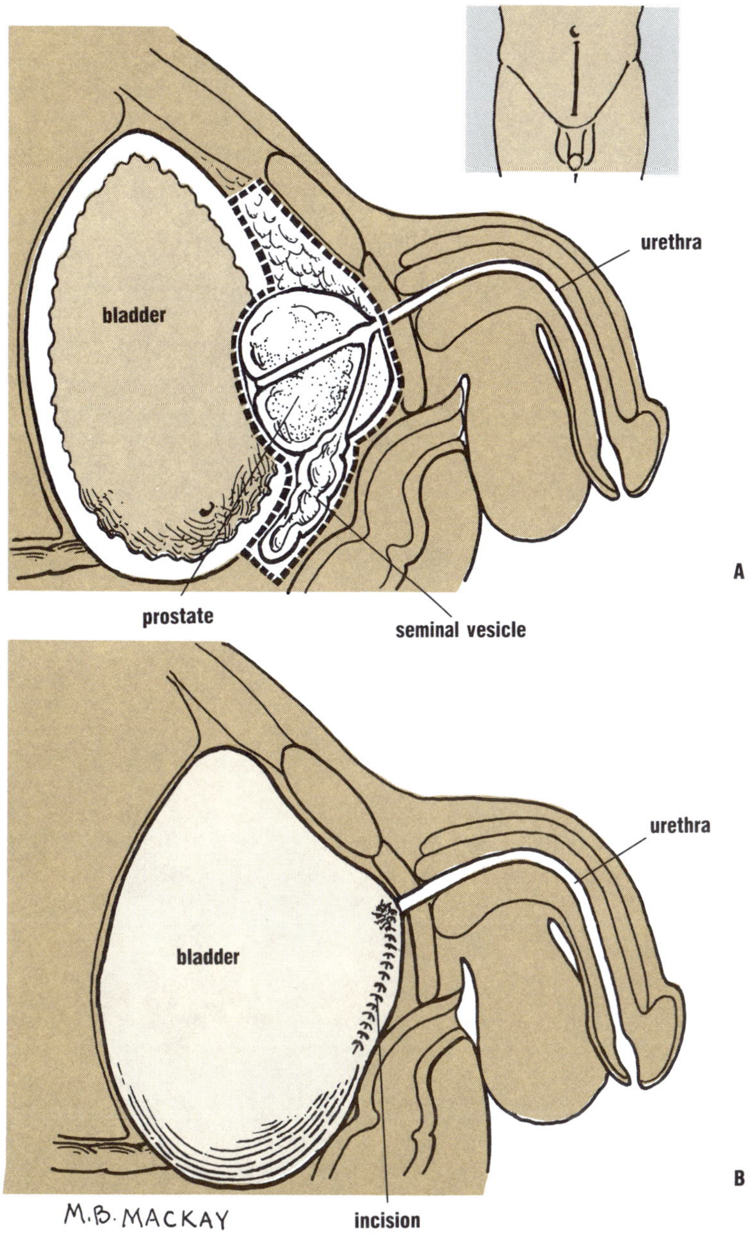

Figure 9.13
Radical prostatectomy for cancer of the prostate. The bladder neck, prostate and seminal vesicles are removed (A), and the urethra is attached directly to the bladder (B).

amount of urine with straining) is common initially, but most patients eventually develop normal control.

With newer surgical techniques, approximately 50 percent of patients who are potent before radical prostatectomy will retain sexual function after surgery.

Difficulty with urinary control and inability to have normal erections frequently persist for many months after radical prostatectomy. The terminal part of the vas deferens and seminal vesicles are removed along with the prostate, and therefore ejaculation does not occur.

If the cancer is detected and treated early, the chances for 10 to 15 years' survival after radical prostatectomy are extremely good. Since cancer of the prostate occurs in the older patient, a relatively normal life span may be expected.

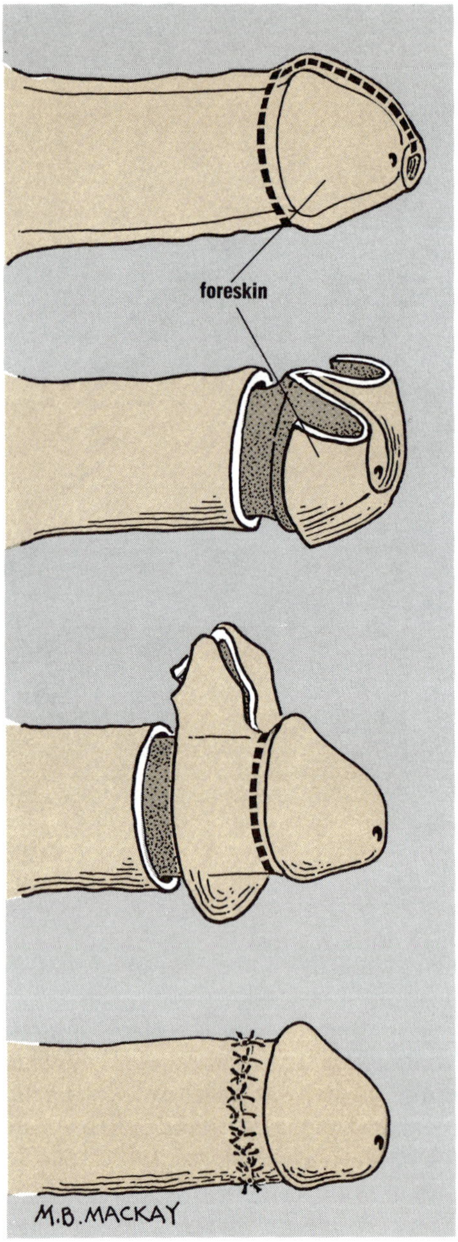

Figure 9.14
Circumcision.

Recent Advances

The technique of preserving the nerves and blood vessels coursing beside the prostate to the penis has increased the possibility for patients to maintain the ability to have erections, and improved the likelihood of normal urinary control following this procedure.

Penis

The penis contains the urethra — the channel for urination and ejaculation. Erection is produced when the blood vessels of the penis become engorged. Erection and ejaculation may be influenced by psychological factors, vascular disease, neurological disorders, glandular disorders, surgical procedures and drug therapy. The major surgical procedures on the penis are circumcision and treatment for impotence.

Circumcision

Circumcision involves the removal of the foreskin from the penis. Some parents choose to have their baby boys circumcised; otherwise, circumcision is usually performed only when narrowing of the foreskin occurs, making retraction impossible and creating hygiene problems and discomfort with erection. Patients are usually given a general anesthetic. The foreskin is cut away and the skin is closed with absorbable stitches (Fig. 9.14). A firm dressing is applied for 48 hours, and the patient can usually go home the same day.

Possible complications are bleeding and infection. The patient may experience pain for up to two weeks, which can be relieved by painkillers. Sexual intercourse should be avoided for three to four weeks.

Sexual Dysfunction (Impotence)

Surgery for male sexual dysfunction has become increasingly common. Psychological factors continue to be the most common cause of impotence, but some factors are amenable to surgery.

The patient is first carefully examined to rule out a congenital defect, and hormone levels and penile blood flow are tested. Assessment of erections which normally occur during sleep is performed by attaching a gauge to the penis.

Non-Surgical Treatment

Psychotherapy is employed if the cause of impotence is psychological. Male hormone (testosterone) may be used, but is primarily helpful only in cases where the testosterone level is low.

Injection of drugs (papaverine and pentolamine) directly into the body of the penis will sometimes stimulate erection. The patient may be taught to administer the injection himself.

Surgical Treatment

A semi-rigid rod of Silastic and Teflon may be surgically implanted into the penis (Fig. 9.15). The resultant semi-rigid penis may be manually bent at the base of the penis when an erection is not desired.

An inflatable prosthesis, which allows erection and flaccidity of the penis, employs a fluid reservoir and valves implanted in the scrotum. Although this technique most closely approaches normal erection, complications and equipment failure are common.

The complications of prosthesis insertion include infection around the prosthesis and breakdown of the skin over the prosthesis, both of which usually require removal of the prosthesis. Repeat operations are very common, due to breakdown of the implanted equipment.

The semi-rigid prosthesis is particularly effective for impotence resulting from surgery or other non-psychological causes.

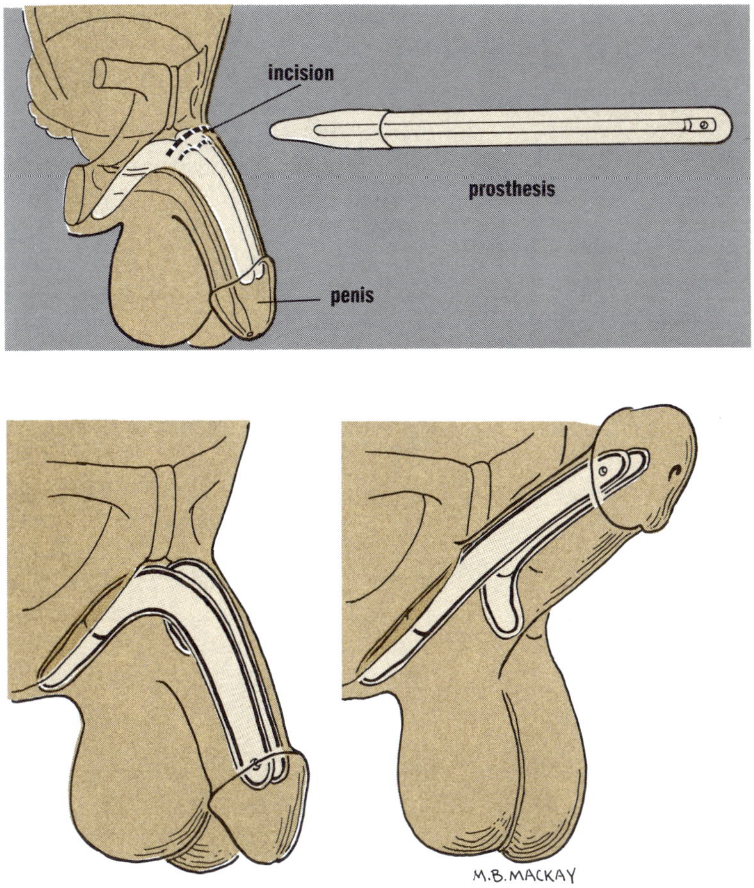

Figure 9.15
Insertion of penile prosthesis. An incision is made at the base of the penis and a semi-rigid prosthesis is inserted. The prosthesis is adjusted manually.

Testes and Scrotum

The scrotum contains the testicles (testes), which are encased in a protective covering and surrounded by a fluid-filled space in which they move freely. The testicles produce sperm and the male hormone, testosterone. The sperm passes from the testicle to the penis via a small tube called the vas deferens, which enters the urethra in the penis through the prostate gland (Fig. 9.11). At ejaculation, the prostate, the seminal vesicles (a structure behind the prostate) and the end of the vas deferens contract, discharging the semen into the urethra. The semen contains sperm and secretions from the seminal vesicles and prostate. These secretions are both the vehicle and nutrition for the sperm.

Minor problems involving the testicles and scrotum are common and usually require no surgical treatment. Testicular tumors, although rare, are almost always malignant, usually occur in young adults, and require immediate removal of the tumor and the involved testicle.

Vasectomy for voluntary sterilization has become the most common surgical procedure on the scrotum; reversal of vasectomy (vasovasostomy) is becoming increasingly common. Vasectomy does not affect the production of testosterone or its secretion into the circulation. It simply interrupts the passage of sperm from the testicle to the urethra.

The most common surgical problems involving the testicles are varicocele and testicular tumors. Another common problem, hydrocele, is covered in Chapter 5.

Varicocele

Varicocele occurs when the veins surrounding the testicle, usually on the left side, become varicosed (Fig. 9.16). The left testicular vein drains directly into the vein of the kidney, so in the standing position the testicular veins normally become distended. These veins may dilate, creating varicose veins.

A varicocele increases the temperature surrounding the testicle, interfering with the normal development and maturation of the sperm. Varicocele is therefore a cause of infertility.

A varicocele feels like "a bag of worms" which distends on standing and collapses on lying down. Diagnosis is made by physical examination or ultrasound. Semen analysis will usually show a decrease in number and mobility of the sperm, with an increase in abnormal forms.

Treatment involves cutting the testicular vein above the groin to stop the collecting veins from filling up on standing. These veins above the groin then drain through small, alternate channels along the vas deferens or to the opposite side.

After varicocele surgery, improvement of semen analysis occurs in up to 70 percent of cases, but may take several months. This improvement does not necessarily guarantee pregnancy, although the chance of pregnancy is significantly improved.

Complications are rare, but varicosities may recur after several years.

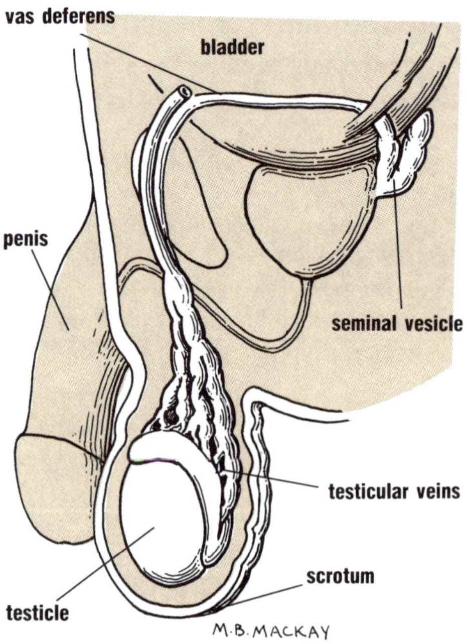

Figure 9.16
Varicocele. The testicular veins become enlarged and distended.

Testicular Tumors

These usually occur in young males and are almost always malignant, requiring immediate surgical removal.

The diagnosis is initially made when a hard lump is felt within the testicle. If hemorrhage has occurred within the tumor, the patient may also complain of a painful swollen testicle. Ultrasound will detect even small tumors. Some tumors also give off a substance that is detectable in the blood (tumor markers), making a blood test useful for both diagnosis and to measure the success of treatment. However, the absence of tumor markers in the blood does not rule out the presence of testicular malignancy.

These tumors spread early via the lymph glands and the bloodstream, so a thorough assessment of spread includes abdominal and pelvic ultrasound, CAT scan and chest X-rays.

Surgical treatment involves an incision high in the groin (inguinal incision), with removal of the testicle, testicular vein, artery and vas deferens. Once the specific type of tumor is identified, certain cases will require a further abdominal exploration and removal of the lymph glands draining the testicle.

Testicular tumors respond dramatically to chemotherapy, and even tumors that have spread beyond the testicle may be cured by these drugs. The earlier the diagnosis, the more effective the treatment is. Patients are therefore seen on a monthly basis postoperatively for a chest X-ray, ultrasound, CAT scan and blood tests.

One particular cell type of testicular tumor, seminoma, is very sensitive to radiation therapy. If detected early, spread of seminoma is virtually stopped with small courses of radiation, so these patients are also carefully assessed at monthly intervals postoperatively.

Tumors confined to the testicle, without evidence of spread, have a 90 percent cure rate. Even tumors with evidence of secondary spread, if detected early, may have more than an 80 percent long-term cure rate with chemotherapy and/or radiation treatment.

If desired, a testicular prosthesis may be inserted into the scrotum following removal of a testicle.

Chemotherapy for testicular tumors may interfere with sperm production; patients wishing to father a child in the future could store sperm in a sperm bank before undergoing chemotherapy.

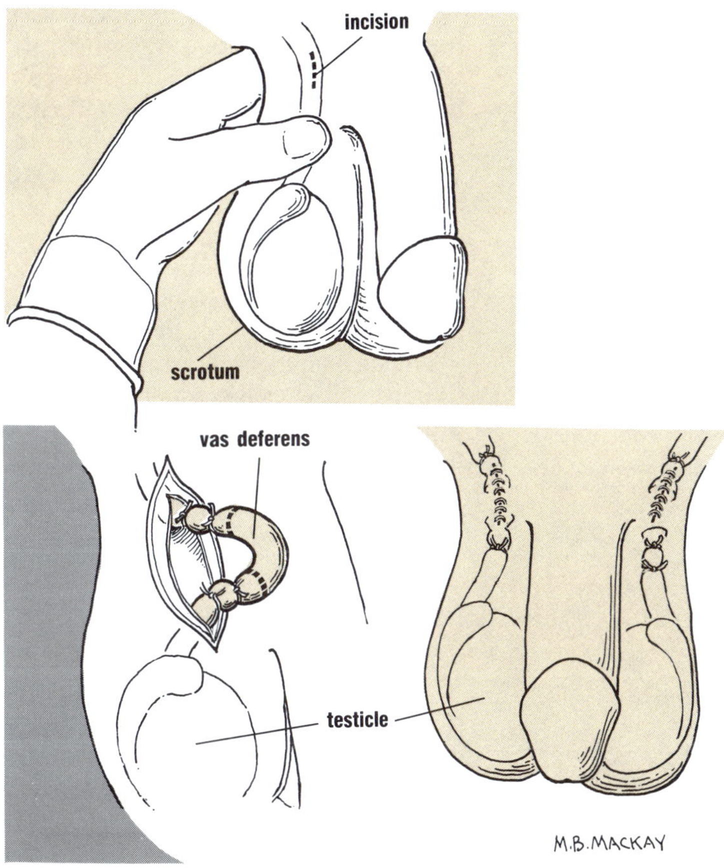

Figure 9.17
Vasectomy. A small piece of vas deferens is cut out and the remaining ends are doubly tied before being replaced in the scrotum.

Vasectomy

Vasectomy is a simple, effective form of sterilization (Fig. 9.17). The operation is very quick, is performed under local anesthetic, and involves cutting out a small piece of vas deferens through a small scrotal incision, and tying off each end. Ejaculation still occurs, but the ejaculate contains only the secretions of the seminal vesicles and the prostate, with no sperm. After the operation, the patient may experience some discomfort for one or two days, which can be relieved with mild painkillers.

A vasectomy should not be considered effective until two semen analyses, done two and three months after surgery, show no viable sperm in the ejaculate. Sexual activity, heavy lifting and strenuous activity should be avoided for two weeks because of the possibility of painful testicular swelling.

The most common complication is bleeding at the operative site, which may occur despite great care. Occasionally, hemorrhage into the scrotum will occur.

Failure of the operation, caused by the vas deferens spontaneously rejoining, occurs in one in 1,000 cases.

Rare cases of impotence following vasectomy are entirely psychological, as there is no interference with the normal hormone production of the testicle.

The development of arthritis or heart disease after vasectomy has been reported in the general press, but has not been substantiated scientifically.

Vasovasostomy

Reversal of vasectomy is usually requested because of marriage breakdown and remarriage. The two ends of the vas deferens are reattached, again allowing the sperm to pass from the testicle to the urethra.

The technique used is an operating microscope or other means of magnification, because the vas and suture material are very small. The surgeon may put a temporary supporting splint within the vas, removing it in two weeks. The patient is usually given a general anesthetic, and goes home the same day.

Factors influencing the success of the operation are the patient's age (patients over age 30 have a decreased chance of success); the number of years since the vasectomy (over seven years decreases success); and the site of the previous vasectomy (the closer to the testicle, the less suitable for repair the vas becomes).

Complications are infrequent, and the success rate in favorable cases is as high as 70 percent. Restoration of sperm production is often delayed for up to four months.

Chapter 10

Otolaryngology

Otolaryngology deals with disease and deformity in the head and neck, except for the eyes and the brain. It includes diseases and disorders of the upper digestive tract, including the mouth, salivary glands and gullet. These conditions involve hearing, balance, taste and smell.

Peter W. Alberti
Professor and Chairman
Department of Otolaryngology
University of Toronto
Otolaryngologist-in-Chief
Toronto General Hospital, Toronto

Mary Ann Williams
Illustrator

Otolaryngologists also treat diseases of the upper respiratory tract, particularly those of the nose, larynx (voice box) and windpipe. They, together with general and plastic surgeons, treat glandular disorders and skin diseases of the head and neck, including many tumors.

Some of the more common procedures performed by otolaryngologists include treatment of infections and allergies of the nasal sinuses, easing blockage of the nose caused by deformity of the nasal partition (septum), treatment of acute infections and fluid in the middle ear, patching holes in the ear drum, removal of tonsils and adenoids, and laryngoscopy.

Nose and Sinuses

The nose is the organ of smell and a very efficient air-conditioner. It is divided into two cavities. The partition between these cavities is called the nasal septum. At the back of the nose the septum is made of bone. At the front of the nose the septum is made of cartilage, which acts as a shock absorber. If the whole septum were made of bone, it would break with every minor blow.

Diseases of the nose usually occur in the sinuses — the many cavities in the facial bones that open into the interior of the nose. The largest sinuses lie immediately beneath the eyes (maxillary sinuses). They give shape to the lower part of the face. Many smaller sinuses (ethmoid sinuses) lie between the eyes and the nose.

The lining of the nose is a mucous membrane containing many mucus-secreting glands and blood vessels. The membrane can shrink or expand to produce more or less mucus. This is part of the "air-conditioning" function of the nose. Dust particles breathed in are caught in the mucus and swallowed harmlessly. In passing along the four-inch-long nasal cavity to the back of the nose, air is warmed to body temperature and is completely humidified. The lining membrane responds quickly to changes in external air temperature and humidity. The normal nose secretes about 1.5 quarts of mucus a day, most of which is swallowed. Because the nose traps dust and pollen, it is a common site of allergic reaction.

The nose may be blocked, may secrete too much fluid, and may be infected. Nasal blockage can be caused by a bony obstruction, by swelling of the lining membrane, or both. The septum may be bent, blocking one or both nasal cavities. This can happen either because it grows that way, or as a result of injury.

Nasal blockage caused by the swelling of the lining membrane has many causes, the most common of which is infection. The common cold, for example, is a viral infection. Bacterial infections can also cause the lining membrane to swell and secrete more mucus to eliminate the infection. Bacterial sinus infection (sinusitis) produces a green or yellow nasal discharge. If the infection persists, it is called chronic sinusitis.

Nasal allergies can also produce chronic swelling of the lining membranes and excessive secretion. The swelling, whether caused by infection or allergies, may become so great that the swollen membranes protrude into the nasal cavity, forming a growth called a nasal polyp.

One of the most common complaints that an otolaryngologist hears is, "Doctor, I can't breathe through my nose, it seems to be blocked." The otolaryngologist asks about the history of the blockage: when it began, whether the patient has allergies or has injured the nose, whether the blockage is worse in certain seasons, whether there is a discharge and, most important, how much difficulty the patient is experiencing from the blocked nose.

The otolaryngologist then uses a bright light and a small instrument called a speculum to examine each nostril in turn. This allows the doctor to see whether the septal is causing an obstruction, whether there is pus or polyps, whether the lining membrane is swollen, whether it is of normal color or inflamed, or whether it shows the distinctive purplish discoloration resulting from using too many nose drops. The doctor may wish to spray the nose with a drug that shrinks swelling of the lining membrane so that there is a better view of the nasal interior.

If the patient has pain in the sinuses, or a green or yellow discharge from the nose, a sinus X-ray will be performed. This shows whether the lining membrane of the sinuses is normal or thickened, or whether there is excessive fluid. If there is a strong history of allergies, the patient may be sent to see an allergy specialist who will do skin tests for specific allergens such as animal dander, house dust, pollens, ragweed or other items.

Sometimes the doctor orders a special laboratory examination called a nasal airflow study. This helps to determine if the obstruction is caused by disease of the lining membrane or by bony obstruction.

An acute bacterial infection such as sinusitis is treated with antibiotics to kill the germs, and decongestant medication to shrink the lining membrane so that the pus can drain. Allergies are often treated by desensitizing injections plus antihistamine pills to control the symptoms. Sometimes nose sprays containing cortisone are used to reduce the effects of a seasonal allergen.

Septoplasty

Correcting nasal obstruction caused by a deformity or malposition of the septum is called septoplasty (Fig. 10.1). Some septal deviation is normal; septoplasty is only performed if the deviated septum is causing an obstruction.

The patient may be admitted to hospital the day before surgery, or on the day of the operation, which is usually undertaken with the patient under general anesthetic.

The surgeon makes a cut into the lining membrane of the septum, near the front of the nose, and lifts the membrane off the septal cartilage. The cartilage is carefully cut and the membrane is lifted from the cartilage on the other side of the septum. The damaged or displaced portion of cartilage is removed and the remaining cartilage is straightened. The incision in the nasal lining membrane is closed with two or three stitches, which are usually the absorbing type which do not require removal. The nasal cavities are then packed with long strips of gauze soaked in petroleum jelly to keep pressure on the lining membrane so that it sticks together where the cartilage has been removed and begins to heal. The septoplasty usually takes about 30 minutes.

Patients can often go home a few hours after surgery, or may remain in hospital overnight. Packs are left in the nose for 24 hours. This is uncomfortable, because they prevent breathing through the nostrils. Otherwise there should be very little pain. When the packs are removed, which is done quickly and without need

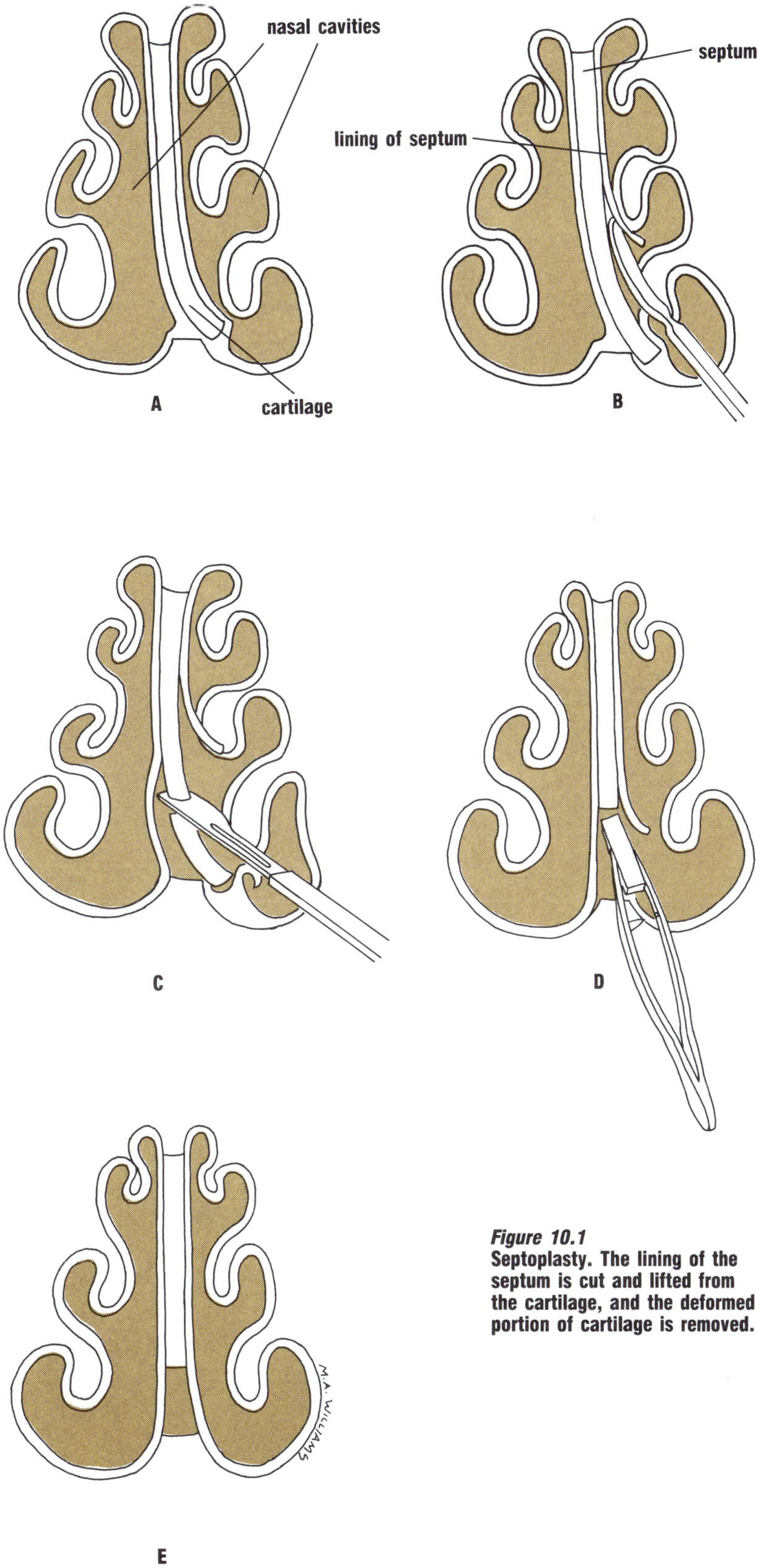

Figure 10.1
Septoplasty. The lining of the septum is cut and lifted from the cartilage, and the deformed portion of cartilage is removed.

for further anesthetic, breathing immediately improves, although it may worsen for about two weeks while postoperative swelling occurs and subsides. Doctors usually advise a week off work after the operation. There are no external bandages, no bruising under the eyes and no need for a cast on the nose.

Complications

Bleeding may occur into the area from which cartilage is removed. If the resulting blood clot is not drained, it will thicken the septum and defeat the purpose of the operation. Even worse, the clot may become infected and produce an abscess, although this is very rare. However, if the nose becomes very blocked in the first two weeks after surgery, the surgeon should be notified at once.

Septal perforation can occur if both sides of the lining membrane of the nose are torn when the cartilage is removed, producing a hole. This is often of no significance. However, it may crust at the edges, producing an obstruction which can defeat the purpose of the procedure.

For three or four weeks after the operation, a certain amount of crusting and scabbing in the nose is common, but this should cause no problem. After a successful septoplasty, breathing through the nose should permanently be much improved.

Recent Advances

About 25 years ago, larger amounts of septum were removed in septoplasties. The initial results were good. However, the external nose was so damaged that later nasal collapse frequently occurred, and septal perforation was common. The present procedure removes less tissue.

Removal of Nasal Polyps (Nasal Polypectomy)

Nasal polyps occur when the extremely swollen lining membrane of the sinuses protrudes into the nasal cavity. The underlying allergy or infection must be treated to prevent recurrence. Nasal polyps sometimes accompany other diseases of the respiratory system, such as asthma. Treatment of the polyps will not cure the asthma; neither will treatment of the asthma cure the polyps.

Nasal polyps can be removed with the patient under local or general anesthetic. The nose is inspected through a speculum. A wire loop, attached to a snare, is inserted and guided around the polyp up to its root in the sinus. The snare is tightened and gently tugged to remove the polyp. This is repeated until all the polyps have been removed. If a polyp hangs right into the back of the nose, it probably starts in the maxillary sinus, which must be opened so the polyp can be removed. Otherwise the polyp will likely recur. (See Caldwell-Luc Operation, page 115.)

If there has been much bleeding at surgery, a pack may be placed in the nose, although this is unusual. After a straightforward nasal polypectomy the patient can usually go home immediately. Blowing the nose or serious exertion should be avoided for a week or so. If the polyps were due to allergies, anti-allergic treatment, including cortisone-containing nose sprays, may be recommended.

Complications

Hemorrhage and infection can occur, although a little blood-stained discharge is common. Any obvious bleeding or signs of infection, such as green or yellow nasal discharge, should be reported to the surgeon at once.

There may be a little crusting in the nose for a week or two after the operation, but then the breathing should be much relieved. The scabs can be softened by rinsing the nose with a little baking soda or salt dissolved in water.

It is sometimes necessary to open the maxillary sinuses and remove diseased tissue or polyps. This is called a Caldwell-

Luc operation, and is performed if there are polyps or a chronic infection in the sinuses, which has not responded to repeated antibiotics or antial lavage.

The Caldwell-Luc Operation

For Caldwell-Luc surgery, the patient is given a general anesthetic. The surgeon makes a cut inside the mouth on the affected side (Fig. 10.2). The lining membrane of the mouth, the muscle of the cheek and all the tissue over the bone in the cheek is carefully lifted off, exposing the thin outer bony wall of the maxillary sinus. A small piece of this cheekbone is removed, and the thickened lining membrane is removed by forceps. Then a drainage opening is made into the nose, and the incision in the mouth is closed with three or four absorbable stitches.

The opening into the cheekbone is usually no larger than the diameter of the finger. It does not need to be replaced and leaves no deformity. As long as the three strong edges of the sinus around the eye socket, the outer wall of the nose and the outermost portion of the cheek are left intact, the sinus will retain its shape.

After the operation there may be a little blood-stained discharge from the nose for up to three or four weeks. Immediately after surgery the nose should not be blown, for fear of blowing air into the soft tissues of the cheek and making it swell. There may be some bruising of the cheek, which looks dramatic but clears very quickly. Otherwise, there should be very little pain. The patient generally goes home after two or three days, or goes home immediately to two or three days of bed rest.

Complications

The complications of the operation are bleeding, infection and numbness of the cheek and teeth. The bleeding may occur

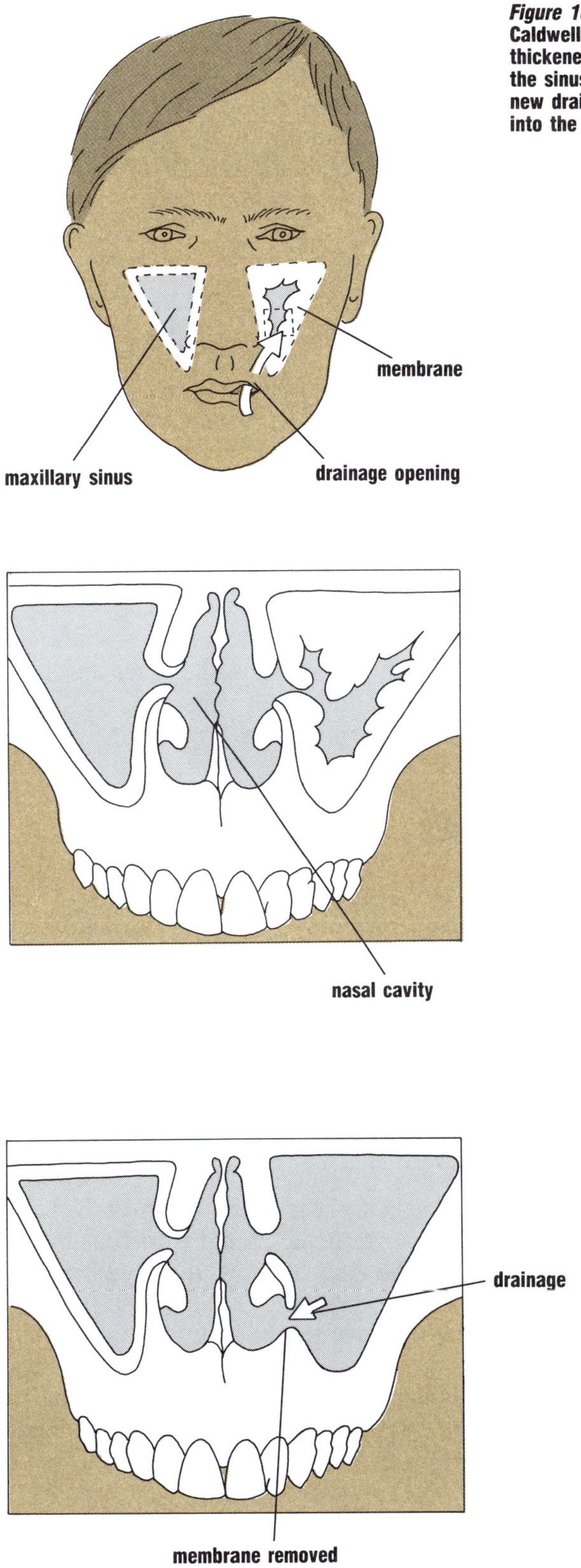

Figure 10.2
Caldwell-Luc operation. The thickened lining membrane of the sinus is removed, and a new drainage opening is made into the nose (arrow).

Case Study: Myringotomy

Myra was used to losing sleep — Jamie had had so many ear infections as an infant. But he was five now, and had missed so much school with ear infections that Myra was really worried about the poor start he'd had.

This morning he had dark circles under his eyes, having woken at 2 a.m. before finally dropping into an uneasy sleep around 4:30. The family doctor had been reluctant to do anything beyond treating each infection promptly, because he, too, said there was a strong chance Jamie would grow out of it.

"Sorry, son, but it's off to the doctor again for us this morning," Myra smiled ruefully at the dark-haired little boy. Dr. Littleton was so used to seeing them that he simply asked, "The usual?" This time Myra told him how worried she was about Jamie's absences from school. Dr. Littleton flipped through Jamie's chart, which by now was thicker than Myra's own.

"Jamie has had three infections so far this winter, and it's only January. He stands a good chance of hearing loss if we let this go on. I'll get you an appointment with Dr. Ricardo, our ear, nose and throat specialist. Let's see what he says."

within 24 hours of surgery and up to 10 days later, and should be reported to the surgeon, though it usually stops without treatment.

Infection is a late and very rare complication, but if it occurs, it causes fever, pain, swelling of the cheek and perhaps discharge of pus from the nose. It must be treated with antibiotics under medical supervision.

Numbness of the teeth beneath the incision line is common after this operation, but usually improves over some months. It occurs because the nerve supply of the teeth generally lies in the incision line.

Numbness of the cheek is much more rare. The nerve supplying the skin of the cheek enters the face through the roof of the maxillary sinus and may be damaged during surgery, producing a feeling of pins and needles over the cheek and a little loss of sensation. It usually disappears without treatment.

Ear

The organs of hearing and balance are contained in the inner ear, or labyrinth. The cochlea is shaped like a snail's shell and forms half of the labyrinth. It converts sound vibrations into a nervous impulse, just like a microphone.

The outer ear, the pinna, catches sound and funnels it into the ear canal. At the base of the ear canal lies the ear drum (tympanic membrane), to which is attached a little bone known as the hammer or malleus. Sound vibrations entering the ear canal set the membrane in motion, vibrating the hammer. The ear drum separates the outer ear from the middle ear, which contains three little bones — the hammer, the anvil and the stirrup (malleus, incus and stapes). Vibrations from the hammer are transmitted to the anvil and through the anvil to the stirrup, which connects with the inner ear.

The ear drum must vibrate freely in response to the minute changes in air pressure produced by soft sounds. To do this, air pressure must be the same on both sides of the ear drum. Even a minor change of air pressure affects hearing, as most people have experienced in an elevator rising or an airplane taking off. To keep the air pressure the same on both sides of the ear drum, the middle ear cavity is connected to the back of the nose by a passage called the eustachian tube. This normally opens on every third or fourth swallow, replenishing the air in the middle ear.

Hearing problems can result from a faulty microphone or a faulty sound-conducting mechanism. The eustachian tube can be blocked, preventing the middle ear from functioning properly; the eardrum can be damaged; or the three small bones can be stuck down by arthritis of their joints, most commonly the joint between the stapes footplate and the inner ear.

Temporary eustachian tube obstruction occurs frequently with a common cold. Chronic obstruction is extremely common in children, where the tube is smaller and thicker than in adults. It is lined by tissue that responds to allergy and infection by swelling and blocking the passageway. In northern winters, up to 30 percent of Grade One children may have blocked eustachian tubes at any given time. Fortunately, they usually clear spontaneously.

Untreated recurring ear infections can eventually cause permanent hearing loss, since the ear drum may gradually become eroded and perforated. Surgery to deal with the after-effects of middle ear infection is one of the most common operations performed in North America today, although perforations of the ear drum are less common than they used to be because ear infections are better treated.

Myringotomy

A blocked eustachian tube causes the air in the middle ear cavity to be absorbed and fluid to be secreted in its place. The

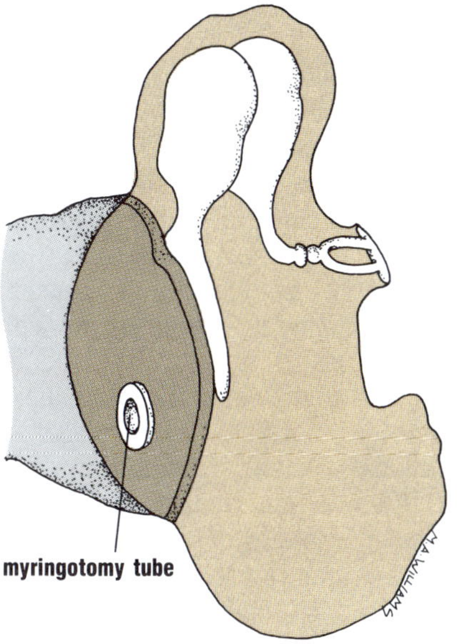

Figure 10.3
Myringotomy with tympanic membrane shunt.

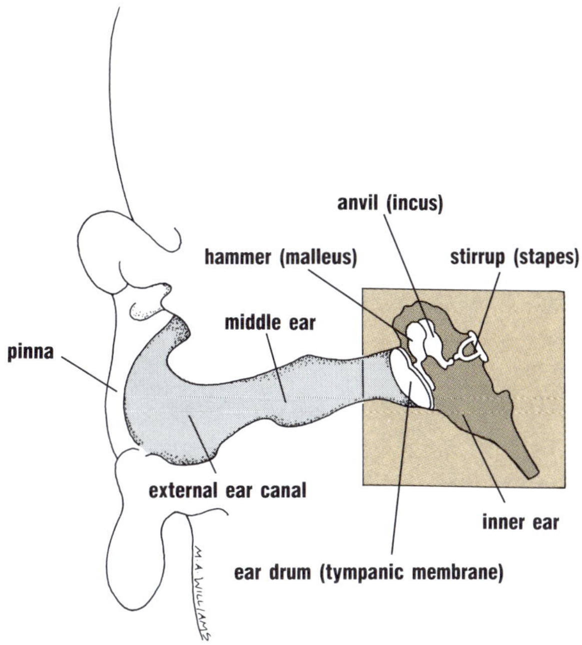

blockages may be caused by enlarged adenoids, allergies, changes in barometric pressure or, much more rarely, a growth in the back of the nose. A blocked eustachian tube usually clears with antibiotic treatment if there is infection, antihistamines if there is an allergy, and occasionally nose drops, particularly if there is a blockage following flying. If the hearing loss persists, further investigation and treatment are needed.

A hearing test is done with an audiometer, a device that measures the sensitivity of hearing at different frequencies. Middle ear pressure is measured by a device called an impedance bridge, to find out if the middle ear is obstructed. The back of the nose must also be inspected for growths which may be causing the problem. These could be nasal polyps, enlarged adenoids in children or, rarely, in adults, cancer.

In a myringotomy, the surgeon makes an incision through the ear drum into the middle ear. Children are given general anesthetic; adults are often given local anesthetic. The surgeon uses an operating microscope, which gives good illumination, stereoscopic vision and a magnified view of the ear drum, so the incision can be made very precisely. A small suction tube, rather like a long, thin, blunted hypodermic needle, is inserted through the incision to suck out the fluid in the middle ear (Fig. 10.3).

What happens next depends on the cause of the blocked eustachian tube. If the condition is chronic, the hearing loss will recur as soon as the hole in the ear drum heals, so a ventilating tube may be inserted through the hole to keep the middle ear aerated while the disease clears up (tympanic membrane shunt). This tube is kept in place until full healing occurs, approximately six months, and is then naturally extruded.

The patient can return home to normal activities right after surgery. Even flying is possible immediately. The ear must be kept dry to prevent infection, and cotton batten smeared with petroleum jelly should be put into the ear when taking a shower. For long-term use an ear mold or plug might be advisable.

This procedure usually restores hearing to normal, with minimal complications. A little blood-stained discharge from the ear is common for the first 24 hours. The hole heals within 48 to 72 hours.

Dr. Ricardo came to his decision very promptly after testing Jamie's hearing. "Mrs. Henderson, I don't think we should wait any longer. Dr. Littleton has obviously kept a close eye on Jamie in the last few years, and since there's been no improvement, I recommend surgical drainage. Depending on how the ear looks, we might put in a drainage tube as well." Myra was relieved that she'd be able to take Jamie home on the same day as the surgery. So was Jamie. He'd never been in hospital and wasn't over-excited about the whole idea. They arrived at the hospital early in the morning, armed with Jamie's favorite toys. Myra was determined to be there the whole time, so that hers would be the first face Jamie would see when he came round from the anesthetic.

Jamie was fairly groggy for a couple of hours after he returned to the room. Myra got him drinks of water and stroked his hair. Later Dr. Ricardo stopped by. "We did put in a tube, Mrs. Henderson. That will just allow the ear to drain until the infection clears. I think you'll notice a difference pretty soon."

Jamie was quite proud of the ear mold that Myra had made for him. Dr. Ricardo had suggested it for the healing period, and Dr. Littleton had recommended that he use it after that for swimming, or when the weather was particularly cold.

Myringoplasty

If, on examining the ear, the doctor finds a perforated ear drum, the size, shape and position of the perforation and the condition of the lining membrane are evaluated to decide on the appropriate treatment. If the membrane is diseased, the operation is less likely to be successful. An audiometric hearing test will also be done.

Non-Surgical Treatment

Perforations can sometimes be healed by stimulating the edges to grow. A chemical is very carefully applied to cauterize the edge of the perforation. Sometimes a surgeon will lay a little piece of paper to cover the perforation, so that tissue will heal over the paper and bridge the hole beneath. This procedure does not work with bigger perforations.

Surgical Treatment

In a myringoplasty, the ear drum is surgically repaired. Tissue is laid across the perforation to serve as a scaffold for the skin to heal across the ear canal surface, and to allow the lining membrane of the middle ear to grow across the inner surface. Some loose fibrous tissue, which covers one of the muscles used for chewing, is often used for bridging. The tissue is taken from the muscle just above the ear in the temple.

The patient is given a general anesthetic, and a little hair is shaved from above the ear so that a clean one-inch incision can be made above the ear, down to the underlying muscle. A small piece of fibrous tissue (fascia) is removed and stored in salt solution until needed. The incision is then closed.

Using an operating microscope, the surgeon inspects the ear canal very carefully, checking the perforation. Using a very fine needle, the surgeon strips the tissue at the edge of the hole, which produces a little bleeding and induces healing across the graft. Then incisions are made to open a flap of skin above the ear drum. The flap, with the ear drum attached, is pulled forward, revealing the under side of the ear drum and the cavity of the middle ear.

The fascia is cut to a size slightly larger than the hole and placed on the inner side of the ear drum. The middle ear is then filled with a gelatin-like sponge material to act as a support for the graft. The sponge material is usually absorbed by the body in a few weeks. The flap of ear drum and ear canal skin are put back in their original position. The graft now lies smoothly on the inner surface of the ear drum and completely covers the hole. The graft is held in place on the outer surface by a pack made of strips of oiled silk and more sponge material.

Following this operation, the patient will stay in the hospital for up to two days. The ear is kept dry, and the packing is left undisturbed for approximately one week. The surgeon then removes the stitches and some of the packing, although some may be left for a longer period. Normal work can be resumed in about a week, although patients who do heavy physical labor should take a two-week break. There is usually very little pain after the operation. The patient should have a good hearing ear and be able to enjoy full activity including flying, swimming and showering without the risk of more infections. About 80 percent of these operations will be successful. In 20 percent of cases, the perforation may not heal or may recur.

Complications

Occasionally a patient may experience temporary dizziness after surgery, ringing in the ears or, rarely, infection of the middle ear or deafness, which may result from inappropriate manipulation of the middle ear bones.

Recent Advances

Originally external skin was used for this operation. Although it healed well, it required constant care and left the ear drum thinner than normal. Grafts used to be placed on the outer surface of the ear drum, which sometimes resulted in skin being trapped under the graft, producing a cyst. The current technique of using fascia (connective tissue found underneath the skin) as a graft placed on the inner surface of ear drum has markedly improved results.

Tonsils and Adenoids

The tonsils and adenoids form a ring around the upper food and breathing passages. The tonsils are situated on each side of the throat at the back of the mouth. The adenoids are located on the back wall of the nose. These large clusters of lymphoid tissue protect the upper end of the breathing and digestive pathways. They are important in early life because they produce antibodies against things with which we come into daily contact. Most everyday environmental allergens are met in the first few months of life, so the prime function of this lymphoid tissue is over by the second birthday. These tissues are at their largest in infancy and gradually shrivel through adolescence. Because they filter germs, they can easily become infected and harbor bacteria.

In a baby or young child, the adenoids are large and the back of the nose is small. The adenoids can block the opening of the eustachian tubes, resulting in ear infections. The tonsils can become infected and cause chronic respiratory infections in children.

Germs are caught in the mouth and grow in the tonsils. The tonsils react by swelling, producing pain, difficulty in swallowing and fever. A single attack of tonsillitis usually goes away on its own, although it may resolve more quickly with antibiotic treatment. If the tonsils become repeatedly infected, however, they become unable to produce antibodies, and may become a reservoir for germs that can live there permanently. If this happens, they should be removed. Removal of tonsils and adenoids remains the most common operation performed in North America.

Tonsillectomy and Adenoidectomy

Diagnosis

Very few tests are made for tonsillitis in children; the history and a physical examination usually reveal the diagnosis. A throat culture may be necessary to find the appropriate antibiotic treatment for acute episodes.

Diagnosis of breathing obstruction by the adenoids is made by placing a shiny spoon or mirror beneath the nose to see whether the mirror fogs up with breathing. If it does not, the nose is blocked. Occasionally an X-ray of the back of the nose is necessary to find out the size of the adenoids. The doctor will also check the palate for defects, because removal of adenoids in children with cleft palates will worsen the speech defect.

Non-Surgical Treatment

The non-surgical treatment of acute tonsillitis is antibiotic treatment. Only when there have been three episodes of tonsillitis a year for two years is surgery usually recommended. Adenoids are usually removed with tonsils, or they may be removed alone to treat chronic ear infections from an obstructed eustachian tube which is not responding to other treatment.

Surgical Treatment

The operation to remove the tonsils is called tonsillectomy. It is done under general anesthetic, and the child usually stays in the hospital for one night after surgery. A plastic tube is passed into the

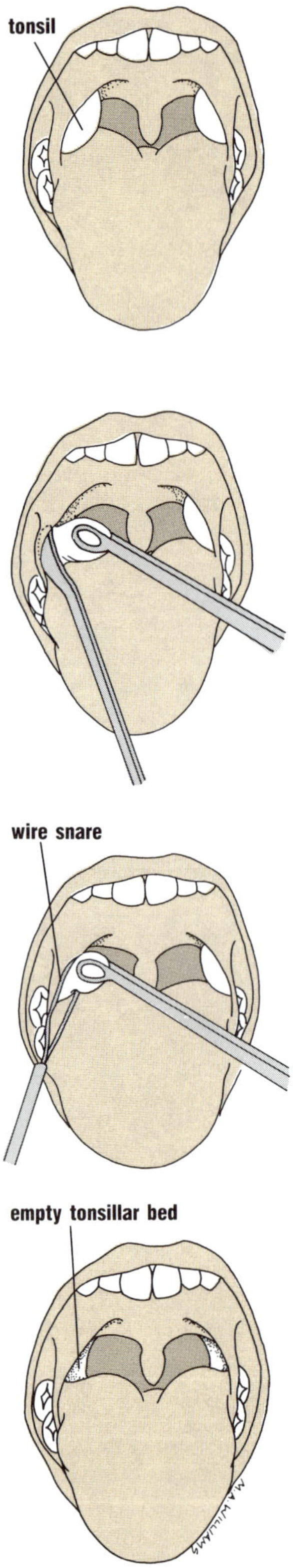

Figure 10.4
Tonsillectomy.

windpipe through the mouth. The child lies flat on his or her back, with a pillow under the shoulders. The mouth is held widely open with a metal retractor. The surgeon picks up the tonsils in a pair of forceps, stretches it and carefully cuts it out, often using a wire snare, which will remove the tonsil and crush blood vessels to help stop bleeding (Fig. 10.4). The tonsil usually separates very smoothly. The blood vessels of the tonsil are clamped and the gap is packed with cotton gauze soaked in adrenalin to reduce bleeding. The procedure is then repeated on the opposite side. The cotton packing is removed and any bleeding points are ligated (sewn up) with black silk. The ligatures look like black specks, and may alarm parents unaware of their existence. They come off about a week later on their own and are swallowed.

In an adenoidectomy, the adenoid is removed with a curette passed up behind the soft palate and hooked over the adenoid, which is then cut out (Fig. 10.5). Bleeding in the adenoid bed is stopped with cotton packs soaked in a medication that helps blood to clot.

The whole operation to remove the tonsils and adenoids takes about 20 minutes. The major concerns are bleeding and pain on swallowing. A scab quickly forms over the raw area where the tonsils and adenoids have been removed, which protects the wound. The more the jaws are moved, the softer the scab becomes. A softer scab makes bleeding less likely when the scab separates about a week after the surgery. For the first day after the operation, feeding is confined to drinks and soft foods like jello and ice cream. Fruit juices (such as apple, orange or tomato) contain acid, which can cause pain. Because of the pain on swallowing, the child may at first refuse to drink, and may become dehydrated. The child must be encouraged to drink.

By the second day the child should begin to chew; chewing gum is very helpful in reducing pain and complications. Depending on the hospital and the physician, the child goes home on the day of the surgery or the day after, but should be kept at home for about 10 days until the scab has separated and the risk of bleeding has passed. Although bed rest used to be recommended for a few days, this can be very difficult for young children. Vigorous exercise should be avoided for about 10 days.

Complications

The complications of this operation are hemorrhage, infection and speech difficulties. Bleeding within 24 hours of surgery is caused when a clot, which forms at the time of surgery, separates off and opens a blood vessel. This does not occur often, but it is the reason for keeping the child in hospital under observation for about 12 hours after surgery. Any clot can thus be discovered and removed before the child is sent home.

Secondary hemorrhage, which happens when the scab separates, occurs between the fifth and tenth day after surgery. The doctor should be notified at once and the child brought back to hospital. It is very rare for major treatment to be necessary at this stage, but the amount of blood can be checked and any clot removed.

Infection is a rare complication. The symptoms are worsening pain and an increase in fever some days after surgery. A little fever in the first 24 to 48 hours after surgery is common, but should completely pass by the end of that time. Later fever indicates an infection and is treated with antibiotics.

A mild speech problem is extremely common after adenoidectomy. If the adenoids were big, before surgery the child was probably talking as if his or her nose were blocked. Removal of a big pad of adenoids can produce exactly the opposite effect. The child may talk as if with a cleft palate, with air escaping from the nose during speech. This is due to the removal of a large obstruction and the stretching of the soft palate during surgery. As the soft palate redevelops its tone, this should disappear. If this symptom is still present two months after surgery, speech therapy may be called for.

After surgery, throat infections should disappear completely. Ear infections should be dramatically reduced, although the operation does not always cure fluid in the ear, for which insertion of a tube through the ear drum may be necessary (see Myringotomy, page 116). The child is often much healthier, grows quickly and is altogether livelier after the tonsils and adenoids have been removed, because the air passages are now open, allowing peaceful sleeping.

Larynx

The larynx is a specialized part of the windpipe situated where the breathing and food passages separate at the back of the throat. Externally it forms the Adam's apple, and closes off the air passage during swallowing so that food and drink do not go down the wrong way. It is also the organ of sound for speech. The larynx contains the vocal cords, which are lined by skin and are thus subject to all the diseases of skin — bruises, corns, polyps and cancer.

The symptom common to all alterations of the vocal cords is hoarseness, commonly found after excessive shouting, or during a cold or other respiratory infection. Persistent hoarseness that lasts for three weeks or more requires detailed investigation. If the examiner cannot see the full length of the vocal cords, or if there is a polyp or an ulcer that does not respond to treatment, then laryngoscopy is called for.

Laryngoscopy

This procedure is performed with the patient under general anesthetic. A large metal tube is passed into the larynx so that the surgeon can examine the vocal cords, usually using a microscope. The required procedure — usually removal of a small piece of tissue, particularly a

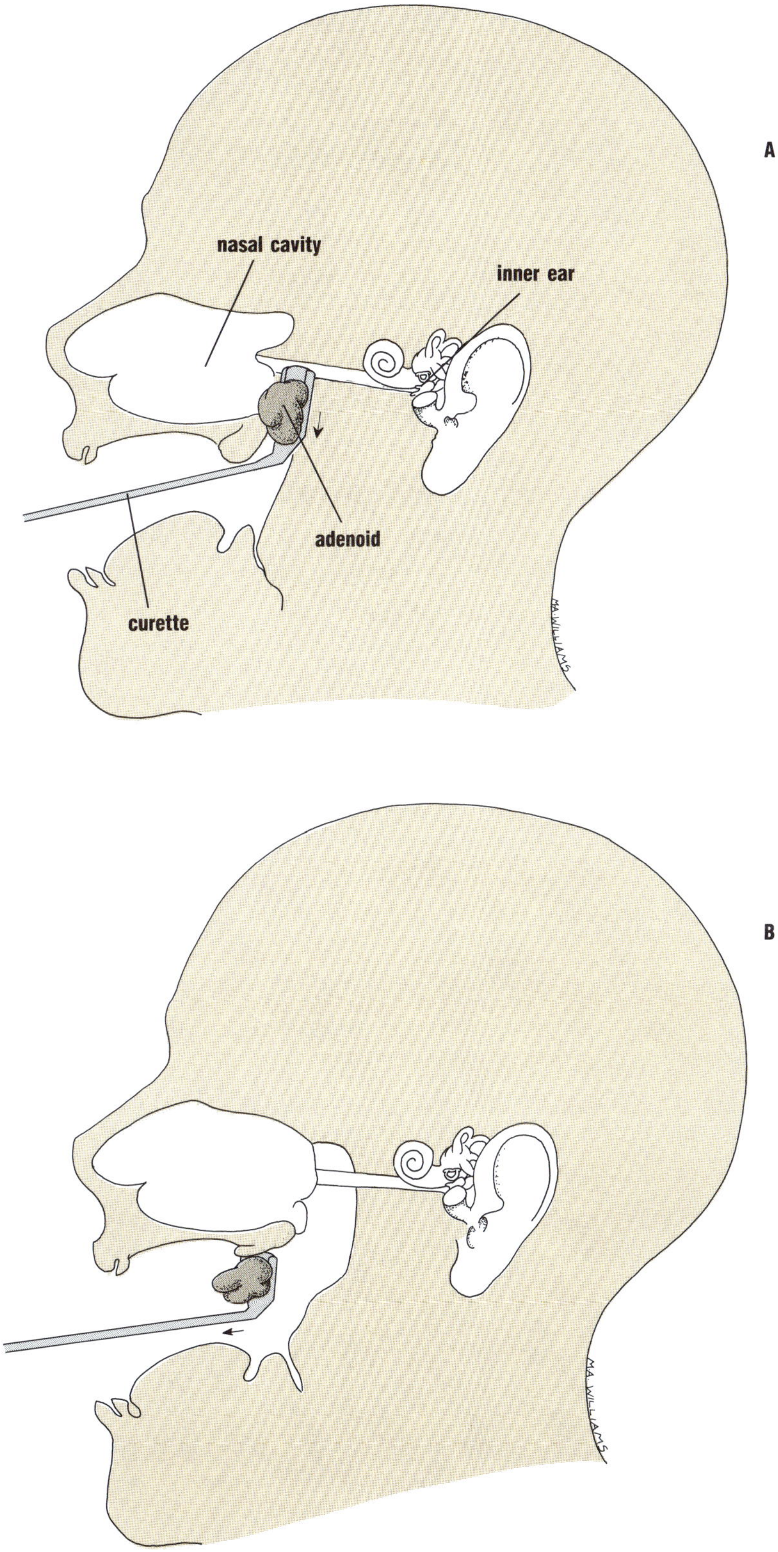

Figure 10.5
Adenoidectomy.

polyp, with forceps, scissors or by laser — is then undertaken.

The patient can usually go home the same day, unless the operation has been extensive, in which case a 24-hour period of observation is advisable, in case swelling of the larynx interferes with breathing.

If no lesion was removed, normal activity can be resumed immediately. If a lesion was removed, the surgeon will usually advise a period of voice rest while the larynx heals.

Complications

Complications of laryngoscopy are unusual, but occur early. At the time of operation the tongue may be bruised, or a tooth may be chipped by the metal tube. Swelling of the larynx may produce some hoarseness and, very rarely, difficulty in breathing. This usually occurs within the observation period in hospital.

Recent Advances

Lasers are now being used to remove lesions in the larynx. Telescopes used to examine the larynx in the doctor's office give a much better view and have quite dramatically reduced the number of laryngoscopies required as the doctor is able to see more of the larynx and perform a more comprehensive examination.

Chapter 11

Ophthalmology

Few fears are as profound as the fear of blindness. The eye is our window on the world; without sight, even routine tasks would become major challenges. The ophthalmologist's role is to prevent blindness whenever possible or, in some cases, cure it.

Clive B. Mortimer

Professor
Department of Ophthalmology
University of Toronto

Ophthalmologist
Toronto General Hospital

Stephen P. Kraft

Assistant Professor
Department of Ophthalmology
University of Toronto

Ophthalmologist
Hospital for Sick Children, Toronto

Linda Wilson-Pauwels
Illustrator
Assistant Professor
Department of Art as Applied to Medicine
University of Toronto

The eye develops before birth as an outgrowth of the brain (Fig. 11.1). The eye has three layers: an outer protective layer (sclera), an intermediate layer of blood vessels (choroid) and the retina, an inner layer of nervous tissue (Fig. 11.2).

The eye can be compared to a camera. Just as the lens is the camera's focusing system, so the cornea and lens are the focusing system of the eye. The camera's diaphragm becomes bigger or smaller, altering focus in the same manner as the colored part of the eye (iris). The camera uses film; the eye uses the retina. When any part of this system malfunctions, the camera doesn't work. In the same way, the eye cannot function without a satisfactory lens and retina system. As the camera is repaired, so, too, can parts of the eye be repaired. In this chapter we describe some of the operations used — cataract removal, repair of retinal detachment, correction of strabismus, and laser surgery for diabetic retinopathy, glaucoma and retinal holes.

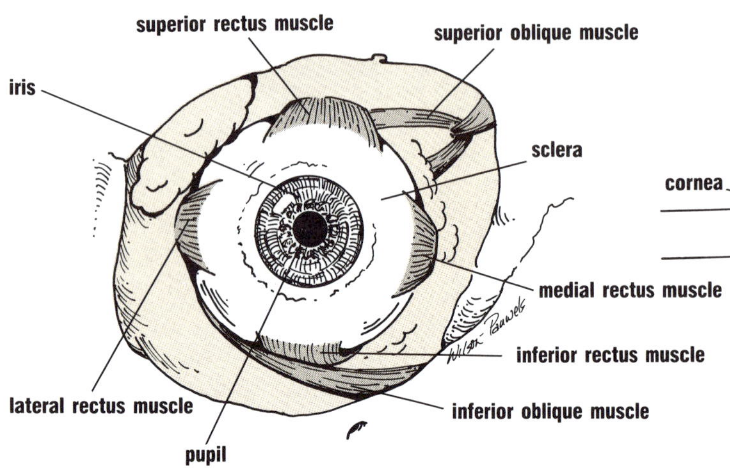

Figure 11.1
Eye and eye muscles. The iris is seen through the transparent cornea.

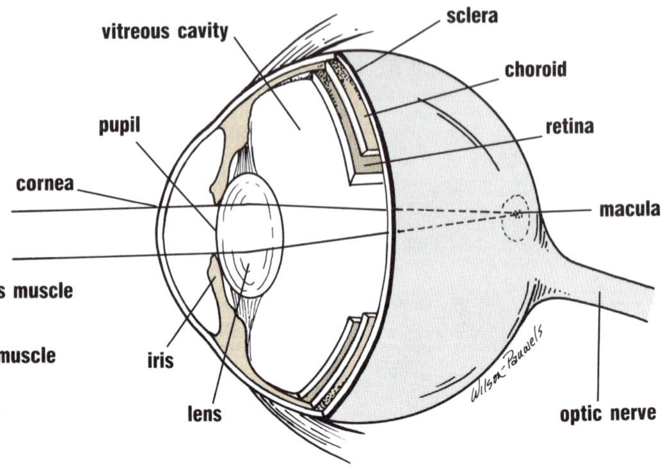

Figure 11.2
Interior structures of the eye.

Cataract Extraction with Implant

Cataract extraction is the most common of all eye operations. Approximately 450,000 cataract extractions are performed in North America every year. A cataract is a clouding of the eye's lens, resulting in a gradual dimming and distortion of vision. The clouding is caused by the absorption of fluid into the lens. This may cause it to swell, or the individual fibers may thicken, distorting light. This is a slow and gradual process, usually affecting both eyes. Cataracts are mostly a consequence of the aging process, or are a result of other diseases, such as diabetes. They can also result from an injury to the eye. Cataracts may occur in children, sometimes as a birth defect.

During cataract surgery the eye's lens is removed. This will change the eye's focusing system radically. The traditional operation for cataracts was simply to remove the lens completely. The patient then had to wear special glasses or contact lenses in order to be able to focus. Now a plastic lens (implant) is made to the patient's prescription and inserted into the eye as a replacement.

The timing of surgery is the patient's decision. When a patient is no longer able to pursue chosen activities because of limited eyesight, surgery is indicated. A person whose eyesight is crucial to his or her work and who wishes to drive, for instance, would probably request early cataract extraction. There is no point waiting for the cataract to thicken. With current technology, the old concept that a cataract should be "ripe" is no longer valid.

Diagnosis

The patient's complaint of blurred vision is the most important factor. Cataracts can be seen without complex equipment, but other tests must be done to ensure that the cataract alone is the cause of decreased vision. The surgeon examines the retina, in particular the central part called the macula (Fig. 11.2), which is responsible for fine vision. No matter how technically satisfactory the cataract extraction, vision may not improve if the macula is no longer healthy. The pressure inside the eye is measured, and the cornea is examined for any condition that could be worsened by surgery.

In some patients the cataract may be so dense that the retina can no longer be seen. In these patients ultrasound examination tells the surgeon whether the retina is in its correct position. In special circumstances more complicated tests may be used to determine the health of the macula. In one test a laser is shone into the eye, and a pattern or grid interferes with the path of the laser (laser interferometry). If the patient can detect the interference in the ray of light, then the retina is probably healthy. Other tests determine the correct power for the lens that will be implanted in the eye. After the operation, virtually all patients will need glasses, either for reading or distance, but the prescription will be much weaker than if they did not have the implanted lens.

Non-Surgical Treatment

There is no effective non-surgical treatment for cataracts. Many medications have been tried, but so far none has retarded cataract development.

Surgical Treatment

Cataract extraction is carried out in the hospital, but many patients can go home the same day. Patients with additional medical problems may have to be admitted, but the hospital stay is usually short.

General or local anesthetic can be used in cataract extractions, although local is more common. When local anesthetic is used, the injection is given around the eye to numb it and prevent it from moving. For most patients this involves one injection, which usually takes full effect after about 10 minutes.

An incision is made where the cornea and the sclera meet (Fig. 11.3). The capsule of the lens is opened — capsulotomy (Fig. 11.4) — and most of the lens is removed. This can be done in several ways. One method uses an ultrasonic probe; the lens is broken into tiny pieces by ultrasonic waves, and the pieces are then removed. Another technique extracts the lens nucleus in one piece (Fig. 11.5). Whichever technique is used, the back surface of the capsule must be kept intact, so that a "bag" remains. The plastic lens is implanted within the bag (Fig. 11.6), the incision is sewn up, and the eye is patched. The whole procedure takes about an hour.

Usually the eye is left patched until the day after surgery. The patient feels some discomfort or pain when the local anesthetic wears off, and a mild painkiller is usually necessary. Some patients feel nauseated, but can usually obtain relief with anti-nausea tablets. Most patients are able to get up and walk around within three hours of surgery. It is sensible to avoid strenuous activity or heavy physical exertion, and one must avoid any injury or direct blow to the eye. Otherwise, normal activities can be resumed. Eye drops are used for two to four weeks, and then in decreasing amounts. The drops reduce swelling and intraocular pressure, and may contain an antibiotic. The eye is usually reddened and irritated for the first two weeks. Some of this irritation is caused by the sutures, which are under the upper lid and can be felt on blinking and eye movement. Absorbable sutures are commonly used, but if suture removal is necessary, it is a very minor, painless procedure.

A typical postoperative routine is a visit to the surgeon on the day after surgery, then visits at two and four weeks, and a final visit about six weeks after the operation.

Improvement in vision is usually gradual, as the eye heals, but some patients have very good vision soon after the operation.

Patients may shop, watch television and keep social engagements within a few days of the operation. It is not wise to indulge in heavy housework or gardening or activities that involve a lot of bending and stooping, but most patients can resume full normal activities after a week, although normal vision will likely not yet have returned.

Case Study: Cataract Extraction with Implant

At age 57, Fred thought life was treating him well. When he'd come to Canada as a young man, he'd scrimped and saved, working overtime to buy his own fruit and vegetable store. He and his wife had worked all hours to build up the business, and now the family owned three large supermarkets. Life was still very busy for Fred, but he wouldn't have it any other way.

He first noticed a problem when he was driving. He did a lot of traveling between stores. For big orders, he'd even do occasional deliveries, but it was getting harder to see the house numbers, and street signs were a bit of a problem, too. The family kidded him about needing glasses — he'd worn them for reading for a few years, but maybe he needed them for distance now as well. When he wasn't so busy, maybe he'd go for an eye test.

Then he noticed that glare bothered him — a lot. It seemed to be much worse with the right eye, so that he found himself closing his right eye when he was totalling a cash register or looking at a scale. His wife mentioned it, but he shrugged it off, until one evening Gloria had to help him up the stairs because he couldn't see the edge of the steps. He went to see the doctor the next day.

Fred thought he'd never been in and out of a doctor's office so fast in his life. Dr. Bergman had taken one look and said, "I'd like you to see an ophthalmologist. I think you have a cataract." Fred was too stunned to ask questions, and Gloria was too scared. They were both thinking the same thing — Fred was going blind.

But after doing several tests, the ophthalmologist, Dr. Blake, was very reassuring. "I'm glad to say, that apart from the cataract, your right eye is healthy, which means that we'll be able to operate." He explained that the operation was not an emergency. It depended on how much Fred wanted to be able to drive, really. They told Dr. Blake about Fred's mild hypertension, diagnosed by Dr. Bergman 18 months earlier. "Yes, Dr. Bergman's letter says you're doing quite well on medication and your blood pressure has been controlled for the past year. That shouldn't be a problem. You'll still be able to have the surgery as an outpatient."

The ophthalmologist then went over the procedure with them step by step, making sure they understood what would happen. They hadn't realized that the lens of Fred's right eye would be replaced by a plastic lens, but Dr. Blake was careful to point out that he'd still be wearing glasses for reading, if not for distance.

Gloria was more nervous than Fred on the day of the surgery. His attitude was, "Let's get it over with," but she knew he hated the thought of surgery.

Fred opted for local anesthetic. He was a bit squeamish about being awake during the operation, but he was told he could go home more quickly that way. Gloria knew that Fred imagined he'd be able to see the scalpel coming down on his eye, so she'd asked Dr. Blake about that. "Actually, Gloria, when you anesthetize the optic nerve, you can't see anything. The sensations are really no worse than having a root canal done."

Fred had continued to take his blood pressure pills as he'd been instructed, and he'd already been to the hospital for blood tests, chest X-rays and a cardiogram. Now, after having some eye drops put in, they were waiting for him to be taken down to the operating room (OR).

Figure 11.3
Incision for cataract surgery.

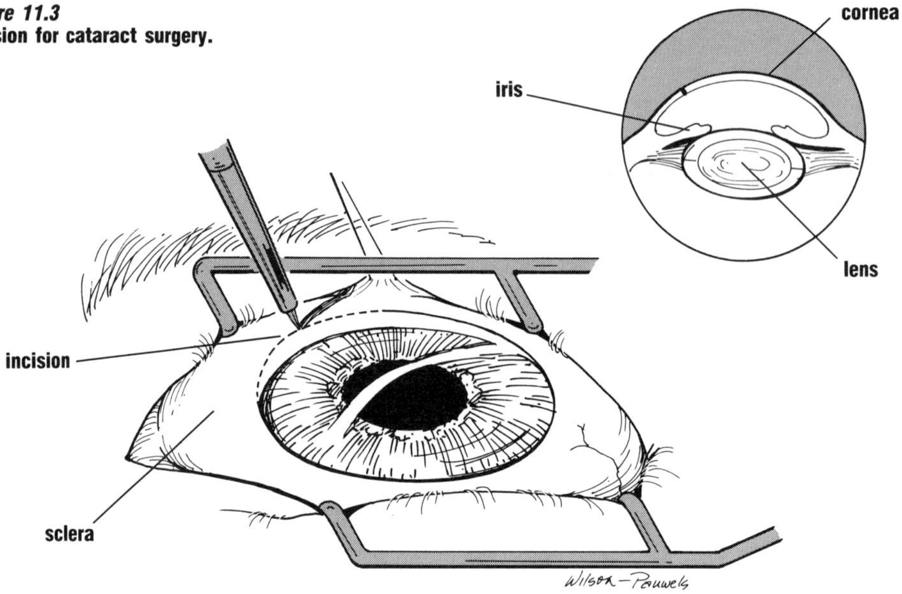

Figure 11.4
Capsulotomy.

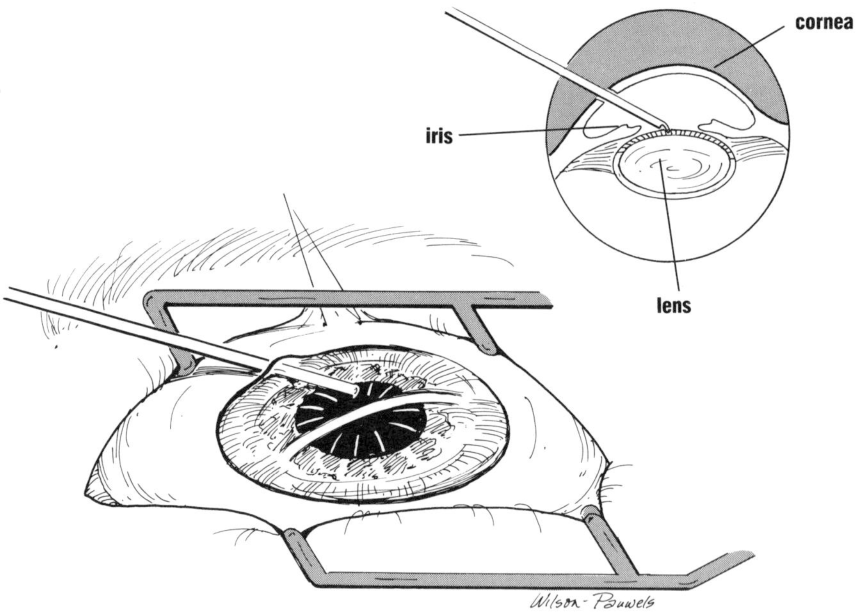

Complications

Complications — persistent inflammation, shifting of the implanted lens, retinal detachment, glaucoma or wound breakdown — occur in about 5 percent of cataract extractions. Major warning signs, which should be immediately reported to the surgeon, are a sudden change in the comfort of the eye or a sudden change in vision.

Recent Advances

Although laser surgery is used for other eye operations, it is not yet possible for

Figure 11.5
Nucleus of lens removed.

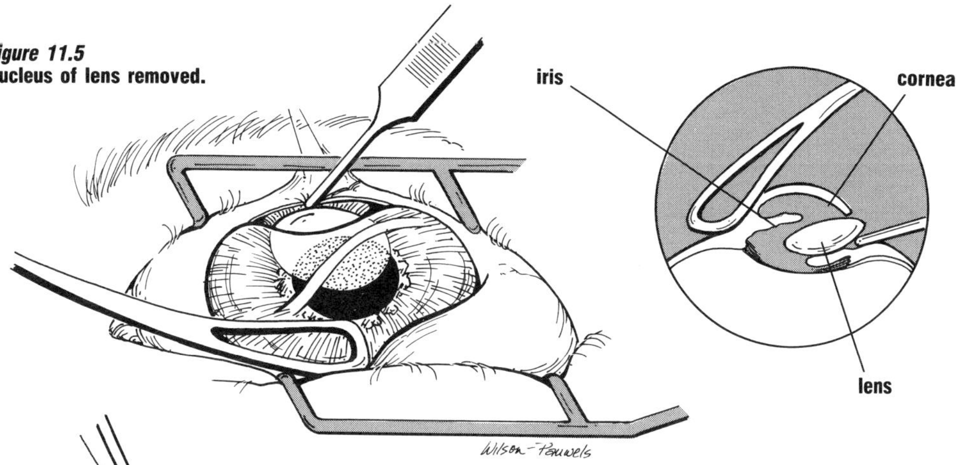

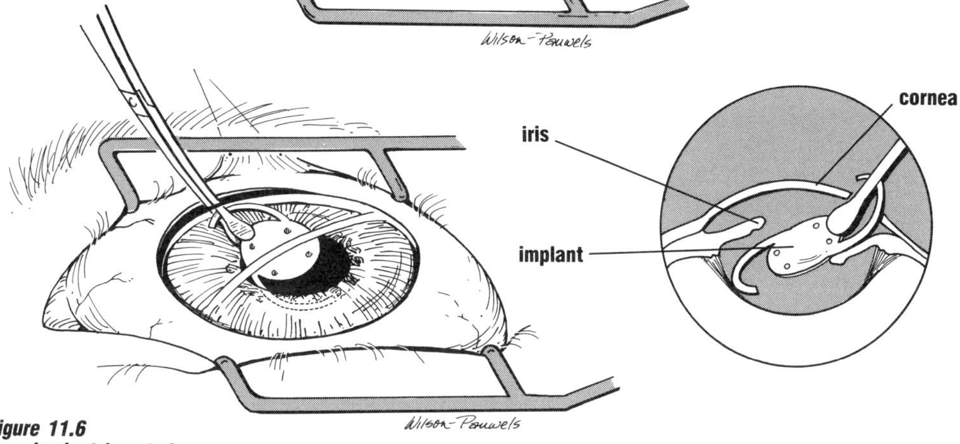

Figure 11.6
Lens implant inserted.

cataract surgery. Lasers have been used to make incisions into the lens and YAG (yttrium aluminum garnet) lasers are used to open a hole in the back of the lens capsule when necessary. Thickening of the lens capsule occurs within two years in approximately 30 percent of patients, and there is a return of hazy vision. The cataract has not returned; rather, the capsule has thickened. The surgeon should be told of any haziness of vision occurring within two or three years of the procedure. A laser opening of the posterior capsule is a painless 10-minute outpatient procedure, and usually restores vision rapidly. (See page 133)

Retinal Detachment

The retina lines the inside of the eye, and is like the bladder in a football (Fig. 11.2). As long as the retina is in its normal position, one has a full field of vision. Should the retina detach from its proper position against the wall of the eye, an area corresponding to that detached area will be missing from the field of vision.

The eye is filled with jelly (vitreous). In youth the jelly is relatively solid and packs the space between the lens and the retina. As part of the aging process, the jelly gradually liquifies and eventually collapses, so that solid vitreous comes to lie at the bottom of the eye, and fluid vitreous at the top. During this collapse, if the vitreous and the retina are attached, the retina may become torn. The fluid vitreous then passes through the retinal hole, separating the retina from the underlying wall of the eye.

Retinal detachment is more common in short-sighted people. It may also occur after an eye injury. It is slightly more common in patients who have had cataract operations, or those with inherited abnormalities of the retina. High-risk patients can often be identified; they should have regular eye examina-

Fred was pretty nervous as he entered the OR. The injection for the local anesthetic was painful, but as the surgeon gently massaged his eye so that the anesthetic would penetrate, he gradually lost sensation around the eye. Then they put a drape over his face. He wasn't aware of very much for the next 30 minutes except the surgeon's hands on his forehead. He even drifted off to sleep for a few minutes. Then they were patching his eye and sending him off to recovery.

As the anesthetic wore off, Fred felt a fair amount of pain, but a couple of mild painkillers relieved it. His ocular pressure was checked, and about three hours after the surgery he was on his way home with a written list of do's and don'ts for the next few weeks, plus some eye drops and some more pain medication. Gloria was very relieved to see him in reasonably good spirits. They had to return to the hospital the next day so that Dr. Blake could check the eye.

The next day all seemed well — the patch was taken off and Dr. Blake said Fred's ocular pressure was normal. His eye was a little uncomfortable. He could feel a slight scratching sensation when it moved, and it ached a bit, but he felt relieved by Dr. Blake's reassurance that all was well. "You'll find that you'll be tearing from that eye quite a bit for twelve to twenty-four hours, but keep using the drops and it should clear up."

After a week Fred's eye felt almost normal, even though he could still feel each movement. He wore dark glasses because glare still bothered him. His eyesight was about the same as it had been before the operation, but Dr. Blake assured him that it would now improve gradually but steadily over the next six to eight weeks, when he'd get his prescription for glasses.

Dr. Blake said he'd likely get a cataract in the other eye, but now that he'd been through the surgery, it didn't worry Fred nearly as much. After two months Fred's vision was 20/20 with glasses and he was able to work and drive.

Case Study: Retinal Detachment

Emily was busy packing clothes for the hospital rummage sale when she could swear she saw a vertical bolt of lightning in the room. But it was a windowless supply cupboard. Was anything wrong with the lights? Oh, well, she was probably tired. Emily took off her glasses and rubbed her eyes. Better call it a day.

Early that evening while writing a letter, Emily suddenly noticed a shower of fine black dots in front of her eyes. Instinctively she wiped the white paper, but the dots weren't there. She took off her glasses, convinced that she must have got ink on them, but the dots weren't there, either. Emily got scared. Sudden flashing lights, black spots in front of her eyes — what was happening? Although it was late on a Friday afternoon, she called her family doctor.

Over the phone Dr. Black seemed to know what was wrong. "Emily, I'm going to call your ophthalmologist right away. I'd like you to go straight to the hospital. Dr. Lee will meet you there."

Dr. Lee was already in the emergency room when Emily arrived. The ophthalmologist, who'd been prescribing Emily's glasses for years, put drops in her eyes and checked her vision. He spent a long time looking at the back of her eye, while asking a lot of questions. Did she get migraine headaches? Could she see the spots even when her eyes were closed? Did she see them with one or both eyes? Emily got the occasional headache from sewing too long late at night, but never migraines. The spots were visible with her eyes open or closed, but only with the left eye. "Emily, we'll have to send you into the city to see an ophthalmologist who specializes in retinal detachment. Your retina is torn, and we have to get it repaired immediately because it's becoming detached."

The weekend was a blur for Emily. Dr. Lee said the surgeon wouldn't be available before Monday, so they admitted her to the local hospital where she spent Saturday in bed. On Sunday they transferred her to the teaching hospital in the city.

tions so that retinal tearing may be anticipated and prevented with laser treatments.

The treatment of retinal detachment, first attempted in the 1930s, was an operation with a very low success rate until the early 1950s, when new methods and materials were introduced. Retinal detachment is relatively rare, affecting one in 2,000 patients who visit ophthalmologists. Nevertheless, when it does occur, it eventually results in total loss of vision if not treated.

Retinal tearing causes the sudden appearance of flashing lights, which are usually vertical or horizontal, colorless, and seen with the eye open or closed. The tear may also cause the sudden occurrence of many fine black floating spots. Patients are remarkably consistent in describing the episode. They liken it to "ink spots on my glasses" or "mud on the windshield." The sudden onset of these symptoms demands immediate attention. Patients should be seen by an ophthalmologist the same day if possible, because if the retinal tear is found before detachment occurs, treatment is greatly simplified — the holes can be sealed with a laser. The time lapse between the formation of a retinal hole and retinal detachment ranges from minutes to months. The most common time frame is probably one to four days.

Diagnosis

When retinal detachment begins, patients may complain that they think they are seeing their nose or that there is a black shadow beside their nose. Typically a curtain is first seen in the lower part of the vision on the side of the nose. The shadow then increases in size, until sight is completely lost.

The length of time between the first loss of vision and surgery is extremely important. Recovery is slower, and the chance of recovery less likely the longer the macula, or point of fine vision, is separated from its blood supply. Any patient who experiences sudden loss of vision or a black shadow in front of the eye should see an ophthalmologist as soon as possible, ideally within the first day. If an ophthalmologist is not available, the diagnosis will usually be made in a hospital emergency department. Approximately 90 percent of all retinal detachments can be repaired with one or more procedures.

At this point, the surgeon must identify all the areas of weakness and tears in the retina so that it can be reattached. Each tear must be repaired, because even one will be enough to allow the retina to re-detach.

The examination is usually done with the patient lying flat in a darkened room. The pupil of the eye is dilated widely so that the retina can be seen more easily. The surgeon then focuses a bright light into the eye. The examination itself is not painful, but it is tedious, often taking 30 minutes or longer. The surgeon may make a diagram of the retina while the examination is carried out.

Other tests may include ultrasound or careful examination of the retina using a special examining contact lens to determine all the possible causes of the retinal detachment. (A few rare retinal detachments are not related to tears in the retina, and these do not usually require surgery.)

Surgical Treatment

On admission to the hospital, the patient may be put to bed to determine whether the retina has a tendency to settle back into position. Under certain circumstances this may make the operation technically easier. For others, immediate surgery is needed. In most hospitals the surgery for retinal detachment is classified as urgent but not an emergency. Before the operation, drops are put into the eye to dilate the pupil so that the eye can be fully examined both before and during surgery. It is also usual to examine the other eye very carefully before the operation.

The operation is usually performed under general anesthetic. An incision is made around the cornea through the membrane covering the eye (conjunctiva). The muscles attached to the eye are exposed and sutured, so that the surgeon can move the eye during the procedure (Fig. 11.7). The surgeon then marks on the outside of the eye those points that correspond to the places where the retina is torn.

The tears in the retina can be closed in several ways. There are two main groups of procedures. The first are called "buckling" procedures (Fig. 11.8), in which a piece of silicone is placed on the outside of the eye. The wall of the eye is then pressed inwards until it meets the point where the retina is torn. Once the outer wall and the retina can be made to touch, the retina is stuck to the underlying structure by laser or a freezing technique (cryotherapy).

The second major group of operations are called "vitrectomy." In this approach the jelly in the eye is cut away, so that there is no longer any traction pulling the retina away from its normal position. The eye is then inflated with air or gas (Fig. 11.9). Once the eye is reinflated, the holes are sealed with laser or cryotherapy.

Some patients need both techniques, to remove the scar tissue from within the vitreous, and to press in the wall of the eye to meet the torn retina. When both procedures need to be performed consecutively, this is called a vitrectomy buckle. Generally, the operation proceeds until all the holes in the retina are closed and the retina is in its normal position. The surgery may take from one to five hours, depending on the complexity of the procedure and the amount of scar tissue to be removed. Once the retina is in position, the freezing or laser is carried out. Then the muscle sutures are removed and the conjunctiva is closed.

The eye is usually left patched until the

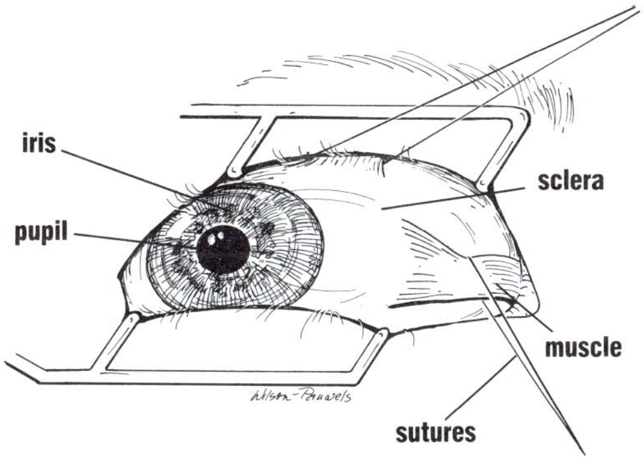

Figure 11.7
Exposing muscles for retinal detachment surgery.

By Monday morning Emily could see a dark shadow in the bottom corner of her vision, near her nose. The surgeon came to see her early, and explained that her retina had torn and was becoming detached, which accounted for the black shadow. He was confident they could repair it, putting to rest her worst fear — that she would be blind. "When we catch them early like this we can operate before the area of detachment becomes too big. That way we can restore vision to what it was before the retina became detached."

Emily couldn't understand what she had been doing that would cause her retina to tear. The surgeon explained that short-sighted people have longer eyeballs, so when the jelly inside the eye collapses as part of the aging process, it might pull part of the retina with it, causing it to tear.

The surgeon spent a long time examining her eye, making a sketch of the retina to show exactly where the holes were.

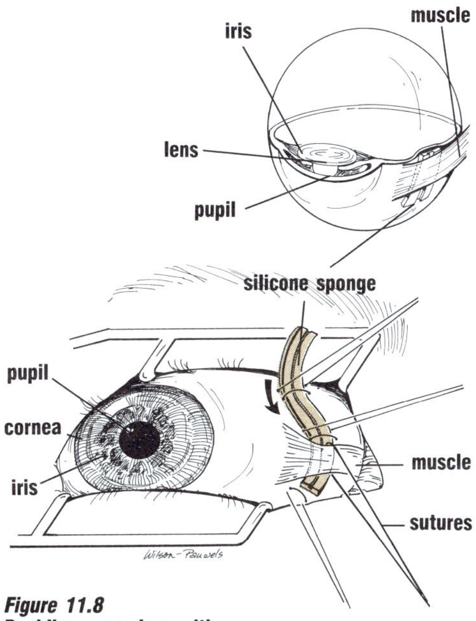

Figure 11.8
Buckling procedure with silicone sponge.

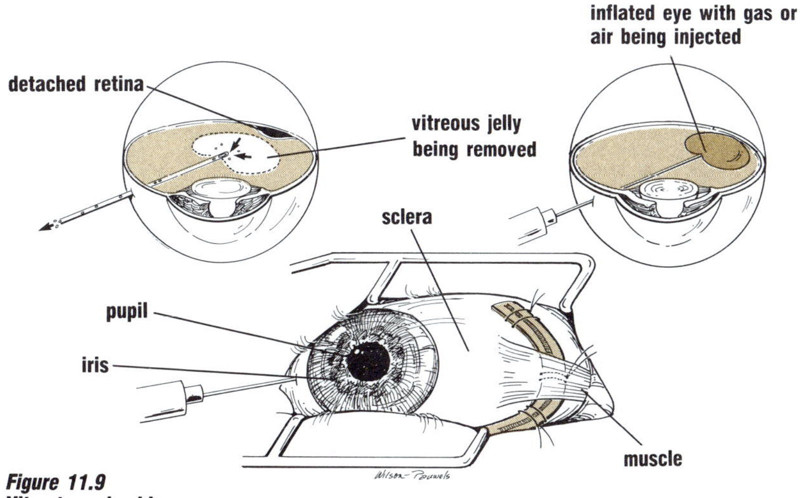

Figure 11.9
Vitrectomy buckle.

Later that day she was taken to the operating room where she was given a general anesthetic. She'd been offered a local, but she felt too nervous to be awake. Emily's daughter had been told that the operation could take up to three hours, so she was very relieved when her mother was wheeled into recovery after only 90 minutes. The surgeon told her that the operation had gone very smoothly. All being well, her mother would be on her way home after about 48 hours.

Emily was most aware of the pain in her eye after the operation. The painkillers helped, but what she really wanted to know was whether her sight had returned. Her eye was patched, so she had to wait until the next day, when the surgeon examined her again. "Everything's where it should be, Emily. The retina has been reattached in the places where it had torn, so your vision should return to normal by six months at the latest."

Emily was given three medications to lessen the secretions from the eye and prevent infection. The surgeon told her there was a 15 percent chance of the retina detaching again, but that the other retina could be prevented from detaching by a painless laser treatment.

She did a fair amount of traveling in the next six weeks; she had to return to the city to see the surgeon every two weeks. At six weeks she felt fine. The pain had gone, the shadow had gone, and the blurry vision she'd had after the surgery had gone. The surgeon told her to make an appointment with her own ophthalmologist at three months, but she'd return to the city to see him once a year for a checkup. Knowing that the risk of further detachment was highest in the first two years after surgery, Emily was only too glad to keep her appointments.

next day. Drops are given three or four times a day, for about three weeks. The drops usually contain atropine (which dilates the pupil and relaxes the muscles of the eye to reduce pain) and cortisone (which reduces the inflammation). In uncomplicated cases the patient can go home within 24 hours if the retina remains attached.

In more complex cases and those requiring vitrectomy, the patient must remain in hospital until it is clear that the retina remains attached. Most patients may get out of bed the next day, but those patients whose eyes have been reinflated with air at the end of the operation may have to lie face downwards to allow the air inside the eye to press on the appropriate part of the retina.

Retinal detachment surgery is not acutely painful, but there is always some discomfort and swelling, which is usually relieved by codeine for 48 to 72 hours. There will be regular follow-up visits to the surgeon to assess the state of the retina. Sutures usually do not need to be removed.

After retinal reattachments, visual recovery is relatively slow. Some side vision will return almost at once. Central vision may take up to six months to recover fully.

Retinal detachment is a worrying experience. Many patients are very anxious during this period. The trauma of sudden vision loss and the uncertainty about the future is stressful to both patient and family. Following successful surgery, activity is restricted for three to four weeks, and moderation should be observed in heavy lifting and physical exertion. After three weeks most patients can resume normal activities, provided there is good evidence of recovery.

Complications

The most common complication is re-detachment of the retina. After an initially satisfactory repair, the retina tears in a new place, or the vitreous jelly shrinks and causes a new tear. Signs and symptoms are the same as the initial detachment, and any sudden change in vision should be reported immediately. Other complications such as hemorrhage, infection or glaucoma may occur, requiring additional treatment.

Recent Advances

Retinal detachment surgery has undergone radical change in the last few years. Recent advances include the use of silicone oil to reattach the retina, metal tacks to pin the retina into position, and methods of deliberately making cuts in the retina to relieve traction and folding.

Laser Surgery

Lasers are used in eye surgery to pass a beam of light through the transparent parts of the eye such as the cornea and lens, so that it can have an effect on other parts of the eye, with little or no need for cutting or anesthetic. Lasers have made eye surgery easier, since most laser treatments can be done in out-patient departments. In most patients a single drop of local anesthetic is all that is needed. Recovery is rapid and the success rate high, but lasers have not yet replaced most conventional surgery.

At present, three different lasers are used routinely for eye surgery — the argon laser, the neodyminium YAG laser and the tunable dye laser.

Argon Laser

The argon laser produces a pure green or blue light, which is focused into the inside of the eye. To achieve the focus, a special examining contact lens is placed on the patient's eye during the treatment, so the laser effects can be seen by the surgeon as the treatment proceeds. The argon laser is used primarily to seal retinal holes and to treat the retinal bleeding that can occur as a complication of diabetes.

Diabetic Retinopathy

Diabetics are prone to a condition called retinopathy, or bleeding within the eye. This bleeding may ultimately cause loss of vision. It is believed to occur because part of the retina becomes deprived of oxygen, and then produces a substance which causes abnormal blood vessels to grow. These vessels tend to bleed.

In laser surgery, the abnormal areas of the retina are destroyed so there will be no tendency for further bleeding. The treatment is called pan retinal photocoagulation (PRP). Two or three sessions per eye are usually needed. Sedation is generally unnecessary, although a local anesthetic is used when the examining contact lens is placed on the patient's eye. The treatment takes 10 to 30 minutes. It is not usually painful, but it is tedious, and the bright light shining into the eye is uncomfortable.

After the treatment, the eye may be patched for several hours. The patient is usually seen a few days later to decide if enough treatment has been carried out. There is no immediate improvement in vision, and one of the long-term side effects of the treatment is to diminish night vision. Diabetic eyes are never cured, but many can be stabilized and vision can be maintained. If the condition is recognized early and treatment is begun, the prospect for maintaining normal vision is improved. There may be long periods when no treatment is required, but retinal examinations must be continued annually throughout the patient's life to check for further bleeding.

Complications of laser treatment are uncommon. Nevertheless, diabetics may be prone to hemorrhage, which can occur during treatment. About 5 percent of patients experience hemorrhage. Particularly after repeated treatments, the eye sometimes becomes sensitive and local anesthetic is needed to completely paralyze the eye before treatment. This occurs in about 10 percent of patients.

Glaucoma

The eye is like a ball, which has fluid running into it and out of it. Glaucoma occurs when the inflow and outflow are no longer balanced, and pressure gradually builds up within the eye (intraocular pressure). One type of glaucoma is characterized by extreme pain, blurred vision, reddening of the eye, and a dilated pupil. Nausea and vomiting may also occur. In other types of glaucoma the symptoms may vary but the long-range effect is to damage the optic nerve, leading to blindness if untreated.

The standard operation for glaucoma used to be drainage, in which a little hole was made in the wall of the eye to allow fluid to drain out more quickly, thus reducing the intraocular pressure. Recently, the argon laser has been used to drain fluid from the eye without surgically cutting a hole in the eye wall. This technique is called trabeculoplasty. It is not appropriate for every case, and certain types of glaucoma cannot be treated in this way.

For trabeculoplasty, a contact lens is placed on the eye. This contact lens has

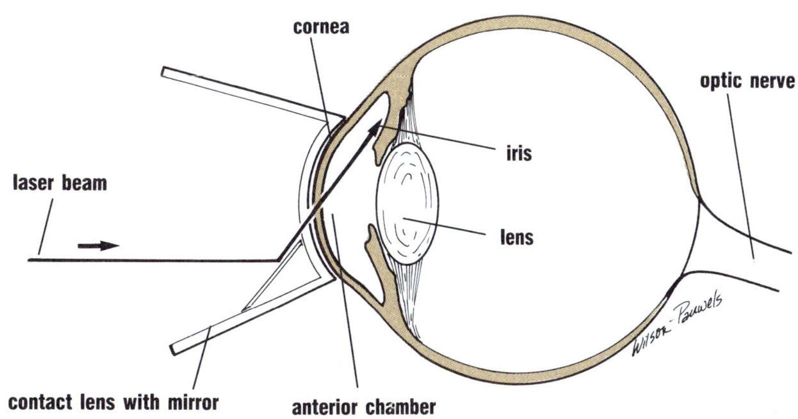

Figure 11.10
Trabeculoplasty. Laser treatment for glaucoma, cross section.

a special mirror which shows the angle of the anterior chamber (Fig. 11.10). Each treatment session consists of 20 to 50 laser shots, each one producing a minute burn within the eye, increasing the space available for fluid to move out of the eye. A few patients will have a small rise in pressure immediately following the treatment. If this occurs, medication is given to reduce the pressure. Regular follow-up determines whether the treatment needs to be repeated. Most patients require more than one treatment per eye to produce permanent control of intraocular pressure. The treatment is usually painless and no anesthetic is required apart from the single drop of anesthetic when the contact lens is inserted.

Complications of trabeculoplasty are rare. Less than 5 percent of patients suffer either hemorrhage or severe rise in pressure immediately after the treatment. Should this occur, admission to hospital may be necessary. Approximately half the patients with a severe rise in pressure may require a conventional drainage operation.

Retinal Holes

The argon laser can also be used to weld the retina to its underlying structure, the choroid (Fig. 11.2), before retinal detachment can take place. This is a relatively simple procedure, comparable to the technique used in diabetic retinopathy, but requiring fewer burns, which are applied only around the tear in the retina. This treatment usually takes no more than 10 minutes and is relatively risk free. The possible complication is failure to prevent retinal detachment or, very rarely, hemorrhage. The treatment is painless. It requires only a drop of local anesthetic for the examining contact lens.

Once the retina has detached, it is no longer possible to treat it with laser alone — the laser can only weld together structures that are still in contact with one another.

Neodyminium YAG Laser

The beam of the neodyminium YAG is infra-red and invisible. It is used in conjunction with a second laser that produces a visible red beam so that the position of the invisible laser can be identified. The YAG laser has two major uses: posterior capsulotomy following a cataract operation, and iridectomy for glaucoma.

As explained in the cataract section, a fine membrane (posterior capsule) is deliberately left in place in a cataract operation. In approximately 30 percent of patients, this membrane may become opaque within two years, causing gradual blurring of vision.

Patients do not have to be admitted to hospital for the YAG laser procedure. A single drop of local anesthetic is used and an examining contact lens is placed on the eye. The laser beam creates an opening in the fine membrane (capsulotomy) through a series of painless shots. Intraocular pressure should be checked within a couple of hours. Vision usually improves within a day.

Complications of this procedure are rare. About 20 percent of patients have a small rise in pressure following the treatment and may require drops to relieve the pressure for one or two days, when the condition usually clears. About 1 percent of patients have a significant rise in pressure that will require treatment for several days with drops and possibly oral drugs. The usual routine is to be checked within one week, when the vision should have returned to previous levels.

The YAG laser may also be used in iridectomies or glaucoma surgery, when a small hole is made in the iris. This procedure used to be done as a surgical operation. It can now be performed with the laser simply, quickly and almost painlessly. Again a drop of local anesthetic is used, an examining contact lens is placed on the eye, and laser shots are fired at the iris, producing a minute explosion that opens a hole in the iris (Fig. 11.11). Most patients hear the noise of the laser but do not feel pain. Complica-

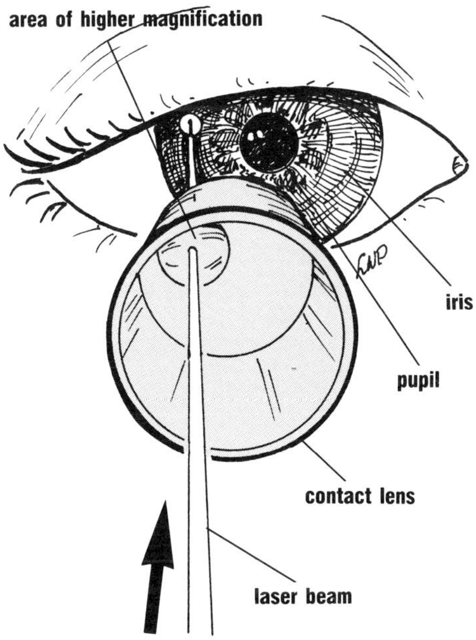

Figure 11.11
Iridectomy using YAG or argon laser.

tions are rare, but include the possibility of hemorrhage or rising intraocular pressure immediately following treatment. Most patients remain at the hospital for two to three hours to ensure that there has been no rise in pressure, and they use drops for a few days. Follow-up within a week is usual.

Tunable Dye Lasers

Different colors are absorbed in different regions of the eye, so one type of treatment may need a red laser, another a green one. The tunable dye laser allows the surgeon to choose the appropriate color for any given problem.

Tunable dye lasers are used to treat macular disease and, in experimental cases, some eye tumors. Macular degeneration is a condition found primarily in the aged. It is a degenerative process that gradually destroys fine central vision. It never leads to blindness, but will remove the ability to drive and to read. Recently, it has become possible to identify patients who have a high probability of developing macular degeneration. Some of these patients can then be treated with the tunable dye laser so that loss of vision is either postponed or prevented.

Recent Advances in Laser Surgery

The next trend in laser surgery may be the introduction of excimer lasers or other ultraviolet lasers to cut the surface of the cornea. Some experiments at the moment suggest that small cuts of the cornea may enable short-sighted patients to see at a distance without glasses. If good results continue, new lasers will be developed for this type of surgery.

Strabismus

Vision is a complex process. When a person looks at an object, rays of light travel from the object to the eyes. These rays are focused onto the rear inner lining of the eye, the retina. The image of the object is created, and the message is sent to the brain for interpretation.

When both eyes are straight and have equal vision, the brain perceives two clear images of the same object, one from each eye. It then creates one unified image of the object. This process is called fusion. Most people who have straight eyes can also see three dimensions. This process is called stereopsis or stereoscopic vision.

If the eyes do not point in the same direction, fusion is prevented. This condition is known as strabismus, or squint, and the misalignment may take the form of a crossed eye, an out-turned eye (''wall-eye'') or an upturned eye (Fig. 11.12).

In cases of strabismus, treatment is first geared to restoring normal vision to both eyes if possible, and then re-aligning them so that they point in the same direction.

Amblyopia (Greek for ''dim sight'') is

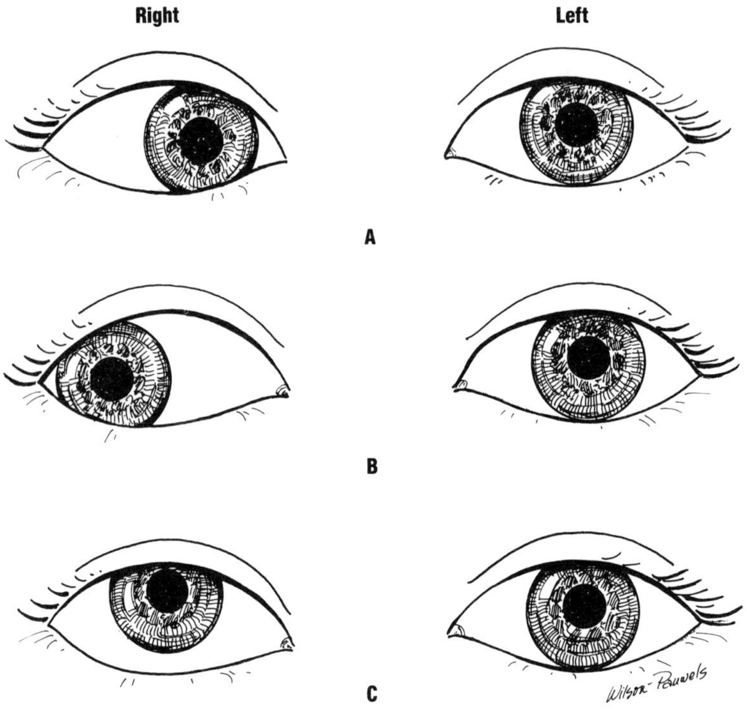

Figure 11.12
Forms of squint. The eye can be inturned, or crossed (A); turned outward, or wall-eyed (B); or upturned (C).

Case Study: Strabismus

Mary's mother had noticed that her five-year-old daughter had a tendency to be "looking at her nose." It seemed one eye was prone to wander — a "lazy eye" as she had heard the condition referred to. Fearing a permanent eye problem, she decided to set up an appointment with the family doctor. The doctor had delivered Susie, so she knew her history well. Both parents wore glasses, and they'd wondered if their children were destined for the same fate. "I think we should get her looked at by an ophthalmologist, Mary," said Dr. Wright.

a decrease in vision due to problems such as extreme far- or near-sightedness, astigmatism, cataracts, drooping eyelids (ptosis) and strabismus. The affected eye can become "lazy," that is, its vision can deteriorate compared to the normal eye. Amblyopia may occur with strabismus, but can also occur in straight eyes. Conversely, in many cases of strabismus, both eyes see equally well and no lazy eye develops.

Approximately 2 percent of the population has ambylopia ("lazy eye"). It is important to diagnose this as early in life as possible, ideally before the child reaches age six or seven. Treatment after this age is painstakingly long and rarely leads to significant recovery. Thus, vision screening tests are usually geared to children aged three to five to detect lazy eyes and strabismus at an age when treatment can still be effective.

Approximately 3 percent of the population have a misalignment of the eyes (strabismus). A further 10 percent have a tendency of one eye to wander under certain conditions, such as fatigue. In many cases the amount of misalignment is small and does not require treatment. However, severe strabismus requires some form of therapy, either surgical or non-surgical.

In adults, the causes of strabismus include neurologic diseases such as strokes, or head injuries that lead to weakness or tightness of eye muscles. Adults who develop strabismus frequently complain of double vision (seeing one object as two) because the eyes are pointing in different directions. They may complain that objects appear to have shifted. Some adults may need to turn or tilt their heads to eliminate double vision. Strabismus due to muscle paralysis can improve or totally resolve on its own. If it persists or only partially recovers treatment is usually required, because the patients have disabling double vision or an abnormal head posture.

Other adults have had their strabismus since childhood. Some have had early surgery or other therapies that have failed. These adults may have none of the above symptoms.

Children can be born with strabismus, but many develop it after several months of life. Strabismus in children may be hereditary or due to birth injuries or illnesses with fever. In addition, any child with strabismus must be thoroughly checked to be sure there is no eye disease present, such as a cataract, because a problem within the eye itself can also cause the eye to wander and become permanently misaligned.

In contrast to adults, young children with strabismus rarely complain of double vision. They are able to "turn off" recognition of the image received by the wandering eyes. This adaptation is known as suppression. It is usually only seen in children who develop strabismus before age five to seven.

Because children often do not complain of vision problems and can develop suppression, parents must look for signs of strabismus. A misalignment may be obvious simply by looking at the child's eyes. Sometimes an eye may wander only intermittently. Other signs include consistent turning or tilting of the head, a tendency to close one eye in bright sunlight, excessive blinking, or a tendency to hold objects very close to the eyes. Nevertheless, some children with strabismus may show no signs at all. For this reason, all children should have complete eye examinations by an ophthalmologist by age three.

Diagnosis

Strabismus should be evaluated by an ophthalmologist. The doctor takes a complete history, asking about the signs and symptoms discussed earlier. A complete eye examination begins with testing the vision in each eye using letter or number charts. The angle of misalignment between the two eyes is measured. Horizontal and vertical movements of the eyes are carefully checked to see if they track together. Finally, the doctor assesses the health of all the structures in the eyes and checks for far- or near-sightedness.

Children up to age three usually cannot cooperate for subjective vision tests, but the doctor can compare the eyes' ability to focus and concentrate on a target, and can detect any loss of vision. Eye diseases and abnormalities of alignment or eye movements can also be diagnosed.

It is normal for infants to have intermittent, random, wandering movements of the eyes during the first few weeks of life. These can include both crossing or out-turning of the eyes. After four months of age, however, constant or recurring misalignment is abnormal and requires medical attention.

Non-Surgical Treatment

The first concern in the treatment of strabismus and amblyopia is to try to restore normal vision to both eyes. If there is a structural problem, such as a cataract or a drooping eyelid, it must be dealt with first. In other cases glasses may be needed to correct focusing problems (far- or near-sightedness, or astigmatism) in one or both eyes.

If these treatments are not required or an eye remains amblyopic ("lazy") even with glasses, the eye with better sight is usually covered with a patch. This forces the lazy eye to "work harder." Patching may be required for only a few days or up to several months or years, depending on how rapidly the lazy eye recovers vision. Sometimes both patching and glasses are required. It has been found that patching the good eye and letting the child play video games is a good way to stimulate the lazy eye!

In some cases, glasses alone will also straighten the eyes. If the child is very far-sighted, for example, the eyes have to work so hard to focus that they may move inward and appear crossed. Glasses help the eyes to focus, and since the eyes no longer have to work to focus, they no longer cross.

Some cases of strabismus can be cured simply by improving the vision of the lazy eye. The eyes may then work together and straighten.

Finally, eye exercises can help patients who have difficulty viewing objects close to their eyes because they cannot turn inward enough. This inability can lead to double vision and headaches. Eye exercises are a form of vision training, known as orthoptics. They are administered by licenced orthoptists who are trained to examine all forms of strabismus under the supervision of an ophthalmologist.

If non-surgical treatment fails to straighten the eyes, surgery is required. However, surgery will not necessarily eliminate the need for glasses. Glasses, exercises or patching may still be needed after surgery.

Surgical Treatment

Each eye has six muscles (Fig. 11.1): four have straight "pulling" actions (left, right, up, down) and two have "twisting" actions. Traditional surgery for

It was a few weeks before they got an appointment with the ophthalmologist. In the meantime, Dr. Wright told Mary to watch for any crossing of Susie's eyes — how frequent, how long, and if it worsened when she was tired.

When they saw Dr. Steinberg, Mary had several pictures with her, and notes on when Susie's eyes appeared crossed. Dr. Steinberg asked a number of questions that worried Mary: had Susie ever hit her head, did she complain of headaches, had she ever had any bad fevers. The answer was no in each case. Seeing Mary's worried expression, Dr. Steinberg explained. "We want to be sure that there's no other problem that we should know about. It looks as though Susie's been pretty healthy, so it's unlikely that we'd find anything like a neurologic problem or internal eye disease. We'll probably find that her eye muscles aren't working the way they should be."

After quite a few tests, where Susie had to look through different colored glasses, read charts and have drops put in so that the doctor could look at the back of her eye, Dr. Steinberg said, "Susie's eyes are healthy, but she's far-sighted. Her vision in her right eye is 20/20, which is normal. In her left eye her vision is 20/50, indicating that the eye is lazy, so we've got to improve that. The first step will be to give her glasses to correct her vision. We want to get that left eye working as much as possible. If we correct her vision, her eye may straighten by itself. If it won't, we'll need to do surgery. In either case, she'll be wearing glasses for a few years at least." He made an appointment for them to return in two months.

At their next visit to Dr. Steinberg, Mary reported that her daughter seemed to be seeing better, but the eye still crossed occasionally, although not as often as before. Susie wasn't too thrilled with the glasses, but she'd worn them because she really could see better with them.

Dr. Steinberg said that Susie's left eye had not improved and was still 20/50. Both Mary and Susie were disappointed, but Dr. Steinberg said this often happened. "We'll try a patch on the right eye for a few weeks." That was even less fun than the glasses. Susie had to wear the patch all day, as well as her glasses. At the next visit the vision in her left eye had improved to 20/25 — but the eye still crossed. "I think we're looking at surgery, was Dr. Steinberg's assessment.

Mary was surprised to find that she could take Susie to the hospital two hours before the surgery, and that she would be able to leave the hospital the same day. Dr. Steinberg was careful to explain that the operation was to straighten her eye — she'd still have to wear glasses. He saw her one more time before the operation, to measure the angle her eyes crossed at, he said, and then the next time they saw him was in the hospital.

strabismus involves strengthening some of these muscles and weakening others, to straighten an eye. A general anesthetic is often required, and surgery can last from 30 minutes to three hours.

Strabismus surgery can be compared to straightening a horse's head with reins. For example, if the horse's head is turned to the left and is to be directed to straight ahead, the rider must loosen the "outer" (left) rein while tightening the "inner" (right) one.

In a similar fashion, eye muscles on opposite sides of an eye can be relaxed or tightened if the eye is not directed straight ahead. If, for example, the right eye is straight while the left eye is crossed, the inner muscle of the left eye can be weakened and the outer muscle strengthened (Fig. 11.13), so that both eyes point in the same direction.

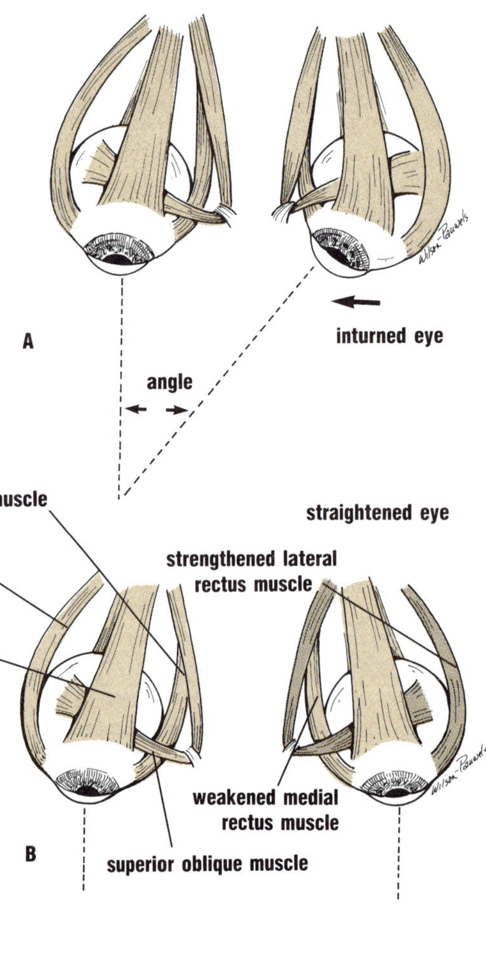

Figure 11.13
Straightening a crossed eye. The inturned left eye (A) is straightened by weakening the inner medial rectus muscle and strengthening the outer lateral rectus muscle, so that both eyes point in the same direction (B).

As a second option, in some cases an operation on the right eye would weaken its inner muscle and strengthen its outer muscle. A third alternative would be to weaken both inner muscles slightly to make the eyes point in the same direction. Any of these three options would allow the two eyes to track together.

Strabismus surgery usually requires a general anesthetic, although it can be done under local anesthetic in some adult patients. Whether a general or local anesthetic is used, the patient usually need not remain in the hospital overnight. If adjustable sutures are inserted (see page 138), the surgery can be completed in the morning and the adjustment done in the late afternoon so that the patient can return home in the evening. However, if the surgery is done in the afternoon, the adjustment is usually carried out the next morning and the patient goes home immediately afterward.

No special medications are given before strabismus surgery. Routine blood tests, a chest X-ray and electrocardiogram a few days before the surgery ensure that the patient is healthy enough to receive the anesthetic. A physical examination is done either by the admitting physician when the patient comes to hospital or by the family doctor in the week preceding surgery.

The general anesthetic commences with an intravenous injection. Once the patient is asleep, a tube is placed into the windpipe so that breathing and anesthesia can be completely and safely controlled.

The surgeon then cuts the two paper-thin tissues that cover the white of the eye (sclera). They are pushed out of the way to enable the surgeon to see the muscles clearly.

The most common weakening procedure involves detaching the muscle from the eye and reattaching it with stitches at a point behind the original point. This procedure reduces the force with which the muscle can rotate the eyeball (Fig. 11.14).

The most common strengthening procedure is to shorten a muscle by cutting out a small section and reattaching the muscle in the same place. The shortened muscle is stiffer and can pull the eye over more effectively (Fig. 11.15).

In traditional strabismus surgery, after the muscles are reattached, the two covering layers of tissue are replaced over the stitches. An ointment containing antibiotic (to prevent infection) and cortisone (to prevent inflammation) is then usually poured onto the eye. Frequently the eye is patched to protect it while the patient recovers from the anesthetic.

After surgery, the patient is observed in a recovery room for about an hour to be sure no problems develop while the anesthetic is wearing off. The patient can usually return home after reaching full alertness and being able to drink.

Patients usually recover quickly after the anesthetic, and can be encouraged to walk around soon after the surgery. The eye may feel uncomfortable due to muscle and tissue swelling and from the stitches on the surface of the eye. Pain can usually be controlled by mild painkillers. If stronger ones are needed, the patient can usually stop taking them within hours or days. Ice water compresses are helpful during the first few hours after surgery to reduce swelling and discomfort.

Patients should not work in dirty or dusty environments for at least a couple of weeks, to reduce the risk of infection. Baths are preferred to showers to reduce irritation from flowing water and shampoo. Otherwise, patients are encouraged to return to their usual lifestyle. Lifting weights and bending over are permitted, although some patients complain of pressure pain around the eye with these activities for a few days after surgery. Patients should not go swimming until the redness and discomfort have disappeared.

The eye can remain red for up to four weeks. Eye medications, either drops or ointment, are often prescribed for a few weeks. These medications generally contain an antibiotic to prevent infection, and cortisone to reduce inflammation. They are used two or three times a day.

The stitches dissolve by the fifth week. The eyelid swelling usually subsides within a few days. Intermittent tearing and sensitivity to wind and cold air can last for several days. Once the eye has healed there are usually no scars visible to the naked eye.

Follow-up appointments are generally scheduled one week, four weeks and three months after the operation. At the first visit, the vision is checked and the eye is examined for signs of infection and inflammation. At the second and third visits the alignment is checked and the eye movements are assessed. By the

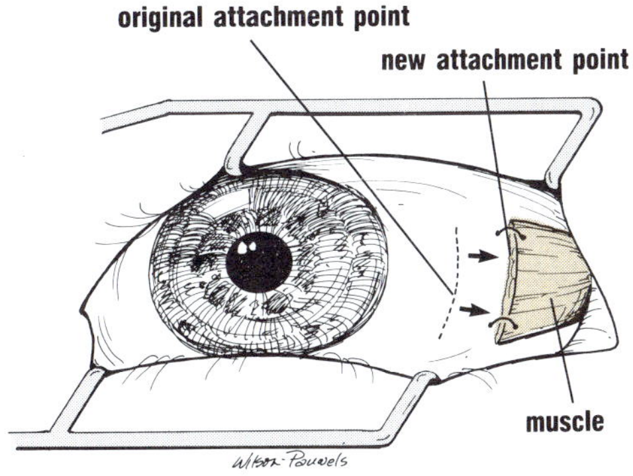

Figure 11.14
Weakening an eye muscle.

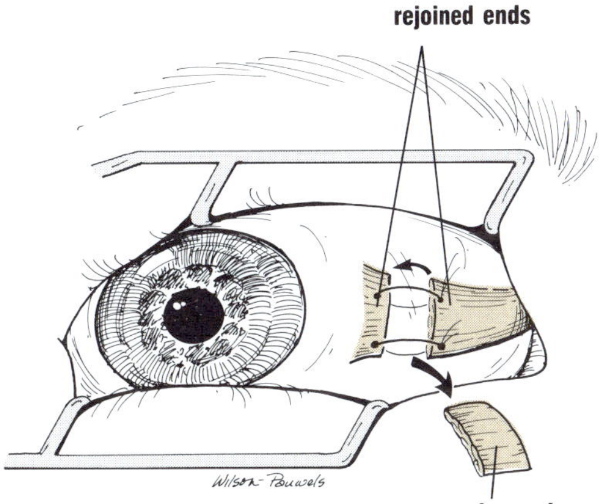

Figure 11.15
Strengthening (shortening) an eye muscle.

Mary and her husband brought Susie to the hospital in the morning. There were blood tests and more examinations, and then Susie was taken to the operating room. The nurses told Mary and Paul that the surgery could take anywhere from one to two hours. Dr. Steinberg had explained that they would adjust the two horizontal muscles in Susie's left eye so that they wouldn't pull the eye inward as much.

When Susie came back to her room after the operation she was very drowsy. Although it was about 24 hours before Susie could open her eye, Mary and Paul were relieved to see that the eye was only a little swollen, although it was quite red and sensitive. Dr. Steinberg had made her put her glasses back on while she was still in the hospital, and she wore a patch on her left eye for a couple of hours, but that was all.

When they went back to see him after a week, he was very encouraging. "The eye's healing nicely. No sign of infection, which is what we check for at this point. Her vision isn't bad with that eye, and so far it seems straight, so we'll see her again in six weeks."

It was about five weeks before the redness cleared from Susie's eye. Dr. Steinberg had warned her mother that she should be careful to avoid injury to the eye, or anything that might irritate or set up an infection. Dr. Steinberg was very pleased with her progress at six weeks. "All healed, — and she's using both eyes together. She'll have to continue with the glasses, which we'll check every three to four months, but there's a good chance that her eye may begin to recover enough that she can do without them in a few years."

Mary was very relieved. The ophthalmologist had told her that some children needed more than one operation, and many needed to wear glasses for life. It seemed that by catching Susie's problem promptly, they had given her eye a chance to develop more normally. "Can we prevent this happening in Michael, Doctor?" she asked. "How old is he — three? A good age to get him checked out by an ophthalmologist. Then if there's a problem, glasses and exercises may be able to correct it before it deteriorates."

third appointment the surgeon can gauge the overall success of the operation.

Strabismus surgery has a high success rate. Patients can return to their normal routine even while the eye tissues are healing. They can watch television, do housework, drive and keep social engagements. They may return to work as soon as the day after surgery, unless they work in a dirty or dusty environment.

Complications

Traditional strabismus surgery has a success rate of about 75 percent, so approximately 25 percent of patients may require a second operation. Adjustable sutures have increased the chances of successfully aligning the eyes at the first operation to 90 percent.

Complications of strabismus surgery include inflammation and infection, which can usually be controlled with eye drops or ointments. Signs of inflammation include increasing soreness and redness, extreme sensitivity to light, and a decrease in vision. An infected eye will discharge pus, the eyelids will be red and swollen, and vision is often decreased.

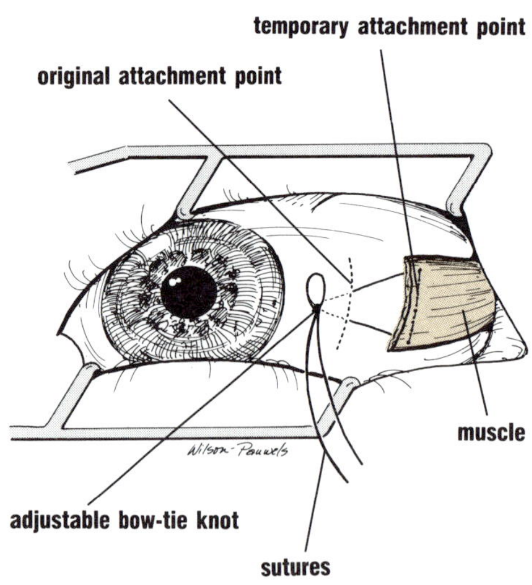

Figure 11.16
Adjustable suture.

Recent Advances

The idea for adjustable sutures was first suggested in 1903. The technique came into widespread use, however, only in the 1970s. When the muscles are reattached at the time of surgery, the stitches are not cut short, but are loosely tied in a bow. The stitches can then be tightened or loosened to move the muscle if necessary at the adjustment (Fig. 11.16), either later that day or the next morning. This allows "fine-tuning" of the eye alignment if the eyes are not yet straight after the surgery.

Adjustable sutures can be used on almost any patient old enough to cooperate (over age eight or nine). The adjustment is done under local anesthetic (eye drops). The patient has to lie still in a reclining chair or on a bed to allow the surgeon and the assistant to adjust the position of the eye muscle. Patients generally do not complain of pain during the adjustment, but they may feel a "pulling" or "pressure" sensation when the muscle is moved or when the surface tissues over the muscle are lifted away. The patient must be alert enough to allow reliable measurement of the eye position before and after any adjustment. The surgeon can then gauge how much the muscle has to be moved from the position it was placed in at surgery.

In 1978, an alternative to strabismus surgery was introduced. The eye muscle is injected with a small quantity of purified botulinum toxin, which weakens the muscle for a few weeks and allows the opposing muscle to strengthen. This method is especially useful for patients with paralyzed eye muscles, or for patients who cannot tolerate the anesthetic required for surgery.

The procedure takes 10 to 15 minutes, and the patient can return to full activity immediately after treatment. In contrast to strabismus surgery, there is no eye redness and the risk of infection or inflammation of the surface tissues is virtually nonexistent. If the initial injection does not straighten the eye, a second injection can be given, or surgery can still be performed on the eye, with the same chance of success had no injection been given.

Chapter 12

Cosmetic Surgery

Walter J. Peters

Associate Professor of Plastic Surgery
University of Toronto

Plastic Surgeon
Wellesley Hospital, Toronto

Valda Glennie
Illustrator

Plastic surgery probably began in India in 700 to 600 B.C., when crude operations for reconstruction of the nose were developed. At that time, nose amputation was a common punishment for certain crimes.

The word "plastic" is derived from the Greek *plasticas*, which means to sculpt or mold. Plastic surgery is concerned primarily with construction or reconstruction, and has nothing to do with plastic materials.

Today, plastic surgeons do both reconstructive and cosmetic surgery. Reconstructive surgery involves repairing damage caused by injury, disease or burns. Cosmetic surgery is done at the patient's request, to change appearance. The two forms of surgery frequently overlap.

During World War I, trench warfare and gunshot wounds resulted in devastating facial injuries. Special treatment centers were organized in Britain, France and the United States. With peace and prosperity came a new branch of plastic surgery — cosmetic surgery. Historically, surgery was performed to treat organic disease; now it was being used to improve the quality of life. Cosmetic surgery was initially regarded as frivolous. Surgeons who performed cosmetic operations were often relegated to the back room, and their surgery was shrouded in secrecy.

World War II changed the scope of plastic surgery again. Gasoline fires (uncommon in World War I) resulted in a phenomenal number of burns. Special centers were again organized, and plastic surgeons made many advances in reconstructive surgery. After the war, cosmetic surgery began to make steady advances. In 1949, about 15,000 cosmetic surgery operations had been performed in North America; today, almost one million cosmetic operations are performed annually.

Scars

Many people think that going to a plastic surgeon means having an operation that will not leave a scar. Unfortunately, this is not true. Whenever the skin is cut, a scar is inevitable, and it can never be totally erased. The plastic surgeon attempts to place these scar lines in natural skin lines or folds if possible, so that they are less noticeable. Despite this care, scars can heal in an unpredictable fashion. People vary greatly in their rate of healing and their reaction to surgery. Some patients heal with very fine scars. In others scars are heavier, and often little can be done to alter them.

When the stitches are removed, most scars are barely noticeable. Over the next four to eight weeks, they usually become redder and wider. As the wound matures, the scar settles and becomes less prominent, but this process can take a full two years. In a minority of patients, scars can remain very noticeable even after two years. Some become red, wide and have a raised surface — they are said to be hypertrophic. Some grow keloids —extensions outside the incision line, which produce further elevation and distortion. The cause of these types of scars is unknown, although they rarely result from surgical or suture technique. Certain patients simply have a tendency to form these scar types.

Scars that the patient finds unacceptable are generally left for one year to allow the scar to mature, before deciding on revision. (Earlier attempts usually result in a recurrence of the original problem.) Many scars become acceptable during the maturation period and will not require revision. Several different techniques of revision are available, but more than one may be needed to revise a scar. Some scars simply cannot be significantly improved, and will revert to their original appearance even after an attempt at revision surgery.

The Aging Face

Skin is the body's protective envelope. It is nearly waterproof, providing a barrier to infection and to the environment. It regulates temperature, allowing heat loss on hot days and providing insulation on cold days.

The thickness of human skin ranges between approximately one-sixteenth of an inch on the upper eyelid area to about one-quarter of an inch on the back area, and has two layers. The outer layer is called the epidermis; the inner layer, the dermis. The epidermis provides a thin but strong outer film, which is about 10 percent of the skin's thickness. The dermis provides the other 90 percent. Its chief constituent and the basis of its structural framework is collagen, spring-like coils that limit stretching. Elastic fibers, which provide tightness, make up about 5 percent of the dermis.

With advancing years, several changes occur in the skin. The collagen becomes looser, weaker and thinner, decreasing skin support. The elastic fibers lose their tension, and the prolonged effects of gravity stretch the skin. Gland secretion is decreased and the skin becomes drier. These processes are hastened by sun exposure. Excessive exposure to sunshine rapidly accelerates the aging process, and these changes may be irreversible. Because the face is usually exposed more than other parts of the body, it is all too often a target for the sun's relentless damage.

In an attempt to prevent the destructive effects of excessive sun exposure, sunscreens and sunblocks have been developed. Sunscreens are designed to screen out the burning rays of the sun, but allow the tanning rays through. Sunblocks decrease both burning and tanning. However, the net effect for both is that they simply lengthen the time required for the sun to cause a burn. The only way to prevent burning is to get out of the sun before that time is reached.

The more effective sunscreening products are those that contain para-aminobenzoic acid (PABA). These preparations are graded according to the degree of protection they offer, using a sunscreen index. The most effective sunblocking compounds are those containing both PABA and titanium dioxide.

Aging generally comes in the mid-thirties, with the sudden appearance of wrinkles around the lower eyelids. Simultaneously, "crow's feet" often appear at the outer corner of the eye. During the early forties, lines from the side of the nose to the mouth (nasolabial folds) deepen, and neck wrinkles begin to appear. With the passage of time, wrinkles and lines deepen and the skin becomes more stretched.

Creams make skin feel better by moisturizing the outer surface. However, no creams, medications, enzymes, collagen substances or other preparations significantly retard the aging process. Similarly, facial exercises, massage, chin supports, ultrasound and other forms of treatment have little permanent effect on the aging process.

Aging, exercise and diet are popular topics today. An individual requesting facial rejuvenation surgery may want to improve his or her self-image and look younger, in response to these concerns. Sometimes the incentive is to remain active and credible in the business world, or to improve one's appearance in public. Most individuals seeking this surgery, however, simply want to change the reflection they see in the mirror.

Many of the aging features in the face can be improved by surgery. The type of operation depends on the way one's face has aged, and the features that are of concern. A suitable candidate for facial cosmetic surgery would have some loose facial skin or puffiness around the eyelids, and would be in good general health, to minimize risk. A patient's suitability for surgery also depends on his or her degree of concern and the expected improvement from the operation. A minor physical irregularity may be of no consequence to one person, but of major significance to another. Plastic surgeons usually question prospective patients closely about why they want the operation. They would advise someone who has recently experienced divorce or widowhood, for example, to wait a year before deciding on surgery. Similarly, if someone's stated wish is to "look twenty years younger," the surgeon may advise postponing surgery until expectations can become a little more practical.

After surgery, the aging process continues. You may turn back the clock with facial surgery, but you don't stop it. The rate of aging differs from person to person — one person may want a facelift redone in eight years, another in five, and many people have a facelift only once. Some patients age more rapidly. Patients with deep lines from sun damage will have poorer results from facelift surgery. Eyelid surgery generally lasts considerably longer than facelift surgery.

Some patients are afraid that their faces will suddenly "drop" again. Although recurrence is highly individualized, it tends to parallel the general aging process. There is no sudden drop.

Facelift

A facelift reduces the looseness of the skin in the lower half of the face and neck. Not everyone is a good candidate for a facelift. The ideal patient is aged 50 to 65, has loose skin in the lower half of the face and neck, is not overweight and is in good general health, with normal blood

Case Study: Facelift

On her fifty-fifth birthday, Mary's husband offered to take her to a very fancy restaurant for dinner. Mary had always enjoyed their active social life, but now she discovered that she didn't want to go out. The reason? Mary was dismayed at how old she was beginning to look. She wasn't overweight, she exercised and watched her diet, but her face was looking jowly, and she had taken to wearing high collars to hide what she called her "turkey neck."

Mary confided in her friend Sarah, whose appearance she had always admired. Sarah revealed that she had had a facelift two years earlier. Mary was astonished — she associated facelifts with taut, drawn skin, not Sarah's natural-looking youthfulness. Sarah described the process and showed Mary the fine scar line around her ear, which Mary had never noticed before.

Mary's husband thought surgery was pretty drastic, especially since his wife was as attractive to him as the day he married her, but he said if it really meant a lot to her, maybe she should find out more about facelifts.

Mary went to Sarah's plastic surgeon. He showed her before and after pictures of other patients, gave her a mirror and asked her to show him exactly what bothered her. Her skin was good except for the looseness, which she pulled tight, saying, "I'd like to get rid of this." The surgeon asked about her general health, especially any heart or bleeding problems, and about her overall circumstances and expectations from surgery. She told him that she enjoyed life in general, that she was pleased with her activities and her involvement in her husband's busy life — all of which made her appearance important to her.

The surgeon agreed that Mary was a good candidate for facial surgery, but cautioned her about expecting too much. Placing his fingers lightly on her cheeks, he lifted her facial tissue gently, telling her to look in the mirror — that's the result she would see after surgery.

It was less dramatic than Mary had hoped for, but she remembered Sarah's natural appearance and decided that was the look for her. After Dr. Webb had ordered some routine lab tests and a chest X-ray, they booked a date for surgery.

The day before surgery, Mary shampooed her hair three times, as Dr. Webb had instructed. On the day of surgery, her sister took her to the hospital, where she was given a gown and started on an IV. Dr. Webb arrived after Mary had been given a light sedative, and he carefully marked the incision lines. Then, beginning on the right side, he gave her heavier sedation, freezing, and made the incision. When that side was finished, he repeated the process on the left.

The whole procedure took 3-1/2 hours. Dr. Webb then applied a padded head dressing. Mary felt a little uncomfortable, but nothing unbearable. Her sister said she looked like a football quarterback who'd been in a fight — the dressing was like a football helmet and her eyes were blackened.

Mary spent about eight hours in the hospital. The nurse elevated the head of her bed to lessen the swelling and bruising, and told her not to talk too much and to eat a soft diet for a couple of days. Mary then went home with a prescription for a mild painkiller, which she needed only for the first 48 hours.

Mary was somewhat dismayed at her appearance the next day when Dr. Webb removed the dressing, but he was pleased with the results. On a scale of one to ten, he said her bruising was about a three, and that it should be gone in about two weeks. Mary was to use ice packs at home for the rest of the day. The stitches would come out at intervals over the next 12 days. Dr. Webb warned that for a few months she'd experience numbness on her cheeks when she applied makeup. Her skin felt tight; this worried Mary a little, but the surgeon assured her that when the swelling went down she would be just fine.

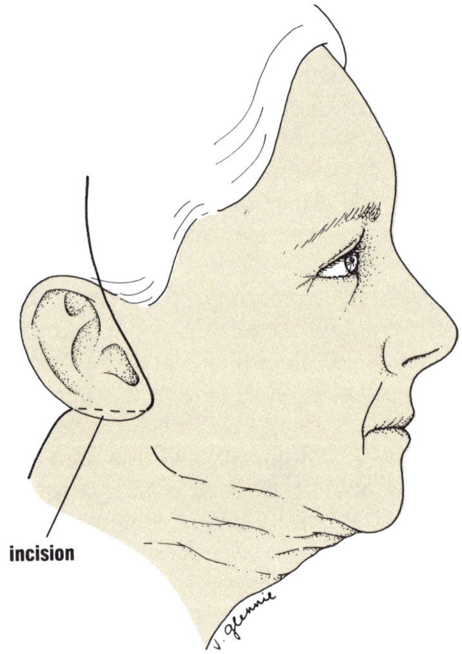

Figure 12.1
Skin incision for facelift.

pressure. The skin should not have excessive sun damage and facial lines should not be deep. Patients who do not satisfy these requirements will generally have limitations from facelift surgery. Similarly, a facelift is not done to prevent aging: the aging process continues before and after surgery.

Patients inquiring about facelifts often indicate their expected improvement by pulling the facial skin taut, but this does not necessarily give an accurate picture of the results. While the neck and jawline may obtain this result, the line from nose to mouth (nasolabial fold) will often not improve to this degree.

A facelift is generally done as an outpatient procedure, using local anesthetic, but with heavy sedation. The surgery lasts three to four hours. The incision lines are marked out, extending from the temple, down in front of the ear, around the base of the ear, across its back surface and down the hairline behind the ear (Fig. 12.1). In some patients a ''forehead lift'' can be done by extending the incisions in the temple upwards and across the scalp behind the hairline.

Local anesthetic is then injected and the incisions are made. The skin is gently separated from the underlying tissues. The facial skin is then moved upwards and back. Excess skin is cut away and the incisions are carefully closed.

Some surgeons are now also tightening the underlying soft tissue of the face and neck in the hope of making the facelift last longer. However, the actual long-term effects of this modification will not be known for several years.

The complications of facelift surgery can include bleeding, which may require drainage. There is usually only minimal discomfort. Temporary cheek numbness lasts about two or three months. Patients may feel mildly depressed for a few days after the operation when the mirror reflects a swollen, bruised, unnatural appearance. The depression usually lifts when the bruising and swelling settle. Damage to the facial nerve is possible, but quite rare.

After a facelift, a patient should not have a tight, stretched appearance. He or she should still retain a ''natural'' but ''well-rested'' look.

''Eyelid Lift'' (Blepharoplasty)

A person's individuality is mirrored in his or her eyes. When medical journals want to render patients unrecognizable in photographs, they put a black bar across the eyes. Drooping upper eyelids and bags below the eyes can give the entire face a constantly tired expression — even in someone with no other signs of aging. Baggy eyelids can occur at any age and for many different reasons. In younger patients, their development tends to be inherited. With increasing age, degenerative changes from normal aging are the most common cause. Much rarer causes are diseases such as allergies, thyroid problems or kidney disease.

The surgery to correct baggy eyelids is called blepharoplasty. The operation was originally done only when vision was significantly impaired, by simply removing extra skin. Today, most of these operations are done for purely aesthetic reasons. It is usually performed to reduce extra skin and puffy, fatty tissue. Each of the three layers — skin, muscle and fat — are corrected.

The operation must be tailored to meet each patient's specific needs. Some patients complain of lines and wrinkles around the eyes when they squint. This occurs in many people over 30, and blepharoplasty will not remove these lines.

Blepharoplasty is usually performed under local anesthetic, but with heavy sedation. The operation takes about two hours, and the patient will likely leave the hospital the same day. Blepharoplasty is frequently done in combination with facelift surgery.

Incision lines are placed so that the final scar will be camouflaged in the normal lid fold of the upper eyelid, and in the natural skin crease below the lash line of the lower lid (Fig. 12.2). Often extra muscle has accumulated; this is carefully removed, along with extra fatty tissue. Excess skin is then cut away. If there is no normal eyelid fold, one can be constructed.

Most patients return home on the day of surgery wearing sunglasses to camouflage the eyelid area. The eyes are not covered with a dressing. Ice packs are applied gently over saline gauze for 15 minutes each hour, until late in the evening, to decrease swelling and bruising. It is helpful to keep the head elevated by sleeping on two pillows for a few days. The minimal amount of pain is usually controlled by mild painkillers, and eyedrops are frequently prescribed for a few days to decrease irritation.

The eyes can be gently patted with a cool wet cloth one day after surgery. A moisturizing ointment containing antibiotic can be applied to the suture line twice daily until after the sutures are removed.

Swelling and bruising are at their worst two to three days after surgery, when they begin to settle. The amount of bruising is difficult to predict, because patients vary so widely in their reactions. Most bruising disappears in 10 to 14 days. With the swelling, the eyes may temporarily tear excessively and be more sensitive to light. The white of the eye may redden. Sutures are usually removed four to six days after surgery.

Makeup can be applied the following week, but contact lenses should be avoided for about 10 days after surgery, unless they can be inserted and removed without traction to the eyelids. When makeup is being applied, numbness may be noticeable for six to eight weeks. The incision lines tend to become more prominent two or three weeks after surgery, but then they begin to fade. They usually blend in well with natural skin lines after two to three months.

A

B

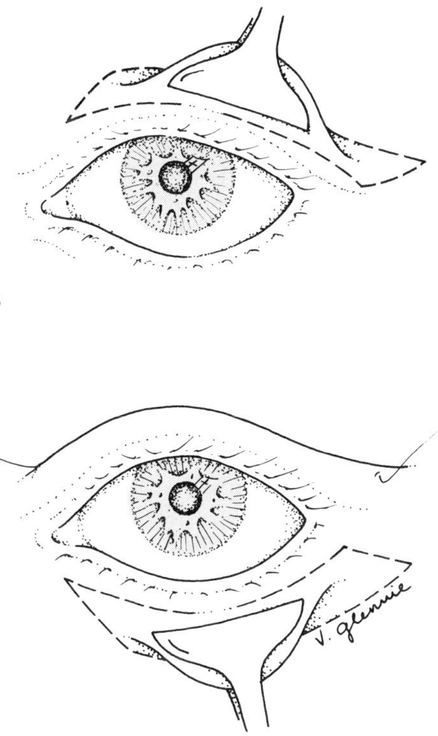

Figure 12.2
Blepharoplasty eyelid surgery. Excess skin, muscle and fat are removed from the upper (A) and lower (B) eyelids.

Case Study: "Lifting" Eyelids

At 54, Marcel had made his mark in the fast-paced world of computer sales. While he was confident in his abilities, the recent remarks about his appearance had been grating on him, especially after the company president put him to work on an important project with a young, aggressive employee. The younger man was always expressing his concern for Marcel's health, telling him to "take it easy — perhaps you'd like me to do that presentation to the client on Monday, give you a chance for a long weekend?" Marcel wasn't about to compromise his professional attitude by such a comment.

Marcel went and slammed a few tennis balls around with some friends, one of whom, a woman, had had eyelid surgery. He had known her for years, and was startled to realize that she was his age. He asked her about the surgery. It seemed so simple that in his usual "let's get it done" fashion, he called the plastic surgeon the next day. The surgeon said, upon seeing Marcel, that he was a good candidate for surgery. Marcel didn't want much — just to stop looking "tired." The rest of his skin was good and his jawline was firm, so the eyelids were the only real concern. He had no health problems. Marcel was somewhat taken aback that he would have to take two weeks off work, but once he had seen before and after pictures of people like himself, he was convinced it would be worth it. So he had the usual lab tests and X-rays, and the date was set for surgery.

The surgery seemed to go quickly, and Marcel felt little discomfort afterwards except that his eyelids felt tight. Marcel knew that the bruising would move down to his cheek with gravity, so he wasn't surprised to see blue, green and finally yellow blotches appearing there over the next two weeks.
The hardest thing for Marcel was to be off work for two weeks and not be allowed to exercise. He knew, too, that he had to avoid harsh sunshine for two months.

When Marcel saw the surgeon two months later for a checkup, all was well. The scars had faded to fine lines, and the surgeon told him they would fade still further until about six months after surgery. Marcel chuckled over the reactions from his colleagues, who in their own fashion complimented him on his youthful appearance.

Reshaping the Nose

While other facial surgery is usually sought to counteract the effect of aging, rhinoplasty (surgery to alter the shape of the nose) is usually requested to counteract the effects of heredity or injury. Because the nose is the most prominent facial feature, its size and shape are readily noticeable, making rhinoplasty one of the most requested cosmetic operations.

Most patients seeking rhinoplasty want their noses made smaller. Not all noses can be equally corrected by rhinoplasty. Specific limitations, such as thick skin or a very thick tip of the nose, may limit the effectiveness of surgery. Rhinoplasty is usually delayed until the patient is 16 years old, to allow the nose to develop fully.

It is extremely important for the patient to define the concerns precisely. Patients must be able to look in a mirror and point to their specific areas of concern. Considerable discussion should then follow between patient and surgeon about the reasonable results and limitations of surgery. The nose must be assessed in relation to the entire face, to obtain the most harmonious relationship.

Rhinoplasty

Candidates for rhinoplasty are treated either as outpatients and given local anesthetic and heavy sedation, or as inpatients and given a general anesthetic. If extensive work on the inside of the nose is necessary — for example, to correct breathing — a general anesthetic is often preferred. A rhinoplasty usually takes about 60-90 minutes.

The nose consists of a tent of skin and soft tissue draped over a bone and cartilage framework. In rhinoplasty this framework is modified to change the shape of the nose (Fig. 12.3). The surgery is usually performed entirely through incisions inside the nostrils, leaving no visible incision marks after surgery. Every nose is different, requiring different surgical techniques. In some instances, a cartilage graft or bone graft may be necessary to achieve the best result.

The nose consists of the tip (cartilage), the dorsum or hump (cartilage and bone) and the nasal bones. The nasal septum is the partition between the nasal cavities. Most candidates for rhinoplasty need alterations in each area. Occasionally, only a partial rhinoplasty is necessary to change the shape in one particular area.

Through incisions inside the nostrils, the skin is first freed up from the underlying skeletal framework. Excess cartilage from the hump and tip is removed or altered, and the nose can then be shortened if necessary. The nasal bones are then broken, to narrow the width of the nose. Sometimes the septum or other structures inside the nose will require surgery to improve breathing.

Immediately after rhinoplasty, a plaster cast or metallic splint is carefully molded to the new structure of the nose. This mold is usually left in place for just over a week, so that the nose sets in the desired shape. The nostrils may be packed to prevent oozing. This may be somewhat uncomfortable; mouth breathing is necessary until packing is removed. A gauze "moustache" dressing is usually applied over the nostrils.

After the operation, ice packs are usually applied over the cheeks for 15 minutes every hour for the rest of the day. The head should be kept elevated (use two pillows when sleeping) for a few days. There may be minor oozing from the nostrils for a day or two after the operation. The moustache dressing is changed once or twice a day and is then removed after two days.

Swelling and bruising are greatest two to three days after surgery. Patients vary greatly in their reactions. If the nasal bones have been broken and reset, black eyes and swelling around the eyes are

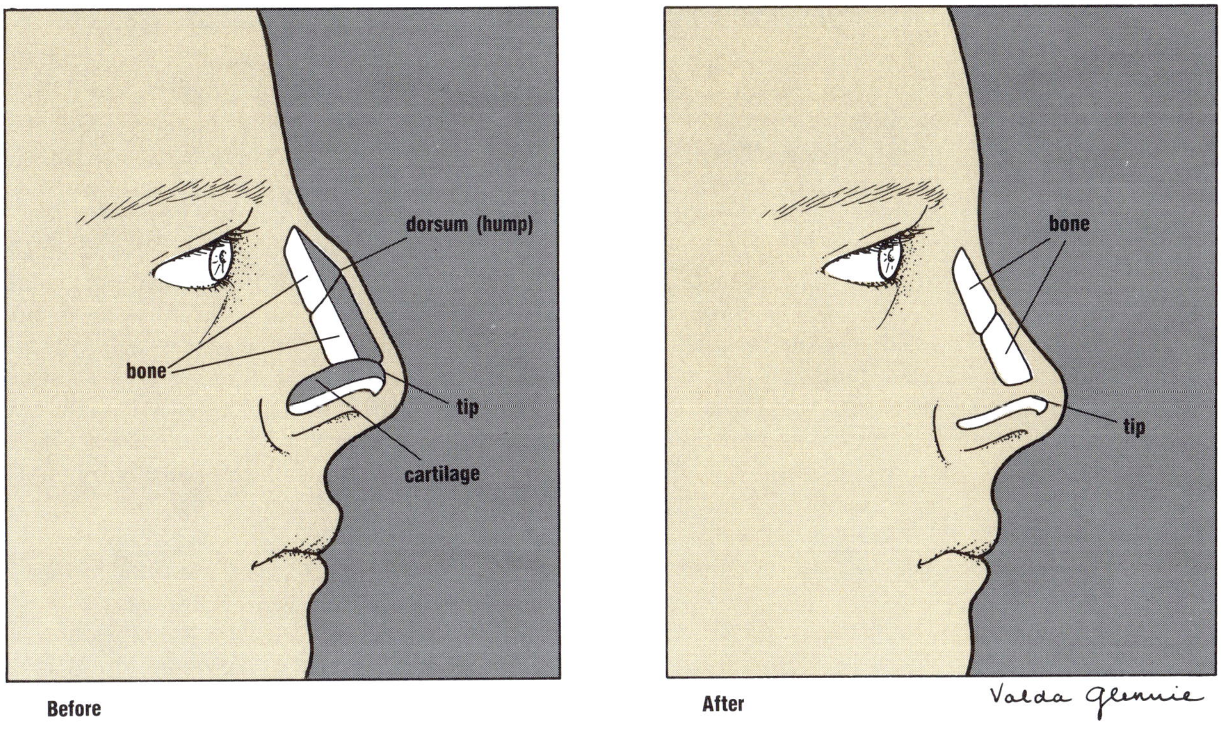

Figure 12.3
Rhinoplasty (reshaping the nose).

common. Lifting, straining and sneezing should be avoided for a week after surgery. The cast must be kept dry.

If packing is used in the nostrils, it is usually removed one or two days after surgery. On the third day, cotton swabs dipped in hydrogen peroxide can be used to cleanse the nostril area and apply a layer of petroleum jelly over the inner nostril, to minimize crust formation. The nose can be quite congested for several weeks after surgery.

About eight or nine days later, the cast is carefully removed from the nose, which will look a little rugged at this point. The sides will be pressed in, where the cast has been molded to hold the reset nasal bones in position. The tip and upper nose may appear quite swollen. The nose will usually need a further week or so before its appearance improves. Patients are advised to remain off work for about two weeks after surgery.

After the cast is removed, patients must avoid any trauma to the nose for a further two weeks, until the healing process has allowed the bone to knit. Gentle blowing of the nose is allowed 10 days after surgery. Harsh sunshine should be avoided for about two months.

The nose can remain tender for many months after surgery, particularly if it is bumped inadvertently. The tip of the nose is often numb for several months. While much of the swelling has gone from the nose two to three weeks after surgery, some swelling remains and slowly settles. The permanent appearance will not be apparent until a year after surgery.

Minor revisions are sometimes necessary to refine a particular area of the nose. These revisions should be delayed for a full year after the original surgery, to allow the tissue to settle in and heal fully.

Many patients requesting rhinoplasty have become preoccupied with the appearance of their noses, so they are often very pleased with the results. They may be surprised when their friends and relatives fail to comment on what they perceive to be a dramatic change — which has actually occurred largely in their self-image.

Reshaping the Breasts

Throughout history, the female breast has been a symbol of femininity. Its size and shape have always been emphasized, and in the past 10 years, new ways have been found to change that size and shape. Many women now go to plastic surgeons to have their breasts made bigger or smaller, or to have a breast reconstructed after mastectomy.

The adult female breast consists of fatty tissue and breast tissue. The breast tissue is composed of about 30 lobules, each of which is attached to a duct which emerges through the nipple. The breast tissue lies underneath the fatty tissue and rests on the pectoralis muscle of the chest.

Breast Reduction

Some women have excessively large breasts, which is known as breast hypertrophy. The tissue in both breasts (sometimes only in one) becomes overdeveloped, for reasons that are still unknown.

The condition usually begins with the onset of puberty, when the breasts may reach enormous proportions. At this age, the distress is psychosocial rather than physical, because patients consider themselves freakish and are often objects of ridicule. Later, however, more physical problems will manifest themselves, because these breasts remain large and may get even larger with childbearing. Heredity plays an important role, but glandular causes are very uncommon.

Apart from the psychological problem of breast hypertrophy, physical symptoms increase with age. The most common symptom is pain in the shoulders, neck or mid- or upper back from the weight of the breasts and from grooves in the shoulders caused by bra straps. In humid weather, skin irritation under the breasts often results in rashes. Pain and tenderness in the breasts themselves can occur, but are not common. Over many years, some women develop a stooped posture. Because of these symptoms, breast reduction surgery is one of the few cosmetic operations fully or partly covered by health insurance plans.

Patients are admitted to hospital the day before surgery, for lab tests and general examinations. Photographs are usually taken before surgery, and the operation is meticulously planned. Breast reduction is considered major surgery, usually performed under general anesthetic, and takes two to four hours. The breast is not only reduced in size but is also lifted and essentially rebuilt (Fig. 12.4). Blood transfusion is rarely necessary.

In earlier breast reduction procedures, the nipples were removed and reapplied as skin grafts. Now the nipple is usually left attached to the breast tissue on a flap (pedicle) and then ''shifted'' to a new position, improving breast appearance and sensation. Excess tissue is removed from either side of the pedicle and from above it.

After the operation a bulky sterile dressing is applied over the breasts, and is usually held in place with the patient's old bra. A drain is left in place along the incision line on each breast to allow drainage of residual fluid after surgery. This drain is usually removed after 48 hours.

The patient usually stays in bed for the first day. Some patients feel nauseated from the anesthetic. Sips of fluid are given initially, building up to a regular diet over 24 hours. An intravenous line provides necessary fluids during that time. There is not much pain, which would tend to occur along the incision line, under the fold of the breast. Painkillers are prescribed as necessary.

The patient is generally up walking and taking a regular diet the day after surgery. She may need pain medication and is encouraged to do deep breathing exercises. Two days after surgery, the drains are removed and the dressing is changed. The patient is usually discharged the fol-

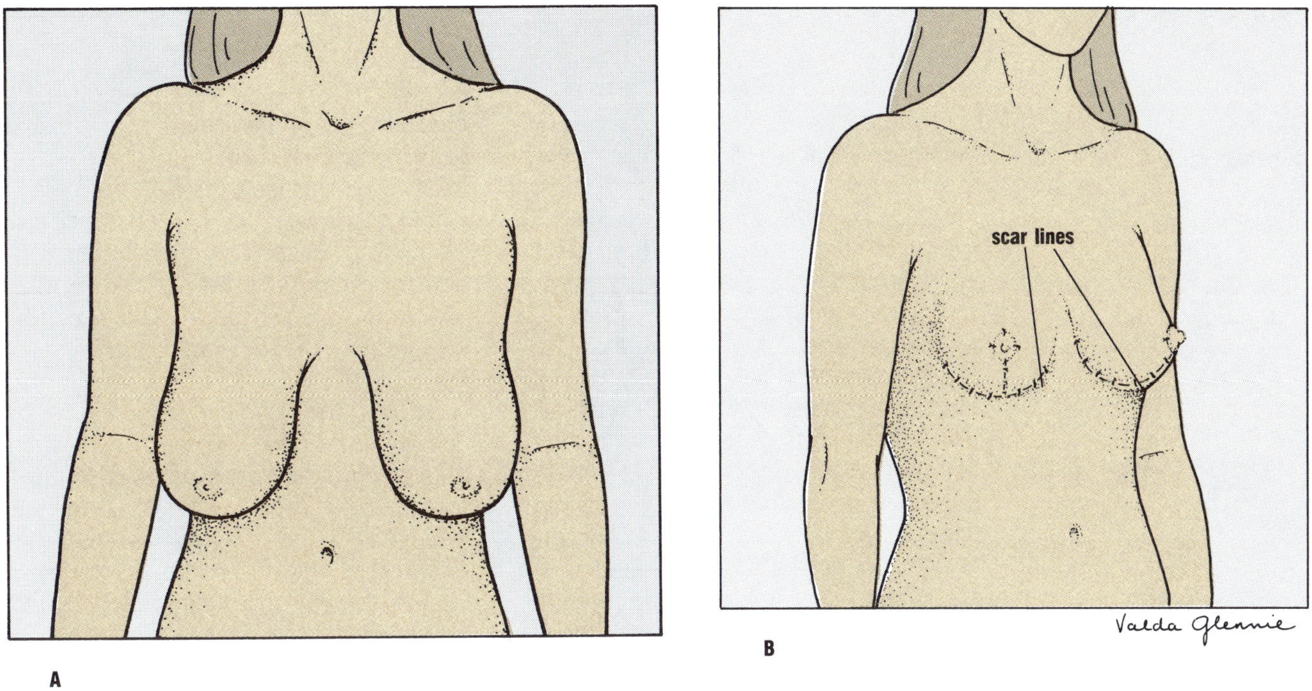

Figure 12.4
Breast reduction, before (A) and after (B), showing the resulting scar lines.

lowing day, with a prescription for mild pain medication (which may not be necessary) and a supply of extra dressings so that she can change them herself at home.

Suture removal usually takes place seven to ten days after surgery. Some surgeons prefer to use dissolving sutures which do not have to be removed. Once the sutures are out, the patient can resume showers and baths. Minor areas of skin irritation may need dressings for a further week, after which patients can be fitted for a new bra.

Three to four weeks off work are the norm after breast reduction surgery. During that time, many women feel weak and easily fatigued. These problems generally disappear about a month after surgery, when full activity, including exercise, can be resumed. Patients are usually advised to wear a bra night and day, except for bathing, until six weeks after surgery.

Complications

With breast reduction surgery, the patient is essentially trading the symptoms of breast enlargement for certain inherent disadvantages, including scars, a possible decrease in nipple sensation, and a possible inability to breast-feed.

The chief disadvantage after surgery is the scarring. Some patients heal with a fine line scar, which may take as long as two years to settle. In other patients the scars remain wider and more noticeable even after that time. The final quality of these scars depends upon the patient's own healing ability.

Nipple sensation is usually retained after surgery, particularly if the nipple has not been removed and reapplied as a skin graft. Most patients with very large breasts have poor nipple sensation before surgery, presumably because the weight of the breast tissue stretched the sensory nerves. Breast-feeding may be possible after surgery, depending on the size of the breast pedicle on which the nipple is retained.

After breast reduction surgery, breasts should not enlarge again, although if a patient gains weight, the breasts may get proportionately bigger. There is no relationship between breast reduction surgery and the development of breast cancer. Theoretically, the likelihood of breast cancer should decrease, because so much breast tissue has been removed by the operation.

Other complications of breast reduction surgery are much less common. Bleeding and infection can occur, as with other forms of surgery. There may be small areas of skin loss (ulceration) due to poor blood supply. These areas heal by themselves. A nipple can be partially lost from impeded blood supply, but complete loss of a nipple would be very rare. These complications, however, are more common in obese patients. Most plastic surgeons recommend that overweight patients lose weight before surgery. Weight loss does not decrease breast size significantly, but it certainly reduces the incidence of postoperative complications.

Breast Lift (Mastopexy)

A mastopexy is a "facelift" of the breasts. It does the same thing for sagging breasts as a properly fitting bra, but is fashioned from the patient's own skin. The operation is similar to that for breast reduction, but no breast tissue is removed — only skin. Mastopexy has disadvantages and complications similar to breast reduction, so the patient must decide if the extent of the resulting scars justifies the improvement from this operation. Patients who are upset by a moderate degree of breast sagging may be even more disturbed by the scars resulting from the mastopexy.

Breast Augmentation

North America has become a very breast-conscious society. Over the years, many purported methods of bust enlargement have appeared. The Sears and Roebuck catalogue of the 1890s advertised "the princess bust developer" and "bust cream or food" concocted by "an eminent French chemist." Today, similar "breast developers" often grace the pages of tabloids. However, no exercise, medication, "bust developer" or lotion has any real effect on the size of the breast. The padded bra can provide the desired outward appearance, but has little effect on the frequently associated feelings of inadequacy.

Before the silastic prosthesis was developed, some women had their breasts enlarged with liquid silicone injections. These injections were performed (often with impure preparations) in places like Mexico and Las Vegas in the early 1950s, often by unqualified practitioners. The medical profession has not used silicone injections for breast enlargement for the past 30 years.

Breast augmentation is done for the patient's psychological need and self-image. Unlike breast reduction, there are no physical symptoms that will be alleviated by breast augmentation. Patients who want this surgery frequently state that they want to "look better," "feel better," or have their "clothes fit better" and be less self-conscious.

Most women who want this operation fall into one of two groups. The larger group is composed of women whose breasts never developed to a size they feel is compatible with the rest of their bodies. The second group feel that their breasts were normal before pregnancy, but then lost substance after delivery. This process is known as involution, and these patients usually want to restore their former state. For both groups, breast augmentation usually results in marked improvement of the patient's self-image.

Breast augmentation became popular only after 1962, when the silicone bag (silastic) prosthesis was developed. This prosthesis has been extensively refined over the years. It is composed of medically approved silicone contained within a sac or envelope, and is compatible with body tissue after implantation. There is no relationship between the use of silastic implants and the development of breast cancer. Today, about 100,000 breast augmentation operations are performed annually in North America.

Women receiving breast augmentation surgery usually do so as outpatients, and frequently have local anesthetic, with heavy sedation. There are three choices for placement of the incisions: in the fold under the breast, around the nipple, or through the armpit. Each of these incision lines tends to be quite inconspicuous — not invisible — after healing; each has its own advantages. Incisions under the breast allow better exposure to control bleeding, which can produce firmness in the breast and often produce more symmetrical results. They also avoid cutting into breast tissue, which is necessary if an incision is made around the nipple. Incisions in the armpit make the scars less conspicuous, but bleeding may be more difficult to control, and symmetry more difficult to achieve.

After the incision is made, a pocket is created underneath the breast tissue. This pocket can be either on top of the pectoralis muscle, or under the pectoralis muscle — on top of the rib cage (subpectoral) (Fig. 12.5). Many surgeons feel that the breasts remain softer if the implant is placed under the muscle, where it is cushioned by the covering muscle layer, although breast appearance is similar in both cases. Implants come in many sizes; some can be adjusted during surgery, to achieve breast symmetry.

After the implantation, the incisions are closed and a supporting bra is put on before the patient leaves the operating room. The operation takes up to two and one-half hours (longer if the implant is placed under the pectoralis muscle). Because the breast gland is not disturbed, the ability to breast-feed is not significantly altered. Sometimes, however, sensation can be decreased.

Patients can be taken home five or six hours after surgery. Because of the sedation, grogginess and nausea may continue that day. Moderate discomfort often lasts for two to three days, and painkillers are usually necessary. There is generally more pain if the implants are placed under the pectoralis muscle.

Patients usually remain off work for one week after surgery. During that time, they should minimize arm movement, particularly lifting or reaching above the head. Patients can have a bath after three days, and wash directly over the breast. A bra is worn day and night for about three weeks. Some surgeons have patients massage the implant regularly after the first week, to help prevent firmness in the breast.

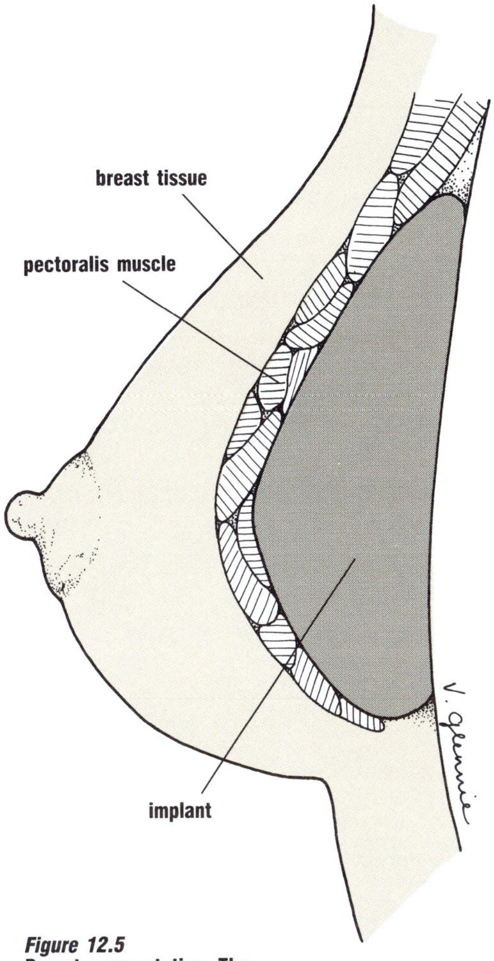

Figure 12.5
Breast augmentation. The implant has been placed underneath the pectoralis muscle (subpectoral).

Case Study: Breast Augmentation

Susan was 33 years old and had two children. Now that her childbearing was over, she wanted to get back in shape, and she was very dissatisfied with the size of her breasts. She thought that after two children her breasts might have enlarged, but they hadn't. She was going back to work and didn't need any holes in her self-confidence. Having read about breast augmentation in several magazine articles, she decided to see a plastic surgeon.

When she saw Dr. Reid, Susan had a number of questions. How was the operation done? Was it painful? What was put in? Could the implant spring a leak? Would it affect breast self-examination afterwards? What were the long-term effects? How would her breasts feel?
Dr. Reid surprised her by answering with a question: "What size are you now and what size would you like to be?" Susan was fairly modest in her requirements. She was a 34A, and would be happy just to be a 34B.

Dr. Reid then answered her questions while finding out about her general health and history. He explained that the implant was a bag of medical silicone which was implanted through a two-inch incision. The silicone implants rarely leaked significantly. There would be no interference with breast self-examination since the implant was placed under the breast tissue. He told her that augmented breasts tended to sag somewhat less than normal, since the implant would hold its shape. The breasts should feel a little firmer than usual.

Susan went to the hospital on the day of surgery fairly nervous, and glad that she would be returning home the same day. Her husband had arranged to leave work early to take her home. After the operation, she was fairly groggy. Dr. Reid warned her to expect pain for about three days and prescribed a moderately strong painkiller. Although Susan found the first few days after the operation quite painful, she healed well. She had her sutures removed nine days later and made an appointment to see him in six months. At this checkup she told him that she was delighted with the way her clothes "fit better" now. Her friends had commented on the difference in her appearance, but weren't sure what to ascribe it to. Some asked if she'd lost weight, because her waistline looked smaller below a fuller bustline. Others noticed her vitality, commenting that going back to work suited her.

Complications

Bleeding can occur after breast augmentation surgery. This is not a common complication, but if it does occur inside the breast pocket it is removed and the implant is replaced.

The most common problem after this type of surgery is excessive firmness in the breasts. A certain amount of scar tissue forms a capsule around the implant. In some patients, this capsule can contract, producing firmness and distortion in the breast. Many surgeons feel that this firmness can be reduced by placing the implant under the pectoralis muscle. Having the patient massage the breast for a few months or longer surgery may also help. Some surgeons have attempted to break down the scar tissue manually by squeezing the breast. This technique is not commonly used today, and cannot be effective if the implant has been placed subpectorally.

If persistent firmness develops, a second operation may be necessary to cut through and release the scar tissue around the implant. But this is necessary in only a minority of patients. Other uncommon complications of breast augmentation include infection and altered nipple sensation, which is a common temporary effect, but usually returns to normal within two to three months.

Chapter 13

Vascular Surgery

F. Michael Ameli
Associate Professor of Surgery
University of Toronto
Vascular Surgeon
Wellesley Hospital, Toronto

Valda Glennie
Illustrator

Hardening of the arteries is as familiar a term as varicose veins. Both are common conditions treated by vascular surgeons—yet one is life-threatening, while the other is often primarily a cosmetic problem.

Vascular surgery treats diseases in the major blood vessels of the body. The two major types of vessels are arteries and veins. Arteries carry the oxygenated blood from the heart and lungs, to all tissues of the body, which use the oxygen. The veins then return the blood to the heart and lungs. The venous system is like a river with minor tributaries called venules, which flow into larger vessels. The largest vessel is the inferior vena cava, which takes the blood back to the heart.

The most common operations performed by vascular surgeons are bypass operations to restore circulation where there is a blockage, repair of enlarged blood vessels (aneurysmal dilatation), repair of the carotid artery leading to the brain to prevent stroke (carotid endarterectomy), and surgery for varicose veins.

Occlusive Vascular Disease

Occlusive vascular disease (narrowed or blocked blood vessels) is caused by atherosclerosis. The inner layer of the blood vessel is damaged due to fatty deposits and a roughening of the surface.

Figure 13.1
Major arteries.

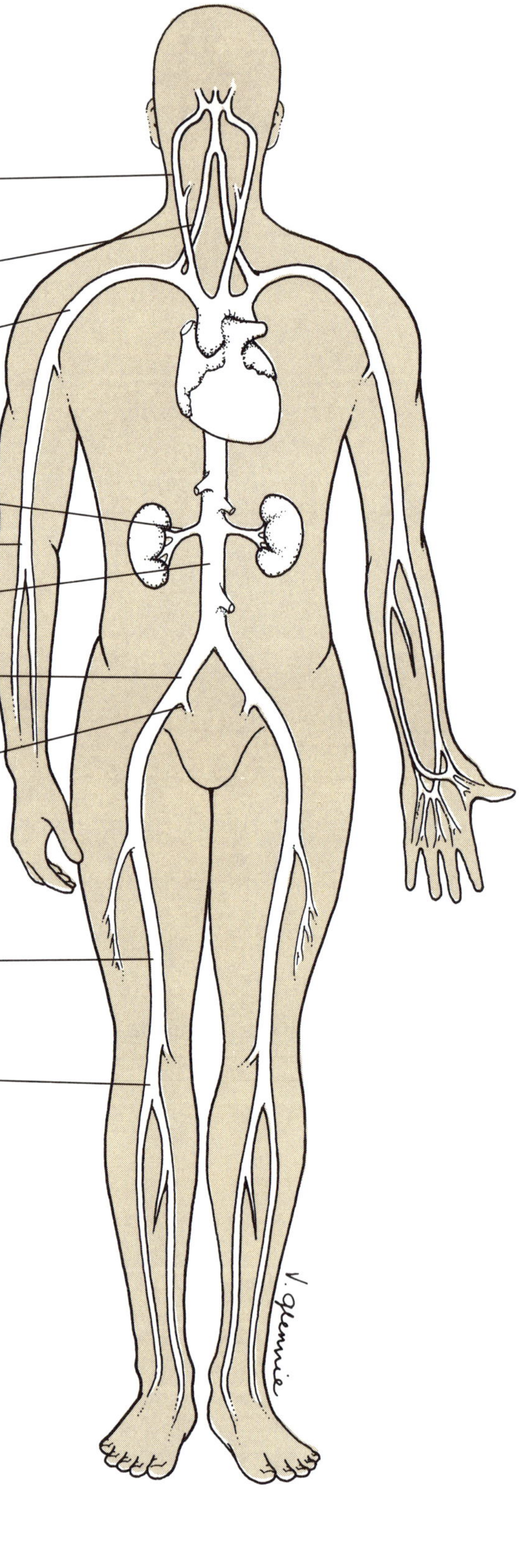

This may cause the vessel wall to ulcerate and lead to clotting (thrombosis), which can narrow or even block the artery. When a clot accumulates and breaks off, the piece of clot that breaks off is called an embolus. Eventually calcium deposits harden the blood vessel, which is why the condition is known as hardening of the arteries.

Atherosclerosis may affect the arteries to the brain, heart, kidney and, most commonly, limbs. There are many contributing factors: blood pressure, diet, diabetes, too much fat in the blood, (hypercholestrolemia) and cigarette smoking. Smoking is the major factor in accelerated atherosclerosis.

Atherosclerosis tends to affect the major vessels where they branch. Narrowing of the aorta (Fig. 13.1), the body's main blood vessel, can lead to intermittent cramping pains in a calf muscle during exercise (claudication). Ten percent of the population over 65 suffers from claudication. In patients who have intermittent claudication, 5 to 10 percent will develop gangrene (death of tissue due to lack of blood), which may necessitate removal of the limb.

Narrowing the aortic branching (bifurcation) is like damming a stream. The effects are felt at the lowest part of the stream — the circulation to the toes or calf muscle. The calf muscle is the major muscle of walking; when it is deprived of adequate blood, the patient experiences pain in the calf.

Atherosclerosis is an aging process that can affect all parts of the arterial tree. The effect depends on the site of the narrowing or blockage, and the number of affected areas. Patients with atherosclerosis are usually over 50 and have gradually developed progressive disease of their arteries as they are subjected to the risk factors, particularly cigarette smoking, over a long period of time (98 percent of patients with narrowed or blocked arteries are smokers). The longer they are subjected to these risks and the older they are, the more likely they are to develop the problem.

Many patients develop leg pain at 65, just when they are retiring. The claudication is relieved by rest, but comes on again as soon as the patient walks. If the calf muscle alone is affected, this can be due to narrowing or blockage of the aortoiliac arteries, or the femoral artery (Fig. 13.1), or a combination of the two. If the cramping is only in the buttock muscle, the patient probably has aortoiliac disease. The severity of the symptoms depends on the location of the disease and the development of collateral circulation — nature's attempt to provide alternative pathways around the narrowed or blocked arteries by opening up new small vessels around the blocked artery.

If the circulation continues to be impaired, the patient is in danger of developing gangrene, which could result in loss of the leg. The symptom of pregangrene is night pain in the toes. The pain is relieved by hanging the leg over the side of the bed or getting up and walking around. When the patient is asleep, the heart pumps less rigorously, and less blood is supplied to the limb. Gravity cannot help to get the blood to the leg because the patient is lying flat. Blood flow is therefore so diminished that it deprives the nerves of blood, and the patient experiences pain.

If the situation worsens, the patient experiences pain at rest, both day and night. The decreased blood supply now also produces numbness. The final pregangrenous stage is ulcers, breaks in the skin that may appear on the toe or foot. Gangrene can set in at this point, appearing as black areas on the toes or forefoot. The tissue usually dies first at the farthest end of the circulation, i.e., the toes.

Occasionally a narrowed area suddenly becomes completely blocked and there is no time for collateral circulation to develop. The symptoms are loss of sensation and movement in the foot and lower leg. Unless something is done very quickly, the patient will lose the leg.

Diagnosis

In most cases the physician will be able to diagnose narrowed or blocked arteries by the patient's history and a physical examination. The physician will feel for the pulse in the affected limb and will listen with the stethoscope for any noises in the arteries that indicate narrowing. Skin changes such as ulcers and gangrene can be seen. Three other tests are also used.

Doppler studies are carried out with an instrument called a pulse volume recorder and Doppler ultrasound to bounce sound waves off the blood vessel. This is a sophisticated way of measuring blood pressure in small vessels. Changes in blood pressure reflect alterations in flow and volume. Doppler ultrasound helps the physician estimate the extent of the disease and find the narrowing or block in the blood vessel. This test involves no incisions or probes, has no side effects and takes approximately 30 minutes.

Transcutaneous Oxygen Pressure Measurement ($PtcO_2$) is a method of measuring skin oxygen by applying a small heated pad (Clarke electrode) to the leg. This indicates the amount of oxygen being delivered by the blood to the skin and is another means of determining the extent of the narrowing or blockage. This test also involves no incisions or probes, has no side effects and takes approximately 30 minutes.

A third procedure, arteriography, is not usually used to make the diagnosis, but helps in planning the type of surgery required. Dye is injected into the blood vessels and X-rays are taken. An artery is punctured, usually in the groin, with a needle or a thin plastic tube (catheter). An iodine solution (which can be seen on X-ray) is injected into the artery. The patient feels a hot sensation when the dye is injected. Reaction to the iodine sometimes occur. They may include nausea, vomiting, itching and hives, but they respond quickly to medication. At the site of the insertion of the needle or catheter there is very often slight bleeding, bruising or soreness.

More serious but rare reactions include loss of blood pressure, irregular heart beat and, very rarely, death. (The incidence of death is approximately one in 10,000.) Occasionally, arteries can become blocked or damaged during the test.

In general arteriography is an essential part of the investigation for a patient who is to undergo surgery. The incidence of complications is very small. A safer dye containing no iodine has recently been developed and is now being used in most centers.

Non-Surgical Treatment

Patients who suffer from intermittent claudication are advised to exercise, reduce their fat intake and, most important, stop smoking. If present, other risk factors such as high blood pressure, diabetes and hyperlipidemia (excess fat in the blood) must be controlled.

Surgical Treatment

Various procedures are used to correct blocked or narrowed arteries affecting the lower limbs.

Transluminal Dilatation

This involves inserting a catheter with a balloon attachment into the femoral artery in the groin. The tip of the catheter is passed through the narrowed area and the balloon is inflated to stretch the area. This method is most useful for narrowed segments less than two inches long and in the larger arteries, particularly in the iliac or external iliac arteries (Fig. 13.1). In carefully selected cases, there is a 95 percent initial success rate. After five years, 90 percent of the arteries remain open. Approximately 10 percent of patients with vascular disease in the lower limbs will be suitable for transluminal dilatation.

Bypass Graft Surgery

Aorto-bifemoral bypass graft is used to save a limb, or when intermittent claudication interferes significantly with a patient's activities. A graft made of Dacron is joined to the aorta via an abdominal incision (Fig. 13.2). The graft is then brought down and joined to the femoral arteries in the groin through two separate groin incisions. The operation takes approximately three hours.

After surgery, the patient is admitted to the intensive care unit for 12 to 24 hours for careful observation of any bleeding, blockage of the graft or problems associated with the heart or kidneys. If all goes well, the patient will return home about eight to ten days after surgery.

It takes six to eight weeks before the patients gets back to normal activity. During this time the patient can be out of bed but must not undertake any strenuous activity such as heavy lifting or excessive exercise. The patient should have help at home for at least the first two weeks after coming out of hospital and should not do any housekeeping or cooking during that time.

If the obstruction is lower down in the femoral or popliteal artery (the femoral artery becomes the popliteal artery at the knee), the femoral popliteal bypass graft is used (Fig. 13.3). This operation is of much lesser magnitude than the aorto-bifemoral bypass graft. It is used primarily for patients who would otherwise lose a limb, and is occasionally recommended for patients with intermittent claudication that is extremely disabling.

The best results are achieved by using the patient's own long saphenous vein (Fig. 13.6), which is taken out and reversed. This vein has valves that allow flow in one direction only; the vein is reversed so that the blood can flow in the other direction. A synthetic plastic material called PTFF (Gortex) is used in patients whose saphenous veins have already been removed in varicose vein operations, but it does not work as well as the patient's own vein.

An incision is made down the inside of the leg from the groin to below the knee. The purpose of this operation is to increase the blood flow to the lower leg, bypassing the obstructed artery. Immediately after surgery, the patient goes to the intensive care unit for 12 hours and is in hospital for about five to seven days. The patient is encouraged to get out of bed and walk during this time, and spends about one month at home before returning to full activity.

Complications

The early complications of all bypass grafts are bleeding and clotting, which would block the graft. This usually occurs where the graft joins the artery. A small amount of bleeding may require no treatment, but if the graft hemorrhages, the surgeon will have to put in more sutures. The risk of bleeding or thrombosis is under 1 percent. After an aorto-bifemoral bypass operation, the overall risk of cardiac and brain complications is significant because the same disease process may affect the blood vessels of the heart and/or brain. Up to 2 percent of patients may die, most likely because of a heart attack or rarely, from a stroke after the operation. The major long-term complication is infection of the graft, which occurs in 1.5 percent of patients. There is a rare risk of losing a limb or paralysis. About 75 percent of men with vascular disease of the aorto-femoral arteries are impotent due to reduced blood supply in the pelvis. After surgery, 30 percent may have improved sexual function, approximately 10 percent are made worse. In 1 to 2 percent of patients, part of the bowel loses its blood supply and must be removed.

After five years, 95 percent of aorto-bifemoral bypass grafts remain open; at ten years, 80 to 85 percent are still open. Overall this operation has low risk, improves walking and saves patients from leg amputation. Patients who continue to smoke, however, will have a much higher chance of recurring thrombosis.

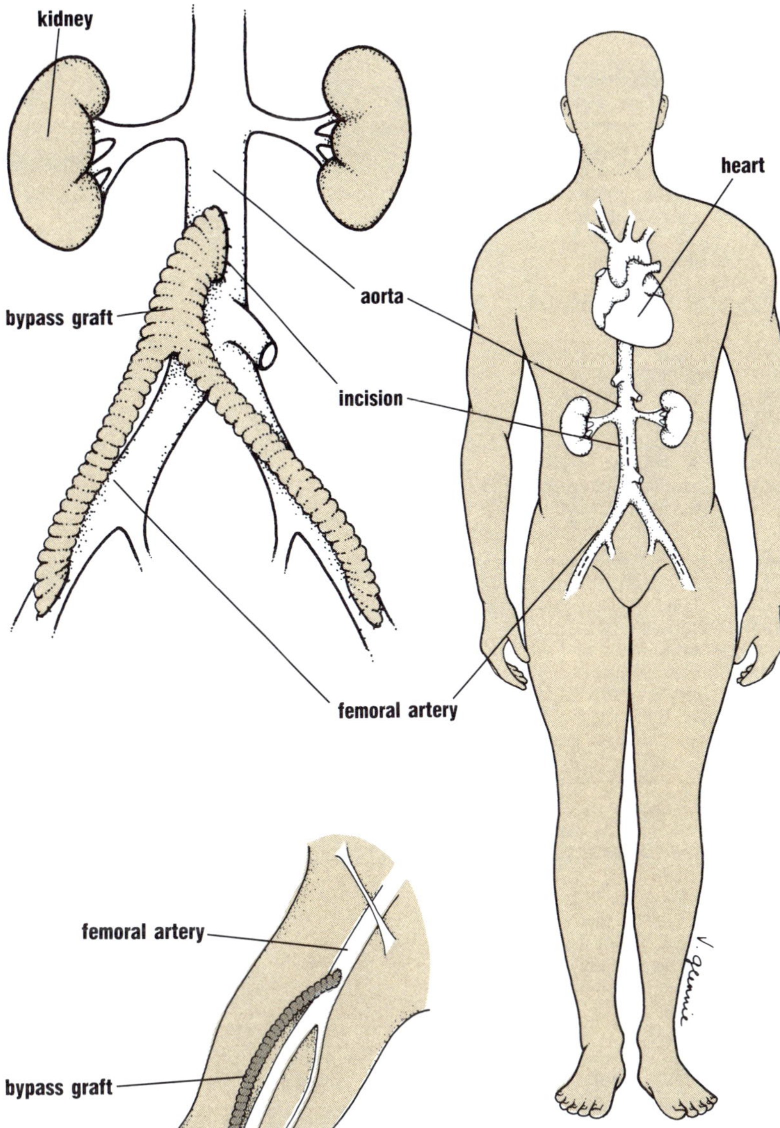

Figure 13.2
Aorto-bifemoral bypass graft.

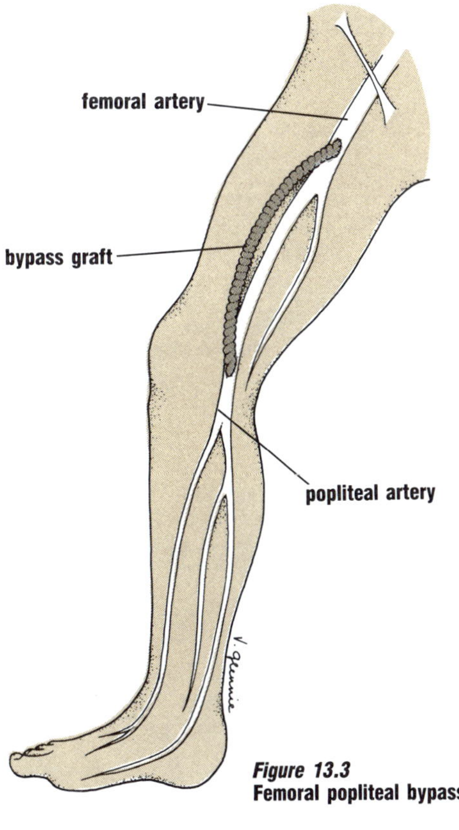

Figure 13.3
Femoral popliteal bypass graft.

Case Study: Abdominal Aortic Aneurysm

At his usual checkup, Harry thought that Dr. Cavanaugh lingered a bit with the stethoscope. And Dr. Cavanaugh didn't deliver his usual sermon about his smoking. "Maybe I've beaten the statistics," Harry thought, as he had recently celebrated his sixty-fifth birthday. "Any pains in your legs or toes, Harry?" That was a new one.

Dr. Cavanaugh pulled up his chair. "I'll come right to the point, Harry. I've heard a sound I don't like in your main artery. It could be a problem. I'd like to be sure, so I'm sending you for an ultrasound and I want you to see a vascular surgeon. His name is Doctor Garcia.

Dr. Garcia didn't mince words. "Your main artery — the abdominal aorta — has an enlarged portion, which is called an aneurysm. It's like a fault in a tire. Unless it's repaired, sooner or later it will blow."
Then he drew Harry a picture to explain where the aneurysm was, and what could be done to repair it. Harry was aghast at the thought of surgery. He'd never been sick a day in his life — why, he didn't feel sick now! "In a way, you're lucky. We can repair your aneurysm before it ruptures. When you get symptoms, that's bad news."

They talked about the risks of the operation, which Dr. Garcia explained was major surgery. He emphasized that there was a very small chance of dying from a heart attack after the operation, and a chance of losing a leg, due to impaired circulation. In your case, you're otherwise healthy, you've got a good few years ahead of you, and I think the chances are very good that you'd weather the surgery well." It was his wife, Doris, who spoke next. "How soon can we get him into hospital, Doctor?"

The complications of a femoral popliteal bypass graft are less serious — the risk of fatal complications is under 0.5 percent. In 10 to 15 percent of patients, the skin incisions will divide a skin nerve, which may produce numbness in the area of the knee or thigh (patients are often concerned that the numbness is caused by circulation problems, which is not the case). Sometimes this numbness will be relieved by other nerves growing into the affected area.

The chance of a femoral popliteal bypass remaining open at five years using a vein bypass is 70 to 80 percent. If a Gortex graft is used, the chance drops to 50 to 60 percent. Again, the most important factor affecting grafts is smoking. If the patient does not stop smoking, the disease process will likely continue, even in the new bypass graft.

Recent Advances

The major thrust of research in bypass grafts is developing new kinds of grafts that remain open longer and have less chance of becoming infected. For femoral popliteal bypass grafts, researchers are trying to find a synthetic graft material that will be as good as the long saphenous vein.

One of the most exciting advances has been the use of lasers to bore out the narrowed areas and the narrowed artery is then dilated. This procedure shows promise, particularly for the narrowed or blocked femoral artery, and will probably be in use within the next few years.

Abdominal Aortic Aneurysm

The abdominal aorta (Fig. 13.1) is the main artery that carries blood to the lower half of the body. In adults it is about six inches long, starting at the renal arteries and dividing just below the belly button into the iliac arteries. An aneurysm is an enlarged portion of an artery. It most commonly occurs in the abdominal aorta, but also occurs in the popliteal and femoral arteries (Fig. 13.1). Normally the abdominal aorta is just under one inch in diameter. When an aneurysm occurs, it enlarges to twice its normal size. Aneurysms occur in 2 percent of people over age 65, but are very rare in patients under age 50. Aneurysm formation is another form of atherosclerosis, or hardening of the arteries. Instead of narrowing, the damaged vessel becomes weak and balloons out. The balloon will eventually break, interrupting the blood circulation and leaking blood into the abdominal cavity. If the patient can be operated on within hours of the rupture, the aneurysm can be repaired. If not, the patient will bleed to death.

Diagnosis

The development of an aneurysm is accelerated by smoking; aneurysms occur three times more frequently in smokers than in non-smokers. Aneurysms occasionally run in families, so a genetic cause has been suspected. Approximately 20 percent of untreated aneurysms will rupture within a year. Over five years, 80 percent of untreated patients will die from rupture.

In 1952 the first attempt was made to reconstruct a vessel affected by an aneurysm. These first reconstructions used aortas taken from accident victims, but they did not work well, and Dacron or Teflon tubes soon replaced them. Today, approximately 13,000 aneurysms are repaired annually in North America.

Initially a patient may describe feeling a pulse in the abdomen, almost like a second heart. When the aneurysm enlarges, it puts pressure on nearby structures, causing sudden abdominal pain, back pain or pain radiating down to the groin. If the aneurysm is leaking or ruptured, depending on the amount of blood loss, the lack of circulation may cause the patient to go into shock and die.

Aneurysms should be repaired before symptoms develop, when mortality and complication rates are much lower.

There are several methods of diagnosing aneurysms. In 50 percent of patients, the calcium deposits in the wall of the aorta will show up on plain X-ray. Doppler ultrasound is a non-invasive examination that can reveal the size of the abdominal aorta and the aneurysm by bouncing sound waves off the blood vessel. Computerized axial tomography (CAT) is a sophisticated method of producing an image of sections of the body. CAT scan gives a great deal more information than ultrasound, but it requires a small amount of radiation and the injection of some dye. It can show the size of the aneurysm, its relationship to the vital arteries leading to the kidneys, and also the condition of other vessels. CAT scan will also show up any other disease in the abdomen, such as a tumor.

Angiography involves injecting dye into the bloodstream. The blood vessels are then examined by X-rays. Digital subtraction angiography is a newer form of angiography using a computer and injecting the dye into the vein. It is less invasive than regular angiography and may be used as an alternative.

Non-Surgical Treatment

In patients who are elderly and have other major medical problems, an aneurysm is not repaired, because the risk of surgery would outweigh the risk of the disease.

Surgical Treatment

This operation requires a general anesthetic and very careful monitoring. Surgery may take up to six hours. Special catheters may be needed to monitor heart function during the procedure. The abdomen is opened and the small and large intestines are carefully moved to the right side of the aorta. The aorta and iliac arteries are exposed (Fig. 13.4), and clamps are applied above and below the aneurysm to decrease the amount of blood loss. The aneurysm is opened and

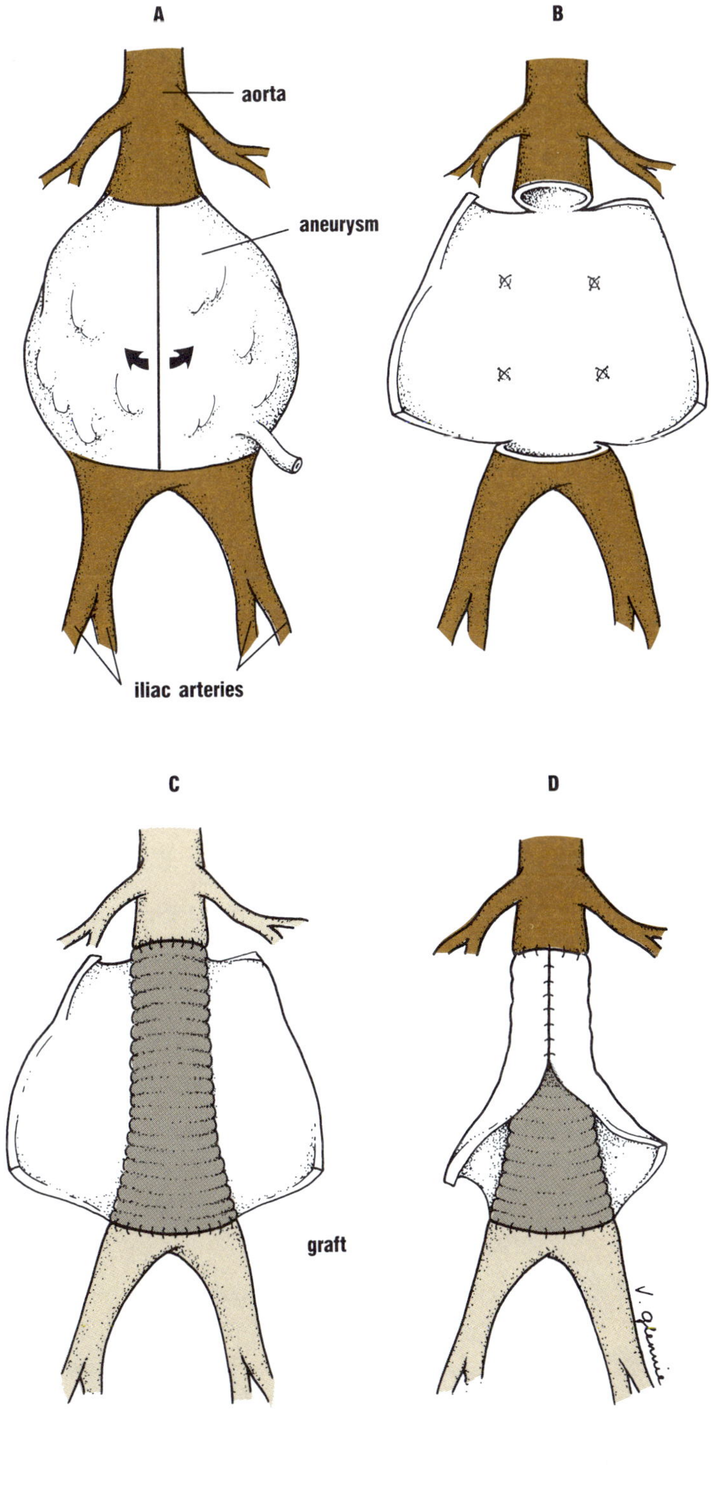

Figure 13.4
Aneurysm repair. The aorta is exposed (A) and the aneurysm is opened (B). After the graft is inserted (C), the wall of the aorta is sewn up to protect it (D).

Dr. Garcia had been very frank with Harry's wife about the risks; she'd wanted to talk to him alone because she wanted to know exactly what Harry's chances were. "During the operation, some people have heart attacks. Sometimes a nerve is damaged. I ought to tell you that three to ten percent of male patients are impotent after the operation, because of nerve damage."

Doris waited outside of the intensive care ward for Dr. Garcia to emerge after the operation. He assured her that the operation had gone smoothly, but that the next twenty-four hours were critical.

Harry spent eight days in the hospital, and Dr. Garcia seemed pleased at the one-month checkup. Harry had at last given up smoking.

a Dacron graft is sewn into position. The wall of the aneurysm is then sewn over the graft to protect it.

Immediately after the operation, the patient is taken to the intensive care unit for 12 to 24 hours. A respirator may be necessary to help breathing, and there is a tube in the patient's nose leading down to the stomach. After three to five days, when the bowels are functioning well, the tube into the stomach is removed and the patient begins drinking fluids, progressing to a solid diet. The usual in-hospital recovery period is eight to twelve days. At home the patient can get up and about, but should not do any housework or chores. The recovery period is gradual; by approximately six weeks the patient is able to go back to full activity.

Complications

Early complications may include bleeding at the point where the graft has been joined to the aorta, which will require a further operation for repair. This is very rare, occurring in only one in 300 patients. The most common complications are related to the heart and lungs, which is why the patient must be in an intensive care unit. If the blood vessels become blocked, and the blood flow to the lower body is cut off, the patient may lose a leg, which occurs in about one in 300 cases. Approximately 70 percent of aneurysm patients have heart disease because of the atherosclerosis and the fact that they are mostly over age 65. The mortality rate for an asymptomatic aneurysm repair (done before symptoms have occurred) is approximately 2 to 4 percent; for a symptomatic aneurysm it is 6 percent, and for a ruptured aneurysm it is 50 percent.

Infection is a later complication of a synthetic graft, occurring in about 1 percent of patients. The graft usually becomes well incorporated into the body, lasting for the patient's lifetime. Another complication arises when nerves are damaged during surgery. As a result, 3 percent of males experience retrograde ejaculation after this operation. Retrograde ejaculation occurs when semen flows into the bladder instead of out of the penis. Three to ten percent of males are impotent. Generally, a patient's life expectancy, ability to work and life-style is the same as anyone of the same age and sex in the general population.

Removal of an abdominal aneurysm is potentially life-saving. Considering that most of these patients are over age 65, death and complication rates are low. Careful selection of patients is essential, but age alone is not a contraindication. Surgeons have operated on many people over age 80 quite safely.

Expectations should, however, be realistic. This is a major operation; it will require a lot of convalescent time, and there are risks involved, although they are small compared to the risks of leaving the aneurysm untreated.

Recent Advances

Aneurysm surgery is only 30 years old, and there have been some dramatic advances in techniques. Improved pre- and postoperative care, in particular devices such as the Swan Ganz catheter, which monitors heart function, has increased positive results. Current research is aimed at a better understanding of the disease's natural history, in the hope of finding methods of prevention. Smoking does increase the risk of aneurysm formation and should be discouraged for this reason. It will be interesting to see whether there is a decrease in aneurysm formation as the smoking population decreases. The most important factor is early, expert treatment once an aneurysm is discovered.

Carotid Artery Stenosis

Four major arteries carry blood to the brain (Fig. 13.5). The two vertebral arteries carry 15 percent of the brain's blood supply to the back part of the brain and are located close to the vertebrae. The two carotid arteries carry 85 percent of the brain's blood supply to the front of the brain and are located in the neck. If any of these arteries narrow or become blocked, the blood supply to that part of the brain is reduced. Small clots can break off from the narrowed and ulcerated carotid artery. If a clot goes to the eye, the patient may experience temporary or, rarely, permanent blindness; if it goes to the brain, it may cause a temporary or permanent stroke.

Stroke is the third leading cause of death in North America. About 20 percent of patients who suffer a stroke die from it. Those who live can be very disabled; 40 percent who have a permanent stroke have experienced a minor stroke in the past from which they recovered.

Narrowing of the carotid artery causes 75 percent of strokes. Over the last 20 years the death rate from stroke has gone down. This decrease is thought to be due to better control of risk factors such as high blood pressure, heart disease and diabetes. Surgical intervention may also be partly responsible for the decrease. Smoking and family history are very important risk factors. Patients with narrowing of the carotid artery tend to have narrowing of arteries elsewhere in the body.

Diagnosis

Since other arteries may also be narrowed, all major arteries must be evaluated, especially those to the heart. The patient may have no symptoms, but there are two common symptoms. Transient ischemic attacks occur when the blood flow to the brain is reduced, causing a temporary stroke (fainting, loss of muscle power) that can last for 20 to 30 minutes. Amaurosis fugax occurs when a small clot goes to the artery of the eye, causing temporary or permanent blindness.

The physician will do a general physical examination, with special attention to the vascular system, feeling the neck pulses and listening to the arteries. If there is narrowing, a "bruit" (noise) will be heard. A patient who has had a transient ischemic attack has a 7 percent per year chance of permanent stroke if left untreated. The diagnosis is made according to the history and physical examination, plus other tests, such as Doppler studies of the carotid arteries (see page 153), CAT scan, (which would reveal any brain damage due to the blood clots breaking off or other possible causes, such as a tumor) and angiography to detect any narrowing or ulceration of the carotid arteries or the blood vessels in the brain.

Non-Surgical Treatment

Blood-thinning drugs such as aspirin (which reduces blood clotting) have been shown to reduce the extent of brain damage, and are currently recommended for patients with vague or no symptoms and also for patients who are not fit for surgery.

Surgical Treatment (Carotid Endarterectomy)

The patient is usually given a general anesthetic, but the operation can be done under local anesthetic. An incision is made in the neck along the course of the carotid artery, and the external, internal and common carotid arteries are carefully exposed (Fig. 13.5). After clamps are applied, the artery is opened and cleaned out. The artery is then carefully sewn up again once the surgeon is sure there is no debris left behind. Sometimes a temporary shunt is used from the common carotid artery into the internal carotid artery, bypassing the opened area during the operation.

Immediately after surgery the patient is taken to the intensive care unit for 12 to 24 hours. Most patients return home within five days. About 1 percent of patients develop a blood clot over the

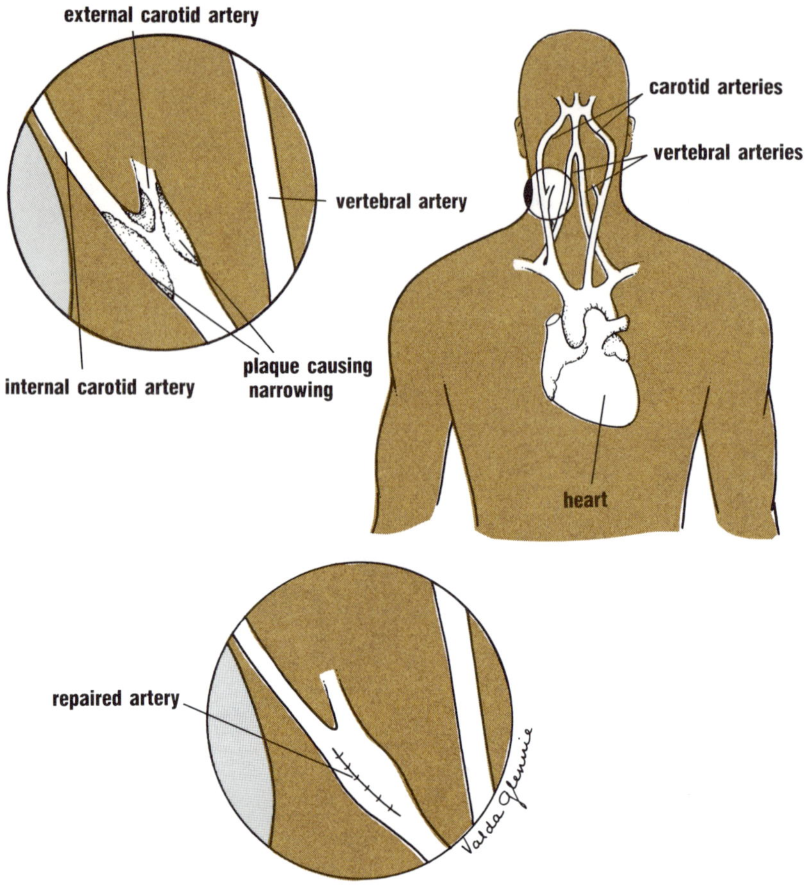

Figure 13.5
Carotid endarterectomy. The carotid artery is opened and cleaned out before being sewn up again.

area of the incision and must have this clot surgically removed. Two percent of patients will have a stroke, mainly because the blood supply to the brain has to be cut off for 10 to 20 minutes while the carotid artery is cleaned out, and small clots can break off and travel to the brain while the arteries are clamped. The risk of stroke in a patient with untreated symptoms is 7 percent per year, whereas the risk of stroke from the surgery is 2 percent, so chances of survival are obviously better with surgery.

Complications

A number of nerves around the carotid artery can be damaged during surgery. If the nerve to the tongue is damaged, when the patient puts the tongue out it may deviate to one side. If the nerve to the voice box is damaged, the patient may become hoarse. Another small nerve supplies the muscles of the lower face; if this nerve is damaged, the patient may have a droop at the corner of the mouth. The chances of these nerves being damaged permanently is 2 percent, although 10 percent of patients experience temporary damage which disappears over a period of a few months. Numbness over the area of the incision is quite common, due to division of the skin nerves.

Long-term complications are related to the underlying hardening of the arteries. Heart attacks are quite common in this group of patients. The original symptoms recur in approximately 3 percent of patients, possibly due to recurrent narrowing of the artery.

Carotid endarterectomy decreases the incidence of stroke, but does not necessarily increase patients' life expectancy, since most of these patients are elderly and have co-existing heart disease. It is most important that patients stop smoking and that their blood pressure be controlled.

Recent Advances

Surgery for asymptomatic carotid narrowing is a controversial subject. At present, Canadian surgeons operate only on those patients who have symptoms, but in the U.S. patients without symptoms are operated on. Research is aimed at controlling the modifiable risk factors, particularly smoking and high blood pressure. Drugs may also become available which can prevent narrowing of the arteries and modify the effects of narrowing on the circulation to the brain.

Varicose Veins

Most of the blood from the lower limbs returns to the heart via veins deep in the leg. The superficial venous system — veins just under the skin — carry only a small amount of blood from the legs to the heart. These veins have valves, which allow blood to flow back in the direction of the heart. The superficial venous system is connected to the deep system by perforating veins, which conduct the blood upwards and inwards. The two main superficial veins are the long and the short saphenous veins. Each joins the deep system at specific sites (junctions) (Fig. 13.6). If the valves become damaged, the superficial veins are exposed to abnormally high pressure, which causes them to become dilated and tortuous (varicose). Valves may be defective or can be damaged by inflammation (phlebitis).

Varicose veins are the most common vascular problem, affecting up to 20 percent of the population. Five women are affected for every one man, and 20 percent of these patients have a family history of varicose veins.

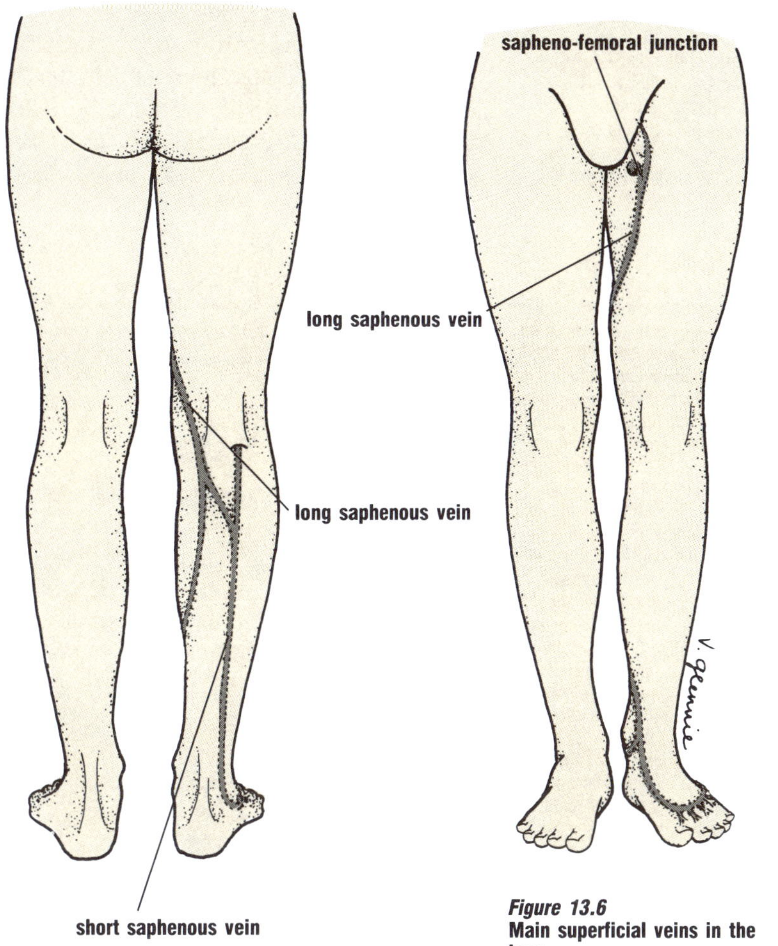

Figure 13.6
Main superficial veins in the legs.

Diagnosis

Women usually notice unsightly varicose veins sooner than men do, because their legs are visible when they wear skirts. Besides the appearance, symptoms may be discomfort, tiredness and heaviness, which is usually worse during menstruation. Male patients, whose legs are usually covered, tend to wait until their varicose veins are very large or complications have set in. Phlebitis (inflammation of the vein) may also occur, which will cause the veins to become red, hard and tender. Superficial phlebitis is not dangerous; the major problem is discomfort. If the valves on the connecting veins between the superficial and deep system become damaged, discoloration around the ankle may result, eventually causing ulcers — breaks in the skin — on the inner side of the ankle.

Varicose veins are usually associated with the long or short saphenous veins.

The diagnosis is based on the patient's history and a physical examination. Family history of varicose veins and the length of time the veins have been in their present condition are important factors in the history. The physician will ask about the relationship of pregnancy to the development of varicose veins and will want to know why the veins bother the patient. The usual concern is cosmetic, but a small percentage of patients have pain from phlebitis, swelling of the ankle, discoloration or ulcers.

The physical examination should take place in good light, with the patient standing and the legs fully exposed. Simple tests can be carried out to determine whether the valves in the communicating veins are damaged. The physician looks at the general configuration of the veins, notes whether the varicosities are associated with the long or short

Case Study: Varicose Veins

Natalie was glad the shift was over. She'd been on her feet all day, to and fro from patients' rooms to the nursing station, and her legs ached, even with the new support stockings she'd bought.

Her doctor, who had seen her through all three of her pregnancies, had said her varicose veins were getting a little more prominent, although they were no threat to her health. "As you know, Natalie, it's not unusual for women to get varicose veins when they're pregnant. Most of these disappear after the baby's born, but some don't. Yours didn't, and with your type of work plus three children, you're bound to experience some aching and prominence of the veins."

The stockings had been some help — she made it through until mid-shift now before she felt she really had to sit down — but she'd taken to elevating her left leg on a box when she was at the nursing station, and always when she was sitting down at home.

Dr. Gifford, a vascular surgeon at her hospital, was sympathetic, but left her in no doubt that 50 percent of surgery on varicose veins was cosmetic. "If there is a problem other than appearance, we can fix it, but there is always the possibility that other veins will become varicose. We treat most veins nowadays with injections and bandaging."

However, when he examined Natalie's left leg, he found what he called "an incompetent valve" in the groin. He spent a long time describing the operation to her, showing how he would inject most of the varicose portions below the valve, on the inner part of her thigh and calf, but that he didn't know if he'd end up stripping the vein. Natalie hoped not. She'd nursed some patients whose veins had seemed in better shape than hers, but who had had them removed, and they complained about the pain afterwards.

Dr. Gifford went into some detail about the procedure and its effects. "We talk about a 15 percent chance of recurrence, but it's actually not recurrence. Once injected, a vein doesn't become varicose again — but other veins may." They talked about the fact that although it could be done as day surgery, she'd have to be off work for two to three weeks, so they booked surgery for a time when they knew she'd be able to arrange it.

Natalie felt a bit odd going into her own hospital as a patient, but soon she was on her way to the operating room. After the surgery, she felt a little nauseous from the anesthetic, and her leg hurt under the snug-fitting bandage, but otherwise she was okay. Her throat was sore from the anesthetic tube and she took a little water.

saphenous system, and whether there is any swelling, discoloration, ulceration or evidence of phlebitis. In most patients the decisions about treatment can be made without further investigation, but more sophisticated tests such as Doppler examination (see page 153) can be carried out if necessary. Venography (injecting dye into the veins for examination by X-ray) should be done only if blood clots are suspected in the deep veins or there is concern about incompetent valves.

Non-Surgical Treatment

Visible veins that appear unsightly but are not abnormally tortuous and dilated need no treatment. Varicose veins that develop during or shortly after pregnancy may go down in time. Very small varicosities do not require treatment, but should be observed. If these enlarge, they can be re-assessed and possibly treated.

Low-pressure stockings may help patients with minor varicosities. If the patient has larger varicose veins, particularly below the knee, well-fitting below-the-knee elastic stockings are helpful, especially for the older patient who does not want either injections or surgery, or for patients who have had a deep venous thrombosis and develop secondary varicose veins.

Compression sclerotherapy is a non-surgical treatment that can be used in most patients with varicose veins, particularly veins below the knee. It involves up to 10 injections of a solution that irritates the lining of the vein, causing the vein to close up. This procedure takes approximately 30 minutes, and the patient need not be admitted to the hospital. Each varicosed area is injected with a small amount of solution. Then small pads are placed over the injection site and taped in place. A rubberized bandage is then worn consistently for two weeks, (a plastic bag is worn over the bandage in the shower).

There can be small complications with compression sclerotherapy. In approximately 5 percent of patients, some discoloration occurs over the vein, due to pigmentation from the clotted blood in the vein. Larger veins tend to be somewhat lumpy for the first few months after injection, but these lumps gradually disappear. The chance of other veins becoming varicosed is about 15 percent over five years, but the procedure can be repeated for these recurrences.

Injections are not nearly as effective without the compression bandage. If injections are given alone the recurrence rate is high. Varicose veins below the knee react much better to compression sclerotherapy than those above the knee, because it is more difficult to get adequate pressure with the bandage higher up the leg.

Surgical Treatment

Sometimes the varicose vein is removed, or stripped. This operation is reserved for those patients who have incompetence of either the long or short saphenous veins. The long vein is involved in 95 percent of cases (Fig. 13.7), and is usually due to incompetence of the first valve in the vein. After a while, all the other valves will become incompetent.

Only 10 percent of patients with varicose veins require surgery. Vascular surgeons are reluctant to remove the long saphenous vein because it can be used in other surgical procedures such as coronary artery bypass or femoral popliteal bypass. However, if the vein is diseased or has incompetent valves, it is usually unsuitable for these other operations and can therefore be removed. Removal causes no problems in the return of blood to the heart, because most of the blood returns via the deep system.

The patient usually comes to the hospital in the morning, having had nothing to eat or drink since midnight the night before. The physician examines the varicosities, marking incision sites. The incisions are small. The groin incision is approximately one inch long and the ankle incision one-half inch long. Where necessary other small incisions are made on the leg. Surgeons prefer to use as few incisions as possible, letting injections and the compression bandage take care of any veins missed at the time of surgery, because this gives the best cosmetic appearance.

The patient is given a general anesthetic and incisions are made in the groin and ankle on the inner side. A plastic stripper (wire) is then passed up the vein from the ankle to the groin. The vein in the groin and its branches are tied off at the saphenofemoral junction (Fig. 13.6). A small plastic head is attached to the stripper and placed underneath the skin. The vein is then stripped or pulled out. Through other small incisions the veins are tied off and/or pulled out. The skin is closed with fine nylon sutures, and a tensor bandage is applied to reduce the bruising. The operation takes approximately 30 minutes.

Immediately after the operation the patient is observed in the recovery room until fully awake, and then is returned to a room. After a few hours the patient can be taken home and is encouraged to move about gradually over the next two days. The incisions are painful, and painkillers are usually required. The patient should not do any housework or other major activities for two weeks. Depending on the amount of surgery required, some patients have their stitches taken out at one week and can then return to work. For other patients, it is a month before they can return to work.

Complications

There are few risks to varicose vein surgery, although all operations with an anesthetic carry some risk. The risk of a major bleed is about one in 1,000, usually due to a stitch slipping from the saphenofemoral junction. Bruising is quite common after this surgery, but gradually disappears over a couple of weeks.

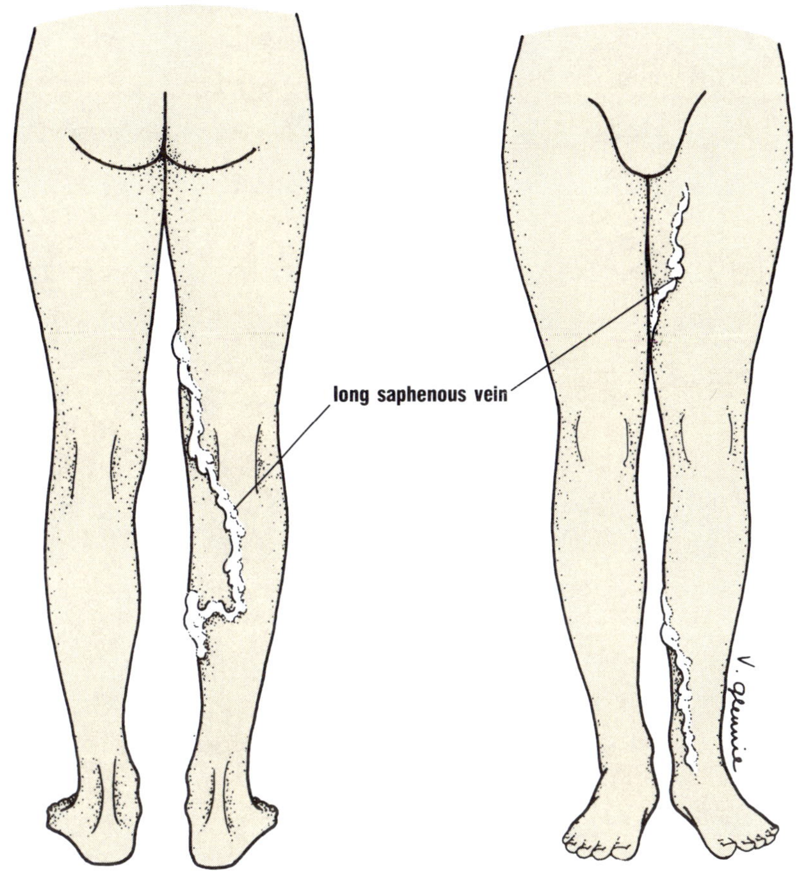

Figure 13.7
Varicose veins affecting the long saphenous system.

Patients may also feel some lumps under the skin; these are blood clots, which will gradually be absorbed into the system. Scars are usually small. They are red at first, but fade to white over six to 12 months. In 2 to 5 percent of patients the skin nerve associated with the vein is damaged and the patient may complain of some numbness around the ankle. This usually does not cause a problem.

Later complications are usually varicosities occurring in other veins. Recurrences cannot happen in a varicose vein that has been surgically removed. The most important factor before surgery is discussing the treatment and the expected results. Patients' expectations are often unrealistic; they must understand that surgery will produce scars, and

Dr. Gifford took the stitches out at the end of a week. The five small scars were red and there were bruises along the vein, but he assured her this was normal for her stage of healing. "I'll see you again at three months, and if there are any small varicosities left, we'll inject them," he told her.

Natalie wasn't sure whether it was the operation or the three weeks off work that did it, but she felt much better on her return to work. Once she got back up to her usual pace, she realized that although she was tired at the end of a shift, her leg didn't ache the way it had done.

that there is a chance of other varicosities developing. Alternatives to surgery should be discussed.

Recent Advances

Over the past 20 years management of varicose veins has gradually become more conservative. Surgery is now done only in selected patients. Future advances will probably involve prevention, better sclerosing solutions and better bandaging techniques.

Chapter 14

Cardiovascular Surgery

Bernard S. Goldman

Professor of Surgery
University of Toronto

Cardiovascular Surgeon
Toronto General Hospital

Hugh E. Scully

Associate Professor of Surgery
University of Toronto

Deputy Surgeon-in-chief
Cardiovascular Surgeon
Toronto General Hospital

Stephen Mader
Illustrator

Heart operations are some of the most publicized types of surgery. Scarcely a week goes by without a television show depicting an inert victim being rushed to the operating room, while surgeons and nurses anxiously watch banks of monitors.

However, although the fear of sudden death is realistic for patients with heart disease, most who undergo surgery are not admitted in an emergency, but to relieve the disabling effects of heart disease.

Advances in Cardiovascular Surgery

Less than a century ago, the leading surgeons of Europe declared that the art and craft of surgery had reached its zenith, and that "He who dared to operate upon the heart would incur the wrath of his colleagues." Thirty years ago, the first open heart surgery was performed. Today, the coronary bypass graft operation alone will probably be performed on almost 200,000 patients in North America, making it the most common of all major surgical procedures. Dramatic progress in the correction of congenital heart defects and disorders of heart valves has also marked these last three decades.

Because the emotional and financial cost of heart surgery is high, and because its growth has been so dramatic, over the years there have been numerous controversies over its value. There is now, however, a consensus on the value of modern heart surgery in the rehabilitation and lifespan of cardiac patients.

The heart is actually a simple muscular pump that primarily responds to nervous impulses and hormones. Each heartbeat is a contraction of the heart muscle that pumps blood through a network of approximately 60,000 miles of blood vessels to reach every cell in the body. In a healthy person at rest, the heart usually pumps four to five quarts of blood per minute. During exercise, this rate may increase four to five times.

The heart contains four chambers. The chambers on the right collect blood without oxygen and pump it to the lungs, which provide oxygen. This blood is then collected in the chambers of the left side of the heart and pumped to the body. Many congenital heart defects involve primarily the right side of the heart and pulmonary (lung) circuits. Most adult coronary and valve disorders involve the left heart (systemic circuit).

The pace of the heart pump depends on the volume of returning blood and the pressure in the peripheral circulation against which it must beat. The volume of blood returning to the heart pump is called "preload," and the pressure in the circulation is the "afterload."

All of the body's muscles and organs receive their nutrition from the blood. The heart must also nourish itself with oxygen and other nutrients via the coronary arteries (Fig. 14.1).

The valves that control the inflow and outflow of blood from the collecting and pumping chambers are thin. They may be deformed at birth, deteriorate with age, become hardened and brittle or be scarred. They may leak, causing an excess volume load upon the heart, or may become obstructed, causing an excess pressure load. In either event, the burden on the heart will ultimately result in symptoms of poor forward output (fatigue, light-headedness, fainting) or backward failure, with increased pressure in the lungs and liver (shortness of breath, abdominal swelling, ankle swelling).

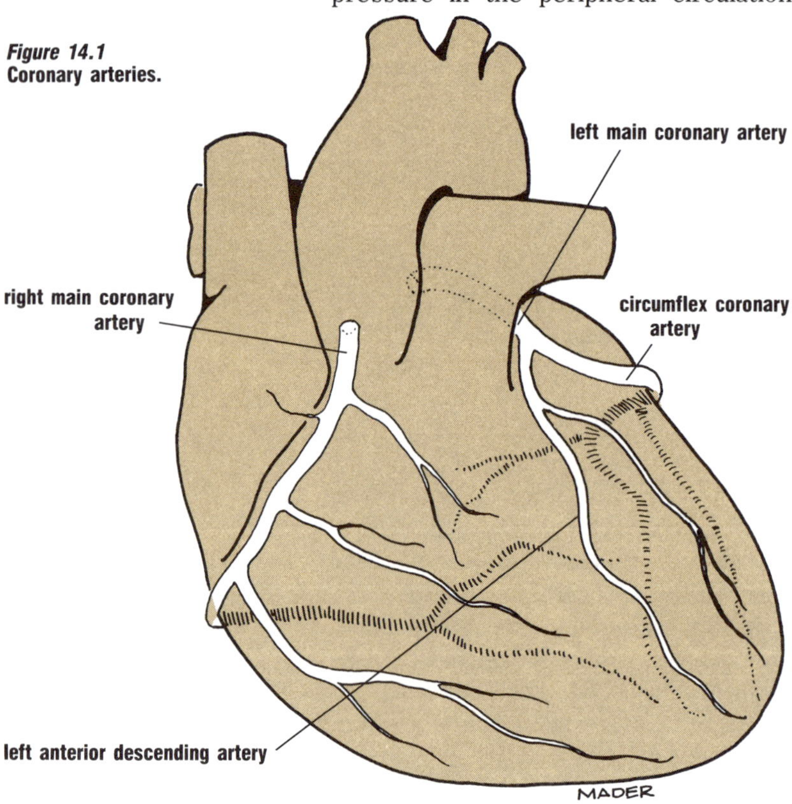

Figure 14.1
Coronary arteries.

Coronary Bypass Graft

The coronary arteries are muscular tubes with a smooth lining that may constrict or dilate, depending on the heart muscle's need for oxygenated blood. Coronary atherosclerosis is the gradual layering of cholesterol and other body fats on the wall of the coronary artery, as a result of hereditary factors or conditions that produce excess cholesterol.

Atherosclerosis can also be aggravated by obesity, smoking and diabetes. The fatty deposit can cause the inner lining of the artery to become swollen and ulcerate, resulting in a blood clot (coronary thrombosis). All of this will narrow the artery's inner diameter (lumen), slowing the blood flow and ultimately obstructing the artery (Fig. 14.2).

When a coronary artery narrows to 60 percent of the inner diameter, there may be a decrease in the velocity and quantity of coronary blood flow, particularly at times when more oxygen is required e.g., when the heart rate or blood pressure increases due to anemia, hyperthyroidism, hypertension, exercise, smoking or stress. The oxygen supply may then be inadequate to meet the oxygen demand from the heart.

Diagnosis

The symptoms and outcome of coronary atherosclerosis may be many and varied. Some patients suffer no symptoms and no consequences; others die without warning. Most commonly patients develop pain in the chest (angina pectoris), which can vary from mild to severe. It may be tolerable or disabling, stable (predictable with effort) or unstable (unpredictable at rest).

These symptoms indicate a poor blood supply to the heart muscle, which may eventually lead to a heart attack (myocardial infarction) — a lack of blood to part of the heart, resulting in damage to the heart muscle. Coronary atherosclerosis can also cause gradual scarring of the heart muscle, which can cause heart failure or irregular heart rhythms. The most difficult condition for patients and physicians to manage is "silent angina" — no symptoms, but evidence on the resting ECG or an exercise stress test of poor coronary blood flow.

The routine electrocardiogram taken at rest is often of little help in assessing coronary blood flow, unless the patient is in pain when the ECG is taken, although it may reveal old or recent heart muscle damage. An electrocardiogram taken during exercise on a treadmill (stress test) may reveal inadequate oxygen supply to the coronary arteries by gradually increasing the demand on the heart muscle. If this test is combined with an intravenous injection of nuclear isotope (thallium 201), areas of heart muscle can be detected that have impaired blood flow during exercise. Abnormalities of contraction in the heart muscle wall can be found by X-ray of the blood vessels

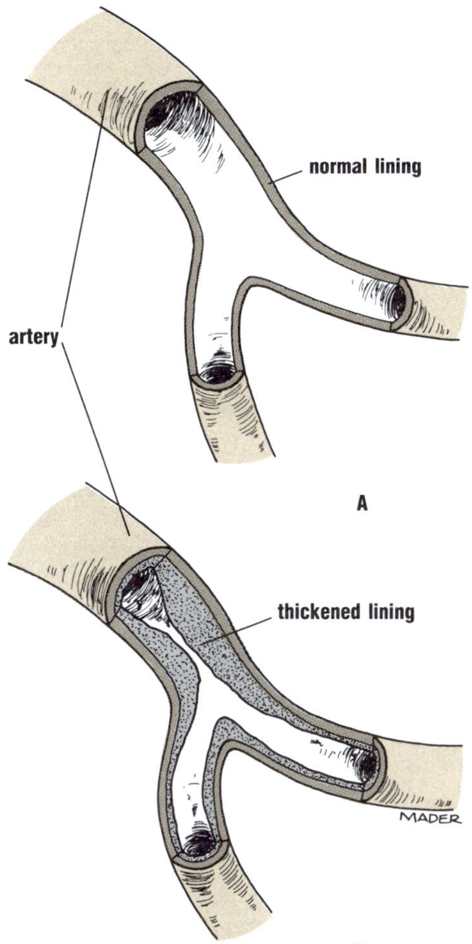

Figure 14.2
Atherosclerosis. A normal artery lining (A) can become thickened with fatty deposits, narrowing the artery's inner diameter, or lumen (B).

(angiogram) or ultrasound pictures (echocardiograms).

The ultimate test for determining the presence and degree of narrowing in the coronary arteries is coronary angiography. This consists of advancing a small tube up into the coronary arteries via a small puncture into an artery in the groin or arm. A dye is then injected that can outline the blood vessels on film. This is not generally a dangerous procedure, but one in 1,000 patients will suffer heart attack or death from it. Patients may also suffer stroke or damage to the artery in the leg.

Normal coronary arteries are found on

Case Study: Coronary Bypass Graft

Rob was 54 when he had his first heart attack. His wife, Margaret, maintained she was the one who had nearly died — of fright. It was what the doctor called a "small" heart attack, meaning it hadn't done a great deal of damage. Rob knew he'd been lucky, so he stopped smoking, something his wife had been trying to get him to do for years. He also enrolled in an exercise program at the local Y, and after a few months he felt better than ever.

But three years later, Rob wasn't feeling so well. Every time he got up to do anything — his jogging, the odd game of squash, even gardening — he was getting pain in his chest. It wasn't the sudden stabbing pain he'd had with the heart attack, more of a squeezing or tightness, but it worried him.

Dr. Jacks referred him for an exercise stress test. "I'd like to see what the ECG says when you've had a bit of exertion, Rob." The exercise stress test a week later showed changes in the electrocardiogram once Rob had been walking the conveyor belt for about five minutes. Dr. Jacks told him that he'd like to try medication for a while, to see if the chest pain decreased. "Am I going to have another heart attack, Doctor?" asked Rob. "I think your coronary arteries aren't pumping enough blood into your heart, Rob. The medication may help. If it doesn't, an angiogram — a kind of heart X-ray — will tell us what we should do next."

Rob worked at his exercise program, took his medication, and went on a low-fat, low-sodium diet. But he had to admit after three months that he was worse, not better. The pills gave him insomnia, which he could have coped with, but he also had no energy. It took the fun out of life. Then, when he discovered that he was impotent, he was back in Dr. Jacks' office. "Isn't there anything else we can do, Doctor?"

Dr. Jacks sent Rob to the local hospital for an angiogram. "This will show us where the problem is, Rob. It may be possible to stretch your arteries a bit with a balloon catheter. If not, I'm afraid we're looking at surgery."

The angiogram told the cardiologist that Rob had a problem in three of his coronary arteries. "If it's one or two, we usually try angioplasty, but in your case I'd recommend surgery." The cardiologist was very straightforward. "Heart disease is unpredictable, but coronary artery bypass is the most commonly performed operation in North America today — because it works. You'll spend a couple of days in intensive care, because this is major surgery, but you'll only be in hospital about a week. Providing all goes well, you could be back at work in six weeks, feeling better than you have done in months." Rob and Margaret left his office with an appointment to see the cardiovascular surgeon the following week.

angiography in 10 percent of patients with symptoms. About 10 percent of patients with symptoms are found to have inoperable coronary artery disease. Severe life-threatening obstructions are found in 15 percent of patients with symptoms, and almost 30 percent have coronary artery narrowing that can be treated with the insertion of a small balloon that is inflated to dilate the artery (angioplasty).

Non-Surgical Treatment

Coronary artery disease is treated surgically or non-surgically, sometimes with a combination of the two, depending on the patient's age, lifestyle, findings at coronary angiography and the condition of the heart muscle wall. In most instances, non-surgical therapy should be tried first in patients who have symptoms (usually angina). This will consist of dietary management to reduce cholesterol intake, weight loss, cessation of smoking, an exercise rehabilitation program, stress reduction and possibly an alteration of life-style and employment. Certain drugs are used to dilate the coronary arteries, reduce high blood pressure, decrease the heart rate and lessen the force of heart muscle contraction, decreasing the heart's oxygen requirements. Associated disorders such as hyperthyroidism, anemia and diabetes should be treated. The value of vitamin E or fad diets is dubious.

Coronary angiography may reveal isolated narrowings in one or two coronary arteries. In such instances, angioplasty may improve coronary blood flow through the diseased segment. Angioplasty involves widening the narrowed segment by inserting an inflatable balloon at the tip of a coronary catheter. It is performed during angiography (Fig. 14.3). Almost 90 percent of narrowed arteries can be dilated, improving not only blood flow but also symptoms. Angioplasty should be performed only by a skilled cardiologist, since there is a 3 to 5 percent risk of damaging the artery, which may require emergency surgery. Furthermore, almost 30 percent of dilated segments may narrow again, necessitating another angioplasty or bypass surgery. Therefore, while angioplasty is useful and relatively simple, there are complications, including a possible recurrence of the problem.

Surgical Treatment

The coronary artery bypass operation was first introduced in 1967. Although there have been periods of doubt and concern about its overusage in the last 20 years, the benefits are now reasonably clear.

A living graft is taken from the lower leg (the saphenous vein), and used as a detour route around the area of arterial narrowing or blockage. This rarely

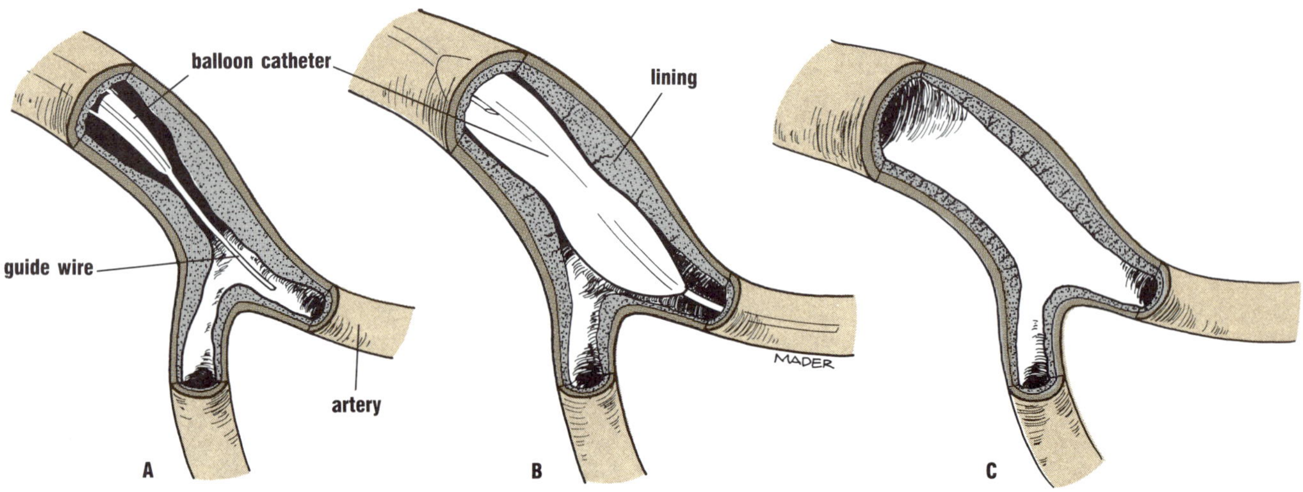

Figure 14.3
Angioplasty. A balloon catheter is inserted into the artery (A) and inflated (B) to improve the lumen (C).

produces any significant problem in the leg, which has many alternative veins. Recently, the artery from inside the chest wall (internal mammary artery) has been used for coronary artery bypass, because the artery size match and the duration of successful function are better than those of the saphenous vein (Fig. 14.4). Veins taken from the arm and synthetic substitutes have been less satisfactory.

Coronary bypass graft surgery has profoundly improved the quality of life for patients with severe angina who do not respond to non-surgical treatment. It has also dramatically improved the lifespan of patients with multiple coronary artery obstructions. In patients with only single or double vessel narrowing and good heart muscle contraction, the coronary artery bypass may significantly improve physical capacity, but may not be better than drugs in improving lifespan.

The prerequisite for bypass graft surgery depends on the coronary anatomy. The artery should be narrowed by atherosclerosis to at least 60 percent of its diameter, with a relatively healthy blood vessel beyond, to which the bypass can be connected. This artery should be serving an area of functioning, unscarred heart muscle or otherwise the bypass would not accomplish anything.

On the day before surgery, patients are usually introduced to the ICU nurse, the physiotherapist and the anesthetist. They also view a teaching videotape that prepares them for the postoperative period. This practice has become common in most hospitals, although the format may differ slightly.

Coronary bypass graft surgery is classified as open heart surgery, although the heart is not actually opened, since the coronary arteries are on the surface. The surgeon exposes the heart by cutting through the breastbone, which is then held open during the operation (Fig. 14.5). The envelope surrounding the heart (pericardium) is opened and the heart is connected by tubes to an external heart-lung pump, which will drain unoxygenated blood and deliver it back to the aorta as oxygenated blood. The artificial heart-lung pump can sustain normal circulation for over four hours, protecting all other vital organs while the bypass graft surgery is performed. The

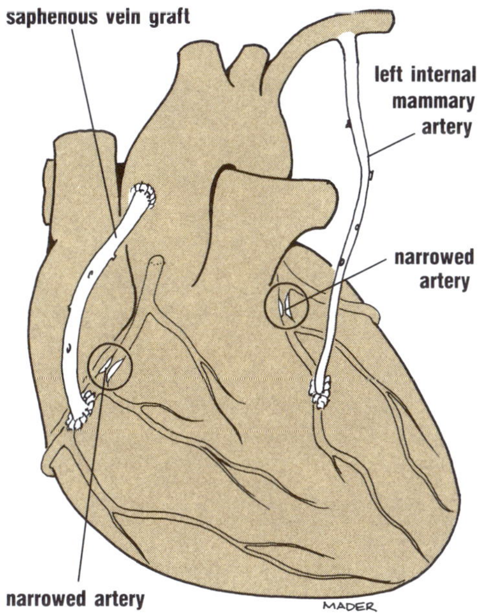

Figure 14.4
Coronary artery bypass. The graft bypasses the diseased portion of the artery.

Dr. Perreault explained to Rob exactly what would happen during the surgery, showing him with diagrams where they'd take the bypass graft from, and where it would go. He described the risks and benefits of the surgery, making it clear that no surgery was risk free, especially heart surgery, but that the benefits were greater than the risks. "In cases like yours, where we've found no other problem, we feel very optimistic."

Rob wanted to know what lay ahead. "The future depends on many things. Because patients live longer now, we are seeing them again for repeat surgery in ten to twelve years. But for that time they've been pain free and able to carry on their normal activities."

Six weeks later, Rob was admitted to the university hospital. Although he was nervous, he'd had enough of feeling disabled. The pain in his chest had been getting worse despite the medication, and there was little he could do now that didn't give him pain.

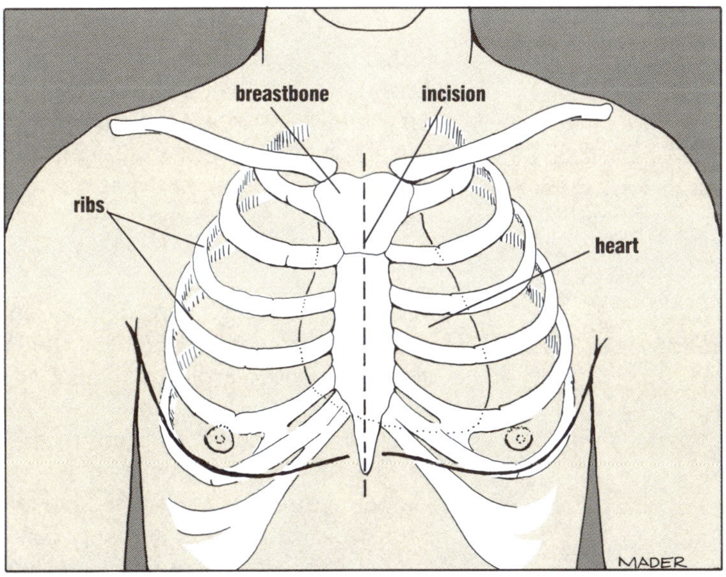

Figure 14.5
Midline incision for open heart surgery.

In addition to visits from Dr. Perreault, the resident, the anesthetist and the physiotherapist, Rob and Margaret were shown a videotape of postoperative care, and Rob was taught exercises that would help clear congestion from his lungs after the operation.

Dr. Perreault performed the surgery. He met with Margaret afterwards to tell her that Rob would be in intensive care for 24 to 48 hours and that he would be on a respirator to give his lungs a rest.

After 24 hours, Rob was moved to the stepdown unit, where the patients were all sitting up. He'd begun his exercises under the watchful eye of the nurse, and secretly rejoiced in every movement. The next day, Rob was back in his regular room and was even taking trips down the corridor.

Dr. Perreault was very helpful. "Physically, I expect him to be very capable once the convalescent period is over. If we can channel his drive into recreation instead of work, he'll do very well." He told Rob the same thing. "There's no evangelist as zealous as a bypass patient, because he feels so much better. But that new energy has to be channeled into healthier ways of living."

Rob waited a full three months before returning to work. His exercise stress test at that time showed considerable improvement, but he would have to continue taking medication. The surgeon was happy with his progress two months after surgery. "The incisions have healed well, and the ECG shows no abnormalities. With care, you should be in good shape for a normal lifespan."

heart is actually stopped during the bypass surgery, by an injection of cold potassium solution which arrests the heart while the bypass graft is being constructed. The heart can be safely stopped for over two hours.

The bypass grafts are sewn to the coronary artery, using fine polypropylene sutures. Small metal clips are often used on side branches of the vein or mammary artery bypass to stop bleeding; these can be seen on the chest X-ray afterwards, as can the stainless-steel wires used to bring the breastbone back together.

After surgery, the patient is usually kept sedated and connected to a breathing machine (ventilator) overnight to keep the lungs expanded and to give the heart a rest. In the early morning, the anesthetist will remove the breathing tube, the physiotherapist will begin instructions on deep breathing and coughing exercises, and the nurse will soon have the patient sitting up and doing some gentle leg and arm exercises. A soft fluid diet is begun. The chest tubes, which drain off excess fluid around the heart and lungs, are usually removed within 48 hours, by which time the patient may have been moved to a secondary intensive care or "stepdown" unit, which is in an area either adjacent to the intensive care unit or adjacent to the regular ward.

In general, most patients with stable angina and good heart muscle function are out of the intensive care unit within 24 hours. However, patients who are elderly, whose cardiac condition is unstable, who have suffered a recent heart attack, have poor cardiac muscle function or are obese or heavy smokers, can expect to spend at least two days in the intensive care unit after surgery. This can be a somewhat distressing experience. Often people feel "out of control" and become depressed at what seems to be lack of progress.

The stepdown unit provides intermediate care between the intensive care unit and return to a regular room on the ward. Patients usually spend only one day in the stepdown unit, but it may be longer if some rhythm disturbance of the heart requires monitoring. Another reason might be the need for intensive physiotherapy, as in a smoker who has difficulty clearing mucus from his or her lungs. Once back in a regular room after 48 or 72 hours, patients are usually quite comfortable and mobile. They are able to go to the bathroom alone, wash, eat regular meals, have company and walk the ward corridors.

Obviously there is some chest discomfort, and the deep breathing exercises are occasionally a chore, especially for smokers. Nonetheless, the midline incision is one of the most comfortable of incisions. The overriding complaint is that of fatigue and difficulty sleeping. Neither are significant and will readjust with time.

Many patients suffer temporary depression. Before discharging patients six to eight days after operation, the convalescent period may be discussed and reinforced with a teaching videotape that covers expectations for the subsequent month. The physiotherapists provide information about activity, exercise and enrolment in a rehabilitation program.

Most patients with sedentary jobs can go back to work after six weeks. Those whose jobs require heavy physical labor can usually return after three months. The extended recovery period actually has very little to do with the heart. It is more related to the overall stress of surgery on the body with some weight loss and aching about the chest wall that eases with gradual healing. There is often some lingering ankle swelling in the leg from which the graft was taken, or some tingling in the left side of the chest where the internal mammary artery has been removed. There is usually an arthritic type of ache in the neck, shoulders and chest wall that is more noticeable rolling over in bed or putting on a sweater.

Although most patients can go directly home, the elderly and infirm often benefit from a week or so in a convalescent hospital.

The first two weeks after discharge

from hospital are an extension of hospital routine at home, focusing on rest and increasing daily activity. Patients should restrict the number of visitors but be encouraged to climb stairs or go for short walks, despite fatigue. In the second two weeks, patients are usually encouraged to go out for longer walks, for a drive or even out for dinner. In the third two weeks, patients should be living essentially a normal life, except for their usual employment. Some may actually wish to drop into their office or workplace, while others may wish to relax at a cottage. There are usually no restrictions on travel, but the incision should be protected from sunburn by a sun-screening agent, swimming should be limited to gentle strokes, and such things as tennis and golf should be avoided until about three months after the operation.

Patients should see their family doctor and/or cardiologist within two to four weeks after surgery, to readjust medications and diet. Most surgeons like to review progress and look at the incisions six to eight weeks after an operation. A stress exercise test is recommended at about three months after surgery to document the degree of improvement, determine the need for continued supplementary medication and allow for some form of exercise prescription or enrollment in a rehabilitation program. Stress exercise testings should then be done annually.

The mortality rate from this operation is low (1 to 3 percent) and more than 60 percent of patients experience marked relief of symptoms. However, while 98 percent of patients survive surgery, not all are totally free of symptoms thereafter: 15 to 25 percent may still require anti-anginal or antihypertensive drugs. All require antiplatelet drugs to keep the blood thin and prevent clotting within the graft. While most patients have a marked increase in their exercise capacity, those who enroll in a supervised exercise rehabilitation program and follow all the usual guidelines for good medical therapy (cessation of smoking, weight and stress reduction) obtain the best results from surgery.

A number of patients may need a repeat angiography and even reoperation. Almost 50 percent of saphenous vein bypasses may obstruct within 10 years, due to new atherosclerosis in the graft. This only happens with 15 percent of internal mammary artery bypasses, which is the reason for increasing use of this bypass. Patients who are operated on at a younger age, those who underwent surgery in the earlier days of bypass grafting, and especially those with a progressive metabolic disorder that results in continued cholesterol deposits, are all more likely to require reoperation.

The vast majority of patients experience a resurgence of vitality, accompanied by a freedom from fear and disabling symptoms. Coronary bypass patients tend to be ''evangelical'' because they feel so much better. Those below retirement age usually go back to their former employment with the security and knowledge that they can once more be self-sufficient. Patients over retirement age are usually able to enjoy their leisure time with increased confidence and physical capacity. However, the expectations for a middle-aged male who undergoes an early bypass graft operation, stops smoking and enrolls in a rehabilitation program is different from those for the elderly patient with a long history of heart disease, several heart attacks and damaged heart muscle. The younger patient's risk of dying from the operation is less than 1 percent, and rehabilitation will be virtually complete. The older patient's risk of dying may exceed five percent, and improvement in function and life-style is sometimes limited. In the public's perception, all bypass operations are the same, but there is a striking difference in operative risk and physical result in different patients. Prospective candidates for this operation should discuss their expectations fully with their cardiologists and/or surgeon before undergoing bypass graft surgery.

Case Study: Heart Valve Surgery

Miriam was always "on the go." In addition to her part-time job, she had always been involved in PTA committees, hospital volunteer groups, neighborhood action groups and political campaigning during election time. At 50, she was a powerhouse of experience. But she found herself beginning to tire in the afternoons, and although she wasn't overweight, she was beginning to puff and pant as she bustled through her day.

When she began to waken at night short of breath, however, Miriam knew that this was something more than her age and busy schedule. She hadn't had regular checkups, and when she went to see Dr. Evans she was asked a lot of questions about her medical history. After listening very carefully to her heart, her doctor asked if she'd ever had an illness with fever as a teenager. "I had the flu pretty badly one time — I remember that because I couldn't go on a school trip. But what's that got to do with me being short of breath now?"

"I picked up a murmur when I was listening to your heart, Miriam. I think you may have had rheumatic fever as a child. It could be causing the problem you're having now. I'd like you to have an ECG so we can check the rhythm of your heart." Dr. Evans made an immediate appointment for her at the laboratory, where she was able to watch the tracing of her heart rhythm on the ECG monitor.

When she was given the appointment with the cardiologist, Miriam still couldn't believe that she had heart trouble. The cardiologist did all of the same examinations as Dr. Evans, including another ECG. He explained that one of the valves in her heart was damaged, and it was now beginning to cause problems. He gave her three different kinds of medication: digitalis to correct her heart rhythm, a diuretic to get rid of the excess fluid in her system, and potassium to replace the natural potassium that the diuretic washed out.

Recent Advances

Although the death rate from cardiovascular disease is decreasing, people are living longer, which eventually means more people with coronary problems. We are now seeing patients in their seventies and eighties requesting coronary bypass surgery for complications of coronary atherosclerosis. Not only are they older, but their heart conditions are more severe and complex. This trend will probably continue, since milder cases will be treated effectively by medication and/or angioplasty.

Repeat coronary artery bypass surgery will become more frequent, as patients return eight to 12 years after their initial operation, looking for another decade of relief and increased activity. Our techniques of protecting heart muscle before, during and after surgery will improve, and the operation will likely be extended to higher-risk patients. At the other end of the scale, patients with failed coronary bypass or inoperable coronary artery disease may anticipate successful rehabilitation with a heart transplant.

In the operating room, we will soon be able to effectively dilate arteries that are not graftable, core out the inside of the narrowed artery by laser technology and then look down the inside of the bypass graft or the artery with an angioscope.

Prevention is still the best cure, but it is unlikely that alterations of diet or smoking alone will rid Western civilization of coronary atherosclerosis within the next few generations.

Heart Valve Surgery

Surgical replacement or repair of diseased heart valves has been practiced since the 1960s. Over 80,000 valve replacement operations are now performed each year all over the world. In North America, 13 people out of every 100,000 undergo valve operations each year.

Some people are born with abnormalities of the valves. For example, approximately 1 percent of people have two cusps or leaflets in the aortic valve instead of three (Fig. 14.6). Some people have rheumatic fever during childhood or adolescence which may damage the valves. Others develop progressive scarring or degeneration of the valves later in life. A severe bacterial infection in the bloodstream may occasionally infect and damage even normal heart valves. Abnormal valves or implanted artificial valves are especially susceptible to damage from bloodstream infections.

If a valve does not close properly, blood may flow backwards. If a valve is constricted or narrowed, it may allow too little blood to pass through. A damaged heart valve may cause part of the heart muscle to thicken and enlarge because it has to work harder to pump the required amount of blood to the body.

These conditions may lead to congestion (accumulation of fluid) in the lungs, or the liver, or both. The increased load on the heart combined with the lung or liver congestion can lead to chronic fatigue, unusual shortness of breath on exertion and, at a more advanced stage, shortness of breath when lying down, plus swelling of the ankles and abdomen. Sometimes patients with narrowing of the aortic valve will experience a tightness or pain in the chest or a feeling of lightheadedness because not enough oxygenated blood is reaching the heart or the brain.

Diagnosis

Heart valve disease is diagnosed by the patient's history of symptoms, a physical examination, and special tests to determine the condition of the heart.

As heart valves open and close, they make characteristic sounds that can be heard through a stethoscope. Diseased valves also make characteristic sounds. These sounds, usually murmurs due to turbulence in flow created by the dis-

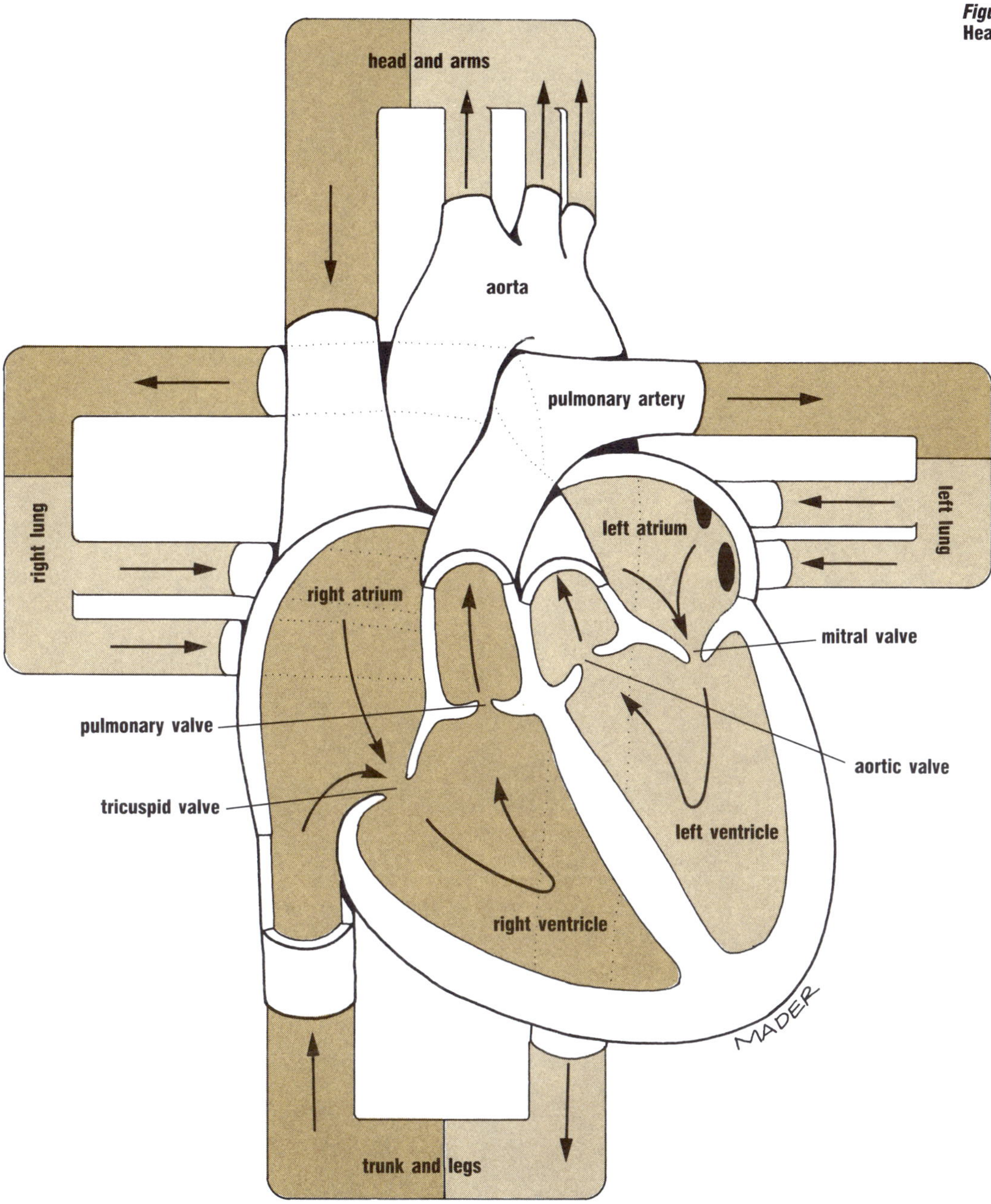

Figure 14.6
Heart valves and chambers.

eased valves, may help the physician reach a diagnosis.

Different tests provide different types of information about the structure and the function of the heart. A chest X-ray gives information about the size of the heart and its chambers, as well as the presence of any congestion in the lungs. An electrocardiogram (ECG) gives important information about enlargement of the heart's pumping chamber as well as about rhythm disturbances which characteristically accompany some types of valvular heart disease. Specialized tests using ultrasound can give valuable information about chamber size and individual valve function. Heart catheterization — special tubes inserted into and around the

For three years that seemed to do the trick, but then the old fatigue and the shortness of breath came back. The cardiologist had changed her medication over the years, but her lungs seemed to be more congested. He recommended a complete examination of her heart, including catheterization, which he explained was the passing of a catheter into her heart to see what was happening to the blood flow.

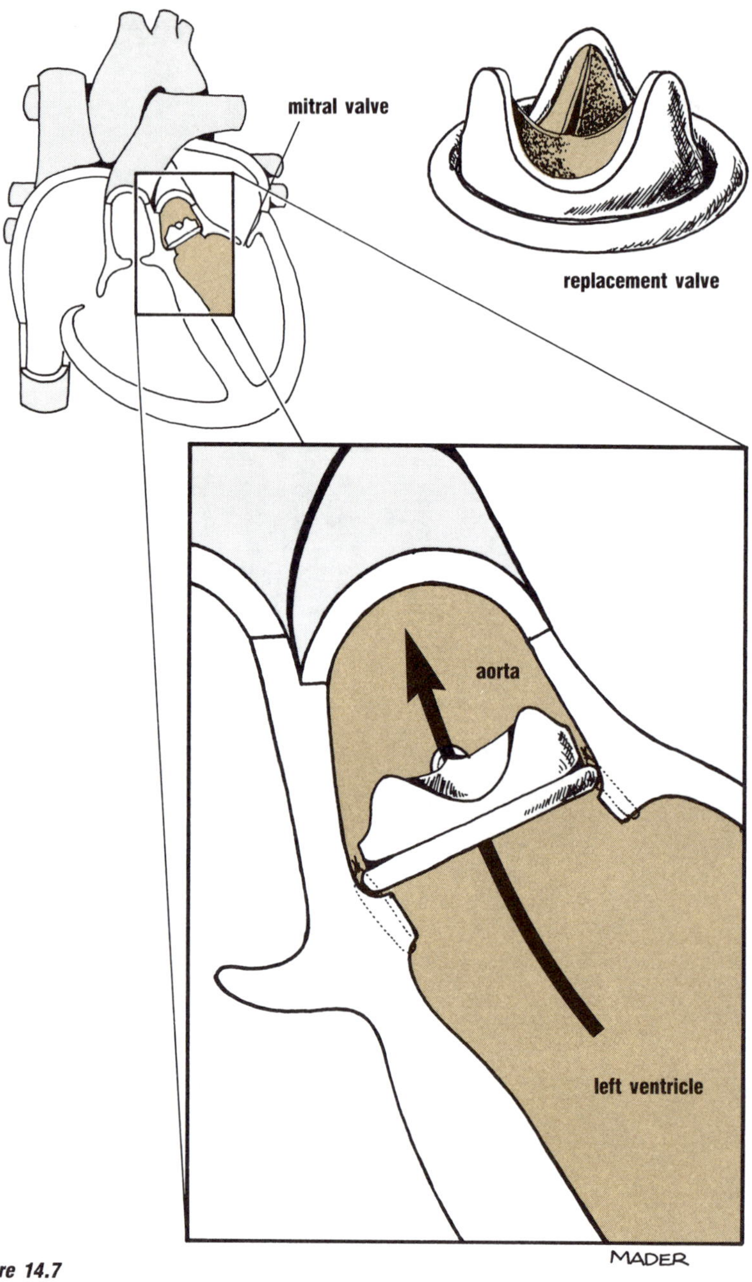

Figure 14.7
Aortic valve replacement (tissue valve). The replacement valve is secured in place with sutures.

heart to measure pressure and inject dye which can be seen on X-ray — is often required to define the extent of valve disease and its effect on the heart. This test will also reveal the presence of any other heart condition, such as coronary artery disease. Using all of these results, the physician establishes a diagnosis and determines if, when and what surgery is necessary.

Non-Surgical Treatment

When all the test results are in, a physician may recommend to a patient that surgical treatment is not immediately necessary. In these circumstances medications to improve the rate, rhythm and contraction of the heart are usually prescribed, and arrangements are made for regular assessment of the patient's heart and general condition. If medications are prescribed, they must be taken as instructed. Taking medication on a regular schedule at the same time every day helps maintain correct levels of the drugs in the body, and helps to remind patients to take the medications.

Surgical Treatment

When surgery is recommended, it should be performed at an early date. Studies have clearly shown that patients with increasingly disabling symptoms from diseased heart valves usually deteriorate rapidly. They become more and more disabled, and if surgery is not performed, often die within 18 months to five years of recommendation of surgery, depending on the nature of the valve disease.

No one relishes the prospect of a major operation such as heart surgery. However, many studies show that 75 to 90 percent of patients undergoing heart valve repair or replacement live 10 years or more after the operation, and feel better than they did before surgery.

The aortic and mitral valves are the most common valves that require surgery. At present it is not usually possible to repair the aortic valve, so it is usually replaced if it develops a problem. However, it is possible to repair the mitral valve. This is particularly true in patients under age 60, and when the valve's degeneration or narrowing is detected early. Since the patient's own valve, satisfactorily repaired, functions significantly better than an artificial valve, every effort is made to repair the valve if possible.

Two types of artificial valves are used for valve replacement today: tissue valves and mechanical valves.

Tissue valves, or bioprosthetic valves, are made either from the aortic valves of pigs or from the pericardium (the sac that enfolds the heart in the chest) of the cow. The animal tissue is treated to preserve the strength of the tissue while assuring that no living cells remain to cause a ''rejection'' reaction (Fig. 14.7).

Human aortic valves (aortic homografts), specially prepared and taken from people who had normal hearts who died for other reasons, may be used to replace the aortic valve.

The major advantage of tissue valves is that patients do not require blood thinners (anticoagulants) after the initial implantation, unless there are other reasons for their use. The major disadvantage is that these valves do not last forever. Approximately 20 to 30 percent fail eight to 10 years from the time of implantation. In younger patients (under age 40, and especially in children), the rate of tissue valve failures appear to be greater, perhaps due to more active metabolism or greater stresses on valves in this more active age group. In patients over age 60, the failure rate appears to be somewhat less. When tissue valves do fail, patients may experience the symptoms that led to surgery in the first place; repeat valve surgery is usually required.

Mechanical valves, by contrast, are entirely manufactured. Their advantage is durability: some mechanical valves have been in place for over 25 years. All mechanical valves have a slight sound, like the click of a small clock, and all patients with mechanical valves require anticoagulants. Structural failure of mechanical valves is very rare, but if one should fail, it must be replaced (Fig. 14.8).

Tissue valves and mechanical valves work equally well. The risk of blood clots forming is approximately the same for patients with tissue valves not taking anticoagulants and patients with mechanical valves taking anticoagulants: just over 1 percent each year. In circumstances with easy access to treatment, the risk of serious bleeding complications from taking anticoagulants has been reduced to approximately 1 percent a year. Therefore, the choice of valves is based on durability, the need for anticoagulants, and the patient's lifestyle, occupation and expectations. Patients who will not or should not take anticoagulants, for example, should receive tissue valves. Patients who will require long-term anticoagulants for other reasons normally receive mechanical valves. There is a general tendency to use mechanical valves more frequently in patients under age 40 and tissue valves in patients over age 60.

The mortality rate for heart valve operations varies from zero to 15 percent, depending on the patient's general health and the stage of his or her heart disease. Patients with aortic valve disease deteriorate more rapidly than patients with mitral valve disease and are often recommended for surgery at an earlier stage when their general condition is better. The risks of aortic valve replacement surgery therefore tend to be lower than for mitral replacement.

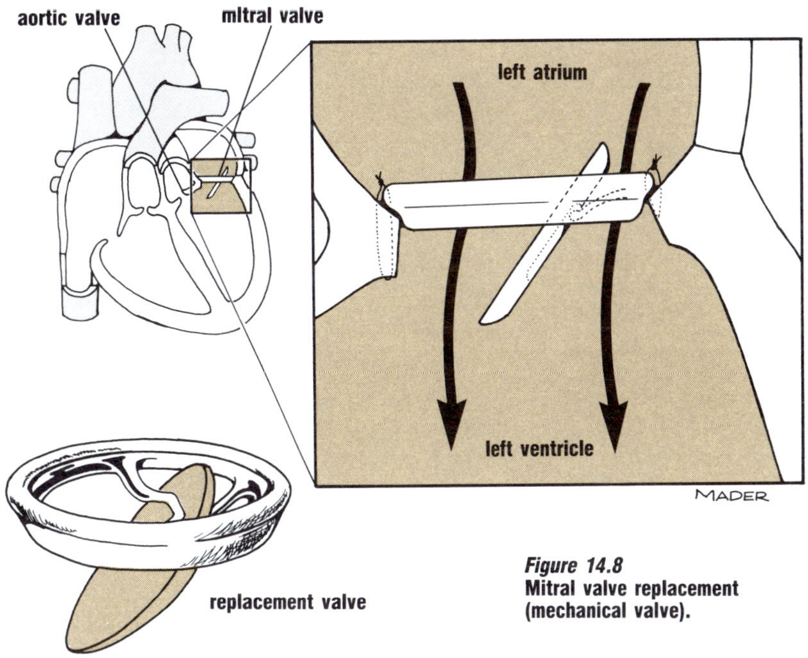

Figure 14.8
Mitral valve replacement (mechanical valve).

Miriam didn't mind the ultrasound pictures that were taken of her heart, but she did find the catheterization scary. The cardiologist had explained that they'd check to see whether the problem was just in the valve, or if any of the arteries were narrowing as well.

When she returned to see him after the tests, he came straight to the point. ''I've discussed your case with my surgical colleague and we agree that surgery seems advisable.''

When Miriam saw the surgeon, he was quite reassuring. ''You probably think that because we use surgery as a last resort, it means you're dying, but that's far from the case. We now have many patients who have lived twenty years after their surgery, and we certainly expect seventy-five percent of our patients to live at least ten years. In your case I'm quite hopeful, because you're in otherwise good condition.'' He ordered the routine preoperative tests such as chest X-ray, urinalysis and blood typing to be done at the local hospital just before she was admitted to the downtown hospital.

Within a few weeks Miriam found herself in the university hospital "taking a course," as she put it, in how to be a heart surgery patient. There were videotapes, classes and exercises to be learned. The surgeon had explained to her that they would try to repair the damaged mitral valve in the heart. If repair wasn't possible, they'd replace the valve, probably with a mechanical one rather than one made from animal tissue.
The operation took three and one-half hours. Miriam would spend the next two days in intensive care.

Miriam left hospital with a Medic-Alert bracelet, anticoagulant medication, a prescription for antibiotics for her next trip to the dentist — and strict instructions to report any infection, however small, to her doctor immediately. She also had a follow-up appointment with the Valve Clinic at the hospital.

She found that within nine months she had returned to her usual activities, and was gradually becoming as busy as ever.

The mortality rate for repair of the mitral or tricuspid valve is less than 1 percent. Aortic valve replacement carries a risk of 1 to 4 percent, again depending on the condition of the valve, the heart, the patient and the complexity of the procedure.

The mortality rate for mitral valve replacement is the same for either tissue or mechanical valve surgery: 4 to 8 percent. The risk of double valve replacement (usually aortic and mitral) is 8 to 12 percent, and the risk of triple valve surgery is 15 percent. The risk of repeat valve surgery is only slightly greater than the risk for a "first-time" valve operation, if the patient is otherwise in good condition.

In general, medications already prescribed should be continued until the time of surgery, unless specifically changed by the physicians. Smokers should stop smoking at least a few weeks before the operation to make the clearing of secretions from the lungs easier after surgery. In hospital, breathing and other exercises are taught for recovery of normal function and activity as soon as possible after surgery.

Like most surgical patients, heart surgery patients are given mild sedatives the night before surgery. These sedatives do not depress the heart action. Special arrangements are often made for patients with diabetes.

Heart operations usually last from three to six hours, depending on their complexity. After surgery, patients are taken to a special cardiac surgical intensive care unit from 12 hours to three or four days, again depending on the complexity of the procedure and the patient's general condition. If the patient has other medical conditions as well, a longer stay in the intensive care unit is likely.

The usual incision used to reach the heart and the great vessels is made down the middle of the chest through the breastbone. This incision in fact produces the least discomfort of the various incisions that can be made in the chest or abdomen. It also provides the best access for the surgical team. Occasionally a surgeon will choose to make an incision in the groin, because it may be preferable to use the artery in the groin for one of the connections to the heart/lung machine. This is often the case in repeat surgery for valve disease. If coronary artery bypasses are being carried out at the same time, there may also be an incision along the inner part of the leg to remove a length of vein for grafting.

Heart surgery uses permanent stitches. The breastbone is brought back together with heavy-gauge wire sutures that also remain in place permanently. These wire sutures show up on chest X-rays, but cause no problems.

Other incisions are usually brought together with absorbable sutures that do not need to be removed. Occasionally skin stitches or clips may be used, which require removal before discharge from hospital.

During heart surgery, a general anesthetic is used. The heart and lungs are placed at complete rest and a heart/lung machine takes over their function. The body temperature is also lowered to reduce the amount of oxygen demanded by the heart and other tissues. The heart itself is cooled further by either cold solution or cold blood, creating a still, quiet field for the surgeon and relaxing the tissues, making the technical aspect of the surgery easier. Once the surgical repairs have been completed, the whole process is reversed. Often the heart starts up in normal rhythm on its own while connected to the heart/lung machine. If it doesn't, it is restarted electrically.

After major surgical incisions there is often some oozing of blood, so clear plastic tubes are left within the chest cavity for drainage. Temporary pacemaker wires are attached to the surface of the heart and brought out through the chest wall to diagnose any disturbances in the rhythm and to provide pacemaker support if necessary. There will be catheters in the veins and arteries of the arms and occasionally the legs, to record pressure and feed in fluids and drugs. Electrodes on the chest wall are attached to a monitor or an oscilloscope which allows the medical staff to monitor the heart's rhythm and rate. A breathing tube in the mouth passes through the vocal chord into the windpipe. It is not painful, but it does prevent talking. This breathing tube is connected to a machine that does much of the work of breathing for the patient, to assure a good level of circulating oxygen, and to allow the heart to rest.

The breathing tube is removed when breathing assistance is no longer required — usually within 12 hours after surgery. The other tubes and intravenous lines will be removed as soon as it is safe to do so. The temporary pacemaker wires are usually left in place until just before discharge from hospital.

As soon as the patient begins to wake up, the nurses and the physiotherapists will begin to apply the exercises the patient learned before surgery, including deep breathing and coughing, as well as gentle arm and leg exercises.

The cardiac surgical intensive care unit can be a confusing and frightening place, but all of the staff are specially trained to care for patients who have undergone cardiac surgery. As much as possible, the staff work to reassure patients and families alike.

After a stay in the intensive care unit, patients are moved to the stepdown unit. Patients usually stay in this unit for a day or so to allow continued monitoring of rhythm, blood pressure, heart rate and other functions. At this stage patients are encouraged to get up and sit in a chair and to go to the bathroom with assistance. They begin taking a fluid and soft diet.

Patients of both sexes are cared for in the same room in both the cardiovascular intensive care unit and the stepdown unit.

Within 48 to 72 hours of the surgery, most patients have been moved back to their rooms, are reasonably comfortable, mobile, able to go to the bathroom alone, wash, cat, have company and go for walks of increasing lengths in the ward corridors. They continue the breathing and other exercises supervised by the physiotherapists and nurses. Both bowel function and appetite usually return on the fourth or fifth day after surgery. Should bowel function not have returned by that time, mild laxatives are given. By the fifth or sixth day after surgery, many patients are increasingly mobile. The incisions are stiff and uncomfortable, but medication can take the edge off the discomfort, to allow increased activity and a sense of well-being.

The usual length of stay in the hospital for straightforward cardiac procedures is six to eight days after surgery. If the patient lives alone or if sufficient support is not available at home, arrangements are made for further convalescence for up to two weeks at a convalescent hospital.

Patients should not drive themselves home. If the trip is long, a stop every hour or so is recommended to allow for a stretch and a short walk. Patients are usually more comfortable lying on the back seat. If travel by bus, train or airplane is necessary, special arrangements can be made.

Complications

As with any major operation, patients undergoing heart valve surgery may develop wound infection (1 percent) or bleeding after surgery, requiring reopening of the incision (approximately 1 percent), but these complications are rarely serious. There are similarly small risks of lung infection. The exercises learned before the operation, the techniques used during surgery and the antibiotics used during and after surgery are all designed to minimize the likelihood of these complications.

There are also some risks specific to heart valve operations. The risk of heart attacks during the surgery is less than 5 percent, and they are usually well tolerated. The other serious and potentially disabling complication is stroke (1 to 2 percent).

Finally, between 2 to 5 percent of patients undergoing valve replacement will require permanent pacemaker implants because of interference with the natural pacemaker, and sometimes because of coronary artery disease.

In the long term, all patients must continue to avoid infection, taking antibiotics when they have colds and other infections, including those acquired through dental work. With these measures the risk of infection of artificial heart valves is less than 1 percent per year. The risk of blood clot formation related to the presence of the artificial valve is approximately 1 percent per year. Bleeding complications in patients taking anticoagulants also occur in about 1 percent of patients.

Anticoagulants do not really "thin" the blood, but are prescribed specifically to prevent thrombosis — the formation of a clot inside a blood vessel or on an artificial device in the heart or the circulation system. Patients who have artificial valves usually take this type of medication. Patients with tissue valves may or may not require anticoagulants. Patients taking anticoagulants normally require blood tests every one or two weeks during the early months after surgery and subsequently every two or three weeks.

Patients taking anticoagulant medication can undertake jogging, swimming, gardening and other exercises quite safely, but heavy contact sports should be avoided. Patients should report to their doctors any excessive headaches, nose bleeds, bloody or tarry stools, pink or red urine, long periods of abdominal pain or painful or swollen joints. The medications should be taken at the same time each day. Except on the advice of a physician, aspirin or aspirin-containing compounds should not be taken at the same time as anticoagulants. Excessive amounts of alcohol should also be avoided.

Patients should wear a Medic-Alert bracelet with the statement that they are taking anticoagulants, plus any other pertinent information (such as the fact that they have an artificial valve). Application forms for Medic-Alert can be obtained from the nursing station in the hospital before discharge.

Patients must tell every dentist and doctor they see at the beginning of each visit that they are taking anticoagulation medications. Some adjustment of the dose may be necessary before excessive dental work. Seemingly simple procedures such as the insertion of an intrauterine device or even an injection into muscle can be hazardous for patients taking anticoagulant medications.

In the immediate period after discharge from hospital, pain medication is prescribed to provide reasonable comfort during increasing levels of activity.

In some patients who have experienced heart muscle damage before surgery, or who require continuing rhythm and rate control, specific heart medications may continue to be necessary. Prescriptions will be arranged at the time of discharge from hospital. These medications should be taken regularly, as directed, and reviewed from time to time during the patient's follow-up visits with his or her local doctor.

Recent Advances

Surgery is now being recommended earlier in the course of heart valve disease, often delaying the need for replacement valves and anticoagulants. Balloon dilation appears to be an exciting possibility for some patients with narrowed or constricted heart valves. Technical advances are being made all the time in the evolution of both tissue and mechanical artificial valves. These advances will allow valves to perform better and last longer.

Cardiac Pacemakers

Written by Jennifer Fraser, R.N.; Head Nurse, Pacemaker Clinic, Toronto General Hospital; Chairperson, Council of Associated Professionals, North American Society of Cardiac Pacing and Electrophysiology.

The first totally implanted pacemaker was an externally rechargeable, nickel-cadmium battery inserted into the heart of a Swedish engineer who had actually assisted in the design of the device. This occurred in Sweden in 1958, and this man is still alive and active. The first battery-driven pacemaker was implanted in the United States the following year. The subsequent 30 years have witnessed breakthroughs in every aspect of cardiac pacing; thousands of lives have been saved and improved through this technology.

The heart is a specialized muscular organ that pumps blood, sending oxygen and nourishment throughout the body. To beat effectively and regularly, the heart has its own "natural pacemaker," or electrical system. A small bundle of specialized cells located in the right upper chamber of the heart produces electrical impulses, causing the heart to contract rhythmically, creating a pulse.

Each person's normal heart rate is different. At rest, the adult rate is usually 60 to 80 beats or contractions per minute, but this can vary for many reasons, such as during exercise, when the working muscles require more blood and oxygen. To handle this demand, the natural pacemaker responds automatically by speeding the heart rate and increasing the total blood supply to the muscles. Through increased nerve impulses and hormonal changes, the heart rate is also altered during times of stress, anxiety and fear. Many diseases and drugs can make the heart rate faster or slower.

However, not every heart functions properly. If the pathway carrying the natural pacemaker signal is blocked by scar tissue, there is a condition known as "heart block." If the heart block is complete, the natural pacemaker signals are not transmitted down the usual pathway and the pumping rate may slow to 30 to 40 beats per minute. In intermittent heart block, a fraction of the natural pacemaker signals are transmitted, making the pulse slow and irregular.

Sometimes the natural pacemaker itself is affected, so that stimulating signals are not produced at the appropriate rate, causing the heart to beat too slowly or irregularly. When this happens the heart does not send sufficient blood to all parts of the body. In some cases the heart may beat too fast and then slow down suddenly. Any of these conditions may require insertion of an artificial pacemaker.

There are many causes for damage to the heart's electrical system. Some people are born with abnormal heart beats that may not require treatment until later years. Sometimes damage occurs after a heart attack or after open heart surgery. Occasionally there seems to be no obvious reason for the disturbance of the pathway.

The physician determines the need for a pacemaker by looking at the tracing from the patient's electrocardiogram (ECG) and the description of symptoms, which often include light-headedness, intermittent dizziness, shortness of breath or blackouts. Occasionally more prolonged monitoring of the ECG in hospital or during normal activity by portable tape (Holter monitoring) is required. Sometimes sophisticated tests are required to provoke the conduction disturbance and confirm the diagnosis.

A pacemaker is a battery-powered stimulating device that sends a steady flow of electrical pulses to the heart. The heart is a unique muscle, because it requires an electrical charge to only a small area to make the entire heart muscle contract.

The artificial pacemaker consists of the pulse generator or battery pack, the wire (lead) and the electrode. The pulse generator is contained in a small metal case about the size of a large pocket watch. Body fluids cannot penetrate the case, so the circuitry and the battery are protected. Early pacemakers had few components and could perform only a specific limited function, such as stimulating a set rate of 70 beats per minute. The newer pacemakers are computer programmed to perform any combination of available functions, of which there may be millions. Most modern pacemakers can be programmed after implantation. A portable device is held over the implanted pacemaker and sends a radio frequency message to the circuitry to alter such functions as rate, output or sensitivity. Programmability often allows the correction of many pacemaker problems that previously required surgery. The patient feels no sensation during programming.

The battery is also contained within the pulse generator package. Most pacemakers are now powered by lithium, which has a potential life-span of about 10 years and, in an ideal situation, could last for 20 years. Unlike a flashlight, a pacemaker battery has a predictable, slow depletion pattern that can be seen on the ECG tracing. Replacement can be planned well before the patient is aware of the need and before any possible emergency might arise.

Most patients receive a "demand" pacemaker system, which remains inactive until the heart rate drops below the pre-set rate. The demand pacemaker then takes over and maintains the pre-set rate until the natural heart beat speeds above it, shutting it off.

The lead — a strong flexible, insulated wire connected to the pacemaker — is the path by which the electrical impulse travels from the pacemaker to stimulate the heart. The far end of the lead, known as the electrode, rests on the inner heart muscle. It is usually made of a highly conductive material and has attached to it small fins, around which tissue will grow within six weeks after implantation, firmly fixing the lead to the inner heart wall.

A pacemaker is generally implanted in an operating room. Surgery takes about an hour and usually requires only local anesthetic. The patient is placed on an operating X-ray table and the surgeon freezes the area under the collarbone. Then a two- to three-inch incision is made. Through this opening, one of the large veins leading to the heart is located, punctured and the lead is inserted down toward the heart while its course is watched on X-ray. The lead enters the right atrium and is swept with the blood flow through the tricuspid valve into the right ventricle. Once the surgeon can see the lead in a satisfactory and stable position, a test electrical current is passed down the lead to assess the amount of current or voltage needed to contract the heart muscle. This amount is known as "threshold." A "pocket" is then created between the skin and the chest muscle under the collar bone. The pacemaker is connected to the lead, placed in the pocket and the incision is closed.

The implantation may vary from surgeon to surgeon and to some degree depends on the patient's condition. However, the recovery period after implantation is usually short. The patient may need ECG monitoring for 24 hours to make sure the new pacemaker is functioning properly. The patient may be instructed to keep the arm on the implant side relatively still for a day. For about six weeks after discharge (until tissue has grown over the electrode) the patient should not do any strenuous physical maneuvers with that arm. After this, however, the patient should be able to return to full activity.

There are very few limitations on a pacemaker wearer. Many are vigorously active in both work and leisure. Activity will not hurt the pacemaker or deplete the battery more quickly, although all pacemaker wearers should receive regular pacemaker checks and report any unusual symptoms, especially those similar to the pre-implant state.

Pacemakers are well shielded against outside electrical interference and properly functioning electrical equipment. Household appliances, including microwave ovens, pose no problem. People who work in areas of unusually high electromagnetic or radio frequency fields should discuss this with their doctor. The patient should avoid leaning over the ignition system of a car, boat or lawn mover while it is running. Normal dentistry should cause no adverse effects, but pacemaker wearers should tell their dentists about the pacemaker. Patients may need to take antibiotics before complicated dental procedures or extractions.

Certain types of physiotherapy including diathermy and ultrasound in the area of the pacemaker may be a problem due to heating and vibration. Likewise, certain activities involving the chest muscle under the pacemaker may temporarily interrupt the pacemaker and sometimes cause dizziness. A programmable pacemaker can usually be adjusted to prevent this.

Theft detectors and airport security systems may temporarily affect pacemakers and will likely alarm the metal detectors. Pacemaker identification cards should be shown at airports to allow a manual security check. Interference with the pacemaker rarely results from something in the environment. The temporary fault is usually caused by a confusion of electrical signals to the pacemaker and is resolved when the outside stimulus is removed.

Pacemaker patients require follow-up care for life. This follow-up may be performed by the individual physician or by a specialized clinic. Hospital pacemaker clinics were established in the mid-1970s to manage the increasing volume of patients, to centralize expensive equipment and to develop sophisticated methods of pacemaker surveillance. Patients usually need an average of three follow-up visits per year.

Telephone monitoring, by which the patient may transmit the ECG from his or her home over the telephone via a small electronic transmitter, allows for a simple pacemaker check without the patient leaving home. It is particularly useful for frail patients or those geographically isolated from medical services.

Pacemaker replacement, when needed, is usually a simpler procedure than the initial insertion. The old incision is opened in the operating room under local anesthetic. The pulse generator and the lead are disconnected and electrical measurements are made to ensure that the lead is still functioning well. If it is, a new pacemaker is connected to the old lead and reinserted in the former pocket. Should there be a problem with the old lead, the surgeon will insert a new lead in a manner similar to the initial implant.

Chapter 15

Microvascular Surgery

Nancy H. McKee

Associate Professor of Surgery
University of Toronto

Plastic Surgeon
Mount Sinai Hospital, Toronto

Kerri Weller
Illustrator

All parts of the body are nourished by the blood. Arteries deliver the blood from the heart; veins carry it back. A portion of the body can be totally separated and then reattached if at least one artery supplying the part and one vein draining it can be reconnected.

The surgeon's ability to repair small blood vessels using a microscope is called microvascular surgery (Figs. 15.1 and 15.2). It includes not only the reattachment of amputated parts such as fingers, but also the transfer of tissues from one part of a patient's body to another.

Advances in Microvascular Surgery

Few events in surgery make front page news, but few surgical operations are as dramatic as replacement of a body part. The first transplants of organs always hit the headlines, no less dramatic are the replacements of severed parts of the body.

Before microvascular surgery, amputated body parts had to be discarded, and the amputation site repaired as a stump. Now, limbs can be replanted. The first successful finger replantation took place in Japan in 1965. Many centers around the world then gained their experience in microvascular surgery by reattaching fingers. Since then, scalp, nose and penis replantations have been performed successfully.

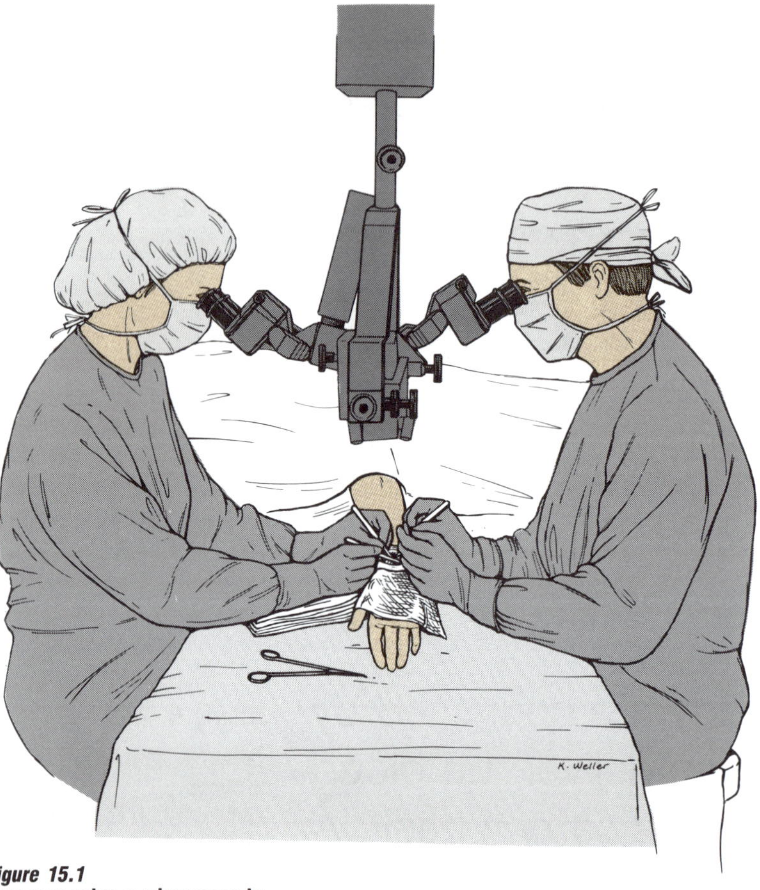

Figure 15.1
Surgeons using a microscope to repair the vital structures of a hand.

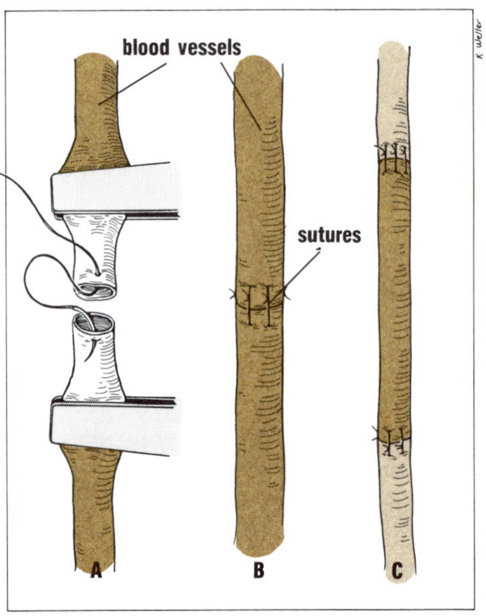

Figure 15.2
Small needles and thread (finer than a human hair) are used to join the ends of a small blood vessel (A and B). Sometimes a spare piece of vein is used to bridge a gap (C).

This new technique also meant that anatomical parts could be severed from their natural place in the body and taken elsewhere where they were more urgently needed. Because the blood vessels could be promptly repaired, the transferred tissue could survive. The first operation of this kind, in 1968, replaced an amputated thumb with a toe (Fig. 15.3).

The body has been carefully explored for other spare parts or "donor sites" — areas from which tissue can be taken without significant loss of appearance or function. There must be at least one reparable artery and vein to restore the necessary blood flow to keep the transferred tissue alive.

Donor sites have been found for skin, muscle, bone and nerve, sometimes in combination (Figs. 15.4 and 15.5). Over 60 donor sites have now been tested. Use of one's own tissue eliminates the chance of the body rejecting foreign tissue. Microvascular surgery enables these repairs to take place in one operation, and the patient's comfort and length of stay in hospital have been significantly improved.

Before microvascular surgery can take place, tests must be done to ensure that the operation will be feasible.

During the operation, the anesthetist carefully monitors the blood pressure and circulation. After the operation, patients are kept under close observation. If either the artery carrying blood into the replanted tissue flap, or the vein leading the blood away from it, become blocked, a further emergency operation will be necessary to save the flap.

One operation can take several hours. Special care is taken to find undamaged vessels in both the donor and recipient areas.

Fingers (and arms) can be suddenly and dramatically amputated. If the parts can be found, there is a good chance that they can be replanted.

The patient should be rushed to the nearest hospital, where the amputated part will be cleansed, wrapped in saline

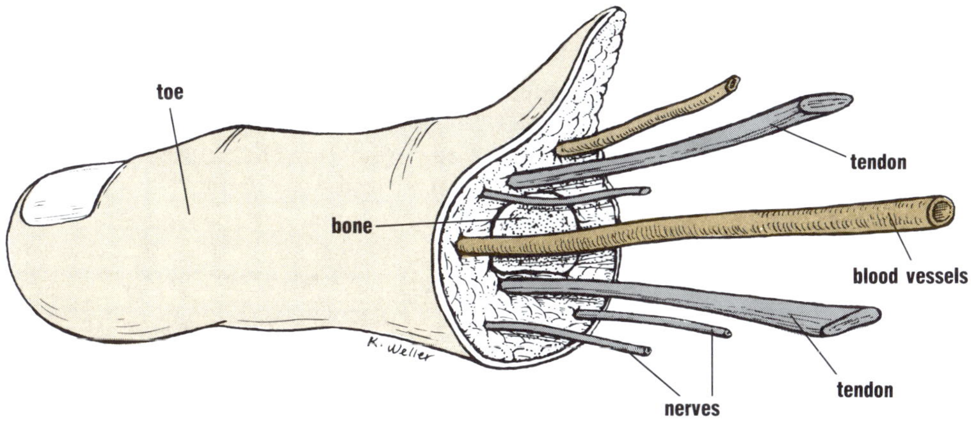

Figure 15.3
Toe flap prepared for transfer to help restore function to a hand.

gauze, and put in a plastic bag containing ice and water. A dressing will be applied to the amputation site. Blood loss must be replaced, and arrangements made for transfer to the nearest replantation center. The nature of the injury, the time that the amputated part has been without blood and has not been cool, the patient's needs and expectations, and the prognosis for overall function must all be taken into account.

Not every amputated finger should be replanted. Single index finger amputations are rarely replanted. A healthy middle finger with normal sensation and mobility will be preferable to a slightly stiff, less-than-normal-feeling replanted index. Amputated thumbs are replanted, if at all feasible, because they represent about 50 percent of hand function.

Surgery may last several hours; the subsequent therapy, for which the patient is going to be responsible, goes on for months and sometimes years. The surgeon and trained occupational and physiotherapists will begin this process, but a lot will have to be done by the patient to achieve the best possible result.

Once a decision is made to proceed with surgery, the amputated part and the patient are promptly transferred to the operating room. Two teams usually work together — one preparing the amputated part, and the other preparing the amputation stump. The amputated part is first cleaned, and dirt and irreversibly injured tissue are removed. The tendons, nerves, veins and arteries are identified, and the bone ends are reunited with wires or screws. Then the tendons, veins, arteries and nerves are repaired, and the skin is closed.

Variations are used in different situations. One of the most common is the necessity to take a short length of a small vein from the front of the wrist or the

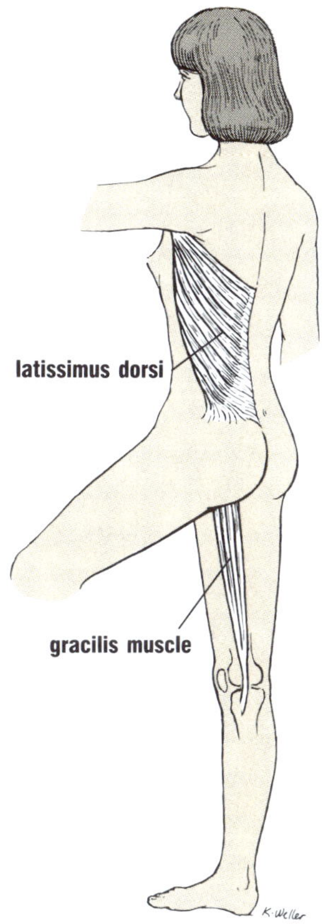

Figure 15.5
Donor muscle sites.

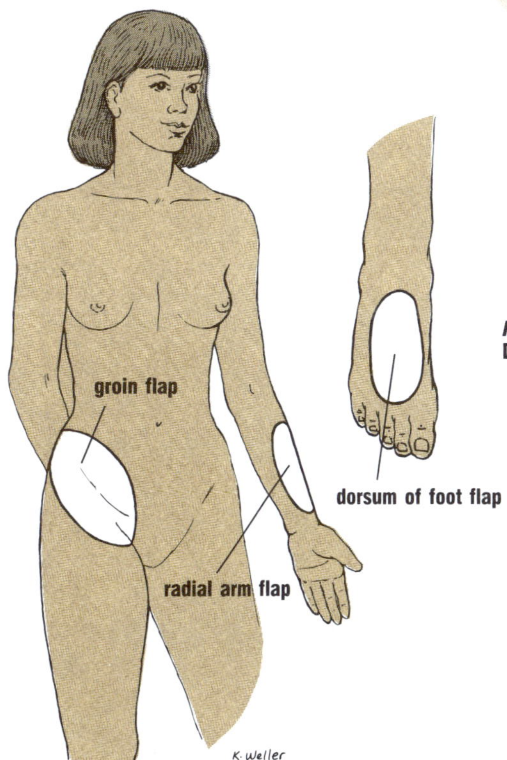

Figure 15.4
Sites for donor skin flaps.

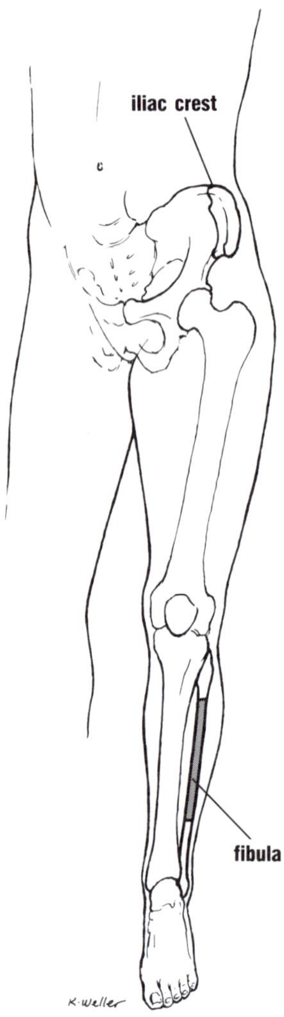

Figure 15.7
Donor bones.

top of the foot to bridge the gap made by the injury.

After the operation, the replanted part is assessed with temperature probes. One temperature-sensitive probe is taped on the replanted part and another on a nearby normal part. A sudden drop in temperature alerts the staff to a serious problem. With each successive day that the replanted part remains pink and warm, the chance of its survival increases.

Once survival has been assured, therapy is started to achieve the best possible function. This involves regaining movement and, in time, retraining the nerves. However, even the best replantation will have less than normal sensation and movement.

Muscle and Bone Transfers

When an injury leaves a limb intact but without movement, occasionally a muscle can be transferred from another part of the body to restore movement (Fig. 15.6). Even bones can be transferred if the blood supply can be re-established (Fig. 15.7). If a portion of a major bone is destroyed by injury or disease, the limb becomes useless. Without a bone transfer, the limb would have to be amputated.

Two donor sites are commonly used for limb reconstruction. The longest is the fibula — the bone that extends from the knee to the ankle, beside the more important tibia. Even after a great length of fibula has been removed, walking, running and jumping can be normal. When the fibula is secured to the bone above and below the defect, and the blood supply is reconnected, the healing proceeds as if there were merely a fracture at either end. With time, and increased use, the fibula assumes the dimensions of the bone that it is replacing.

Another donor site is the pelvic bone (iliac crest), which can bridge shorter defects in curved bones. Its shape is especially suited for reconstructing a large defect of the jaw, most commonly lost to cancer.

Conclusion

There has now been almost a quarter century of replantations and grafts, and our own bodies continue to be the best source of spare parts. Surgeons dream of "spare parts banks." The surgical techniques are ready but we have yet to overcome all the problems of rejection.

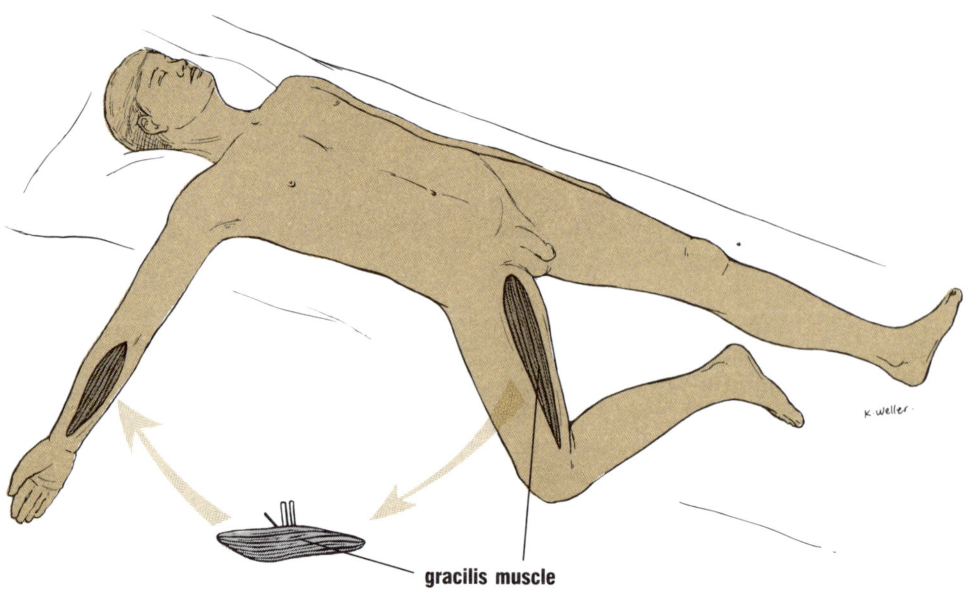

Figure 15.6
Gracilis muscle en route from the leg to the arm to restore finger movement.

Chapter 16

Orthopedic Surgery: Pediatric

Robert B. Salter
Professor of Surgery
University of Toronto
Orthopedic Surgeon
Hospital for Sick Children, Toronto

Margot Mackay
Illustrator,
Associate Professor
Department of Art as Applied to Medicine
University of Toronto

While the history of disorders and injuries of the musculoskeletal system dates back centuries, the specialty of orthopedics is relatively young. In 1741 Nicolos Andry, a professor of medicine in Paris, coined the term "orthopedia" from the Greek words *orthos* (straight) and *pais* (child), to emphasize that many deformities in adults have their origin in childhood.

The present scope of orthopedics includes all ages, but the orthopedist who treats children is particularly concerned with preventing future deformity as the child grows and develops.

Growth of Bones

During childhood, long bones like the thigh bone (femur) grow from a disc-shaped structure of cartilage near each end of the bone (Fig. 16.1). This cartilage, which is called the epiphyseal plate, multiplies continuously throughout the growing years, adding to the length of the bone.

Certain genetic disorders, glandular diseases or biochemical disturbances affect all growth plates and may cause stunted growth of the limbs and spine (dwarfism). Local diseases, such as bone

Dr. Robert B. Salter is grateful to Williams and Wilkins Publishing Company of Baltimore for their kind permission to use some of the illustrations from his book, *Textbook of Disorders and Injuries of the Musculoskeletal System,** Second Edition, 1983, as models for line drawings.

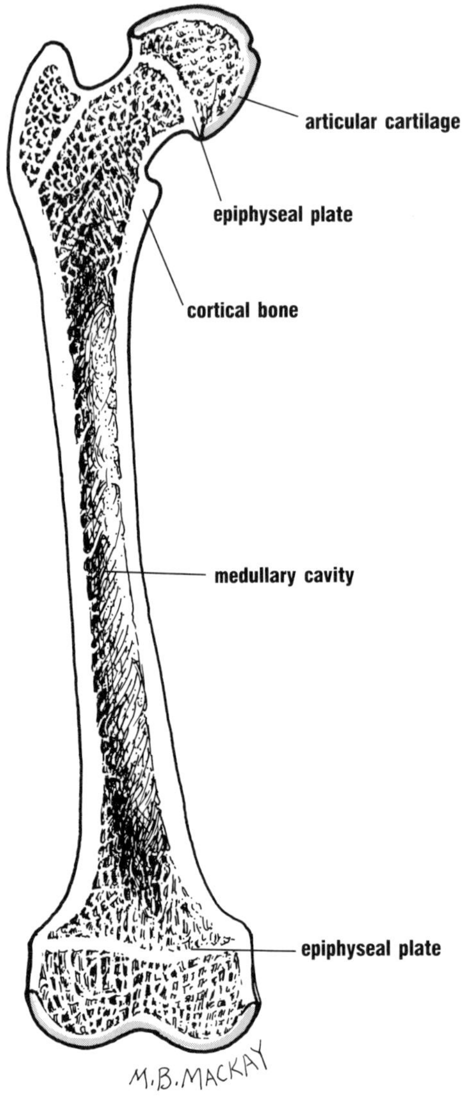

Figure 16.1
A child's femur (thigh bone) during growth.

infections or fractures, affect the growth plate in only one bone, and may cause that bone to become crooked or stop growing prematurely, causing a discrepancy in limb length.

Children's bones also grow in width as new layers of bone are produced by the soft-tissue covering of bone (periosteum), rather like the bark of a tree.

Like other living tissue, bone responds to use by becoming thicker and stronger. It can form new bone to heal a fracture. Without use (as with prolonged immobilization in a cast), bone becomes thinner and weaker.

Diagnosis

A child is most likely to see an orthopedic surgeon at the suggestion of the family physician or pediatrician, who will continue to coordinate the child's total health care. If an orthopedic consultation has been arranged for a child, the parent should write down the following to assist the surgeon in making a diagnosis: chief complaint or concern; when the symptoms began; type of onset (sudden or gradual); severity; constancy (constant or intermittent); progression; activities that aggravate it and those that relieve it; relation to any injury or other incident in the past; any associated symptoms.

The most common complaints that bring a child to an orthopedic surgeon are pain, decrease in function, and appearance. The surgeon will carry out a systematic physical examination and will probably order X-rays or other tests. The amount of radiation involved is so slight that it does not pose a risk, and lead shields protect the child's ovaries or testicles if X-rays of the pelvis and hips are taken.

The orthopedist may also order laboratory examination of certain body fluids such as blood, urine and joint fluid, or a biopsy of tissue. It is now also possible for the orthopedic surgeon to see inside the larger joints (especially the knee) using an arthroscope to make an accurate diagnosis of disorders and injuries within the joints. (See page 206.)

Non-Surgical Treatment of Disorders and Injuries

Orthopedic surgeons generally treat 90 percent of children with disorders and injuries of the musculoskeletal system by non-surgical methods, which may involve any or all of the following:

Psychological Considerations

Every child who is old enough to understand will require sympathetic understanding as well as assurance that everything possible will be done to help him or her. For children with minor disorders, or with musculoskeletal variations of normal, the only treatment needed may be reassurance. However, this requires both time and skill — a child's concern is often greater than we might realize.

Therapeutic Drugs

No drug will accelerate the normal healing of injured musculoskeletal tissues, or will make a weak muscle stronger, a lax ligament tighter, a stiff joint mobile or a deformed bone straight. Nevertheless, certain types of drugs have an important place in treating musculoskeletal disorders. Analgesics relieve pain, antibiotics cure infection, corticosteroids reduce inflammation, vitamin C treats scurvy and vitamin D treats rickets. But the underlying causes of all of these conditions must also be treated.

Rest

For centuries it was thought — on the basis of experience rather than research — that total body rest was necessary for certain severe disorders and injuries of the musculoskeletal system. However, prolonged and continuous bed rest can cause muscle wasting, bone thinning, increased loss of calcium in the urine, blood clots in large veins (rare in children) and pressure sores. Bed-ridden patients should therefore be encouraged to exercise their good limbs and, whenever possible, should be helped from their bed to a chair for at least part of each day.

Local rest for an affected limb may be provided by simply preventing a limb's usual function.

Traction is another form of rest for a limb, to maintain the length of the limb and the alignment of unstable fractures. It can also relieve painful muscle spasm associated with joint inflammation or injury, and stretch soft tissues that have become shortened by a deformity or dislocation. Immobilization in a cast is used to maintain or stabilize the position of a fracture or a dislocation.

Support

Patients with muscle weakness and joint instability can be helped by braces. Braces can transmit movement to the weak part of the limb from some other muscle group. If the muscles that bend the fingers are paralyzed, for instance, a brace can be worn that will cause the fingers to bend when the wrist is bent upward. Braces can also prevent unwanted motion while allowing desired motion, as in a leg brace that will immobilize a limb while permitting walking (Fig. 16.2). Loose joints in the feet occasionally require temporary support by arch supports and sole wedges in the shoes. Mild soft-tissue injuries may be given temporary support by adhesive tape strapping.

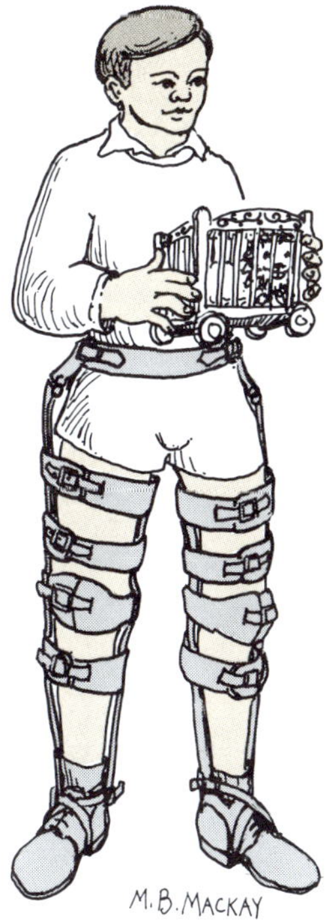

Figure 16.2
To treat weak or unstable lower limbs, braces can prevent unwanted motion while permitting desired motion. Braces can be metallic (A) or plastic (B), which are usually lighter and more acceptable cosmetically.

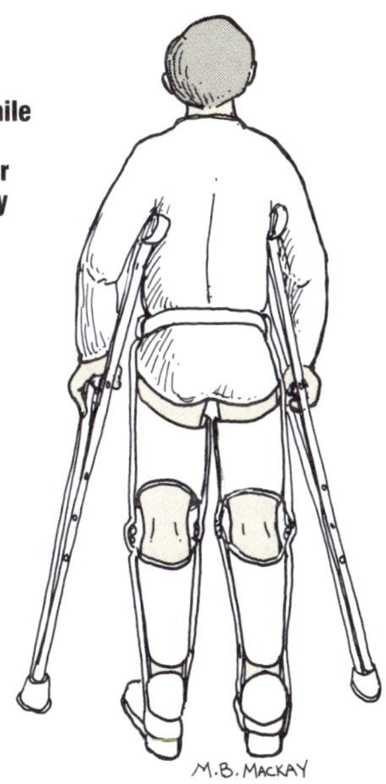

A

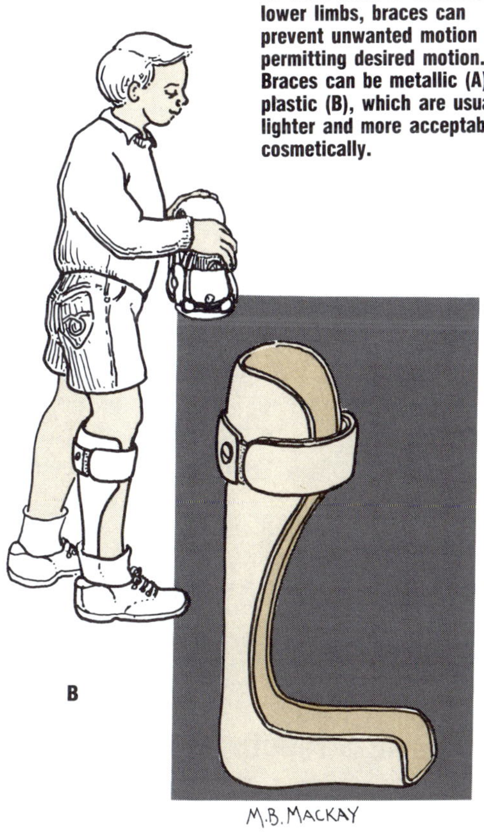

B

Prevention and Correction of Deformity

When the development of a joint deformity can be anticipated, as in paralysis or arthritis, it is frequently possible to prevent the deformity by intermittent immobilization in a removable splint. The joint is immobilized intermittently (perhaps at night) to prevent the deformity. Gradual correction of certain twisting deformities in growing long bones is possible over some months by wearing splints at night to transmit corrective forces to the growth plates.

Physiotherapy and Occupational Therapy

The aims of these closely related forms of treatment are to regain and maintain joint motion, to increase muscle strength and to improve musculoskeletal function. Physio and occupational therapy are carried out by trained therapists at the request of the child's physician or surgeon.

Joint Motion

The safest method of regaining motion in a painful stiff joint is active movement (by the patient's own muscle action), which is directed by a physiotherapist. The pain that arises at each end of the range of motion causes the patient to stop the action, thus protecting the joint from being forced. Movement of such a joint by the therapist (passive movement) is potentially dangerous, especially if it is forceful, because it may irritate and injure the joint, resulting in more stiffness. However, passive movement can help maintain joint motion to prevent deformity if a joint is paralyzed. Passive movement can also help stretch shortened muscles.

Muscle Strengthening

A muscle is strengthened only by active exercise. Even when a limb is immobilized, as in a cast, muscles can be strengthened by static exercises (muscle contraction without moving the joint). Dynamic exercises (producing joint motion) increase muscle strength and help to regain motion. Muscle exercises performed against progressively increasing resistance are particularly effective for increasing strength. When a muscle has an intact nerve supply but is not functioning following an injury or operation, it can be stimulated to contract by electric current.

Improvement of Musculoskeletal Function

Functional training involves coordinating muscles in skilful and purposeful activity, such as walking, going up and down stairs, dressing and eating. This training is supervised by an occupational therapist, who also encourages purposeful manual activities (including handicrafts) to improve coordinated hand function and provide interesting and absorbing mental diversion.

Orthopedic Manipulation

The aims of orthopedic manipulation are to correct deformity in a fractured bone or a dislocated joint and, to a lesser extent, to regain motion in a stiff joint. The majority of fractures and dislocations can be treated by manipulating the parts into satisfactory position under local or general anesthetic. This is called closed reduction, and it can also be used to treat many congenital dislocations, at least in very young children. Joint deformities due to shortening of the muscle and joint capsule can often be gradually corrected by repeated gentle stretching of these tight tissues.

Continuous Passive Motion (CPM)

The author's research has shown that joints heal more quickly if they are moved continuously right after an operation. CPM machines have been devised which move the joints continuously day and night at a rate of approximately one cycle per minute for at least one week, starting when the surgery is completed while the patient is still under general anesthetic (Fig. 16.3). After this the patient can usually maintain an excellent range of motion by active exercise.

Surgical Treatment

The aims of surgical operations for musculoskeletal conditions include relief of pain, improvement of function and mobility, and the prevention or correction of deformity. The operations involve various combinations of repair, release (the cutting of deforming tissue such as tendons, joint capsules or scar tissue), resection (removal of tissue), reconstruction and replacement of tissues.

Three of the most common conditions for which a child may require orthopedic surgery are clubfoot, congenital dislocation of the hip, and curvature of the spine (scoliosis).

Clubfoot

The normal human foot can be placed on the ground so that the weight is taken evenly on the heel and sole. A clubfoot is a congenital abnormality that turns the forefoot and the heel inward (Fig. 16.4). The degree of severity — mild, moderate or severe — is better assessed by feeling the foot's rigidity or resistance than by its appearance.

Clubfoot is found in two out of every 1,000 live births. Boys are affected twice as often as girls. In half of those affected, both feet are deformed. The abnormality is inherited in only 10 percent of children; in the rest, the clubfoot deformity appears inexplicably.

A patient with an uncorrected clubfoot cannot place the heel and sole of the foot flat and must bear weight on the top of the outer side of the foot. Normal pain-free walking is impossible. The main underlying abnormality is a shortness and tightness of muscles, tendons, ligaments and joint capsule on the inner side and back of the foot and ankle. Despite treatment, these structures may become short and tight again as the child grows, and the deformities may recur.

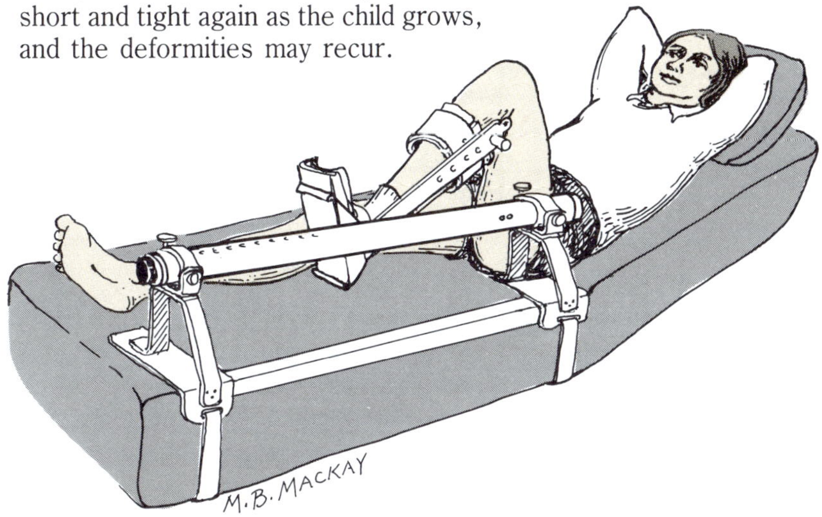

Figure 16.3
A continuous passive motion device. The device can be removed from the bed and attached to a crutch when the patient is out of bed.

The physician or surgeon must be able to differentiate a true clubfoot from muscle paralysis or malformation, or a less severe deformity in which only the forefoot is turned inward (metatarsus varus). An accurate assessment can be made by a special type of X-ray examination.

Non-Surgical Treatment

The initial treatment of a child's clubfoot should begin on the very first day of life, because with each passing week the

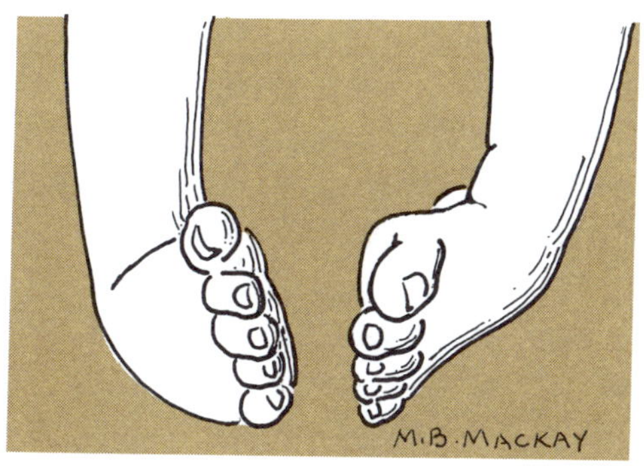

Figure 16.4
Moderately severe congenital clubfoot deformity in a newborn infant.

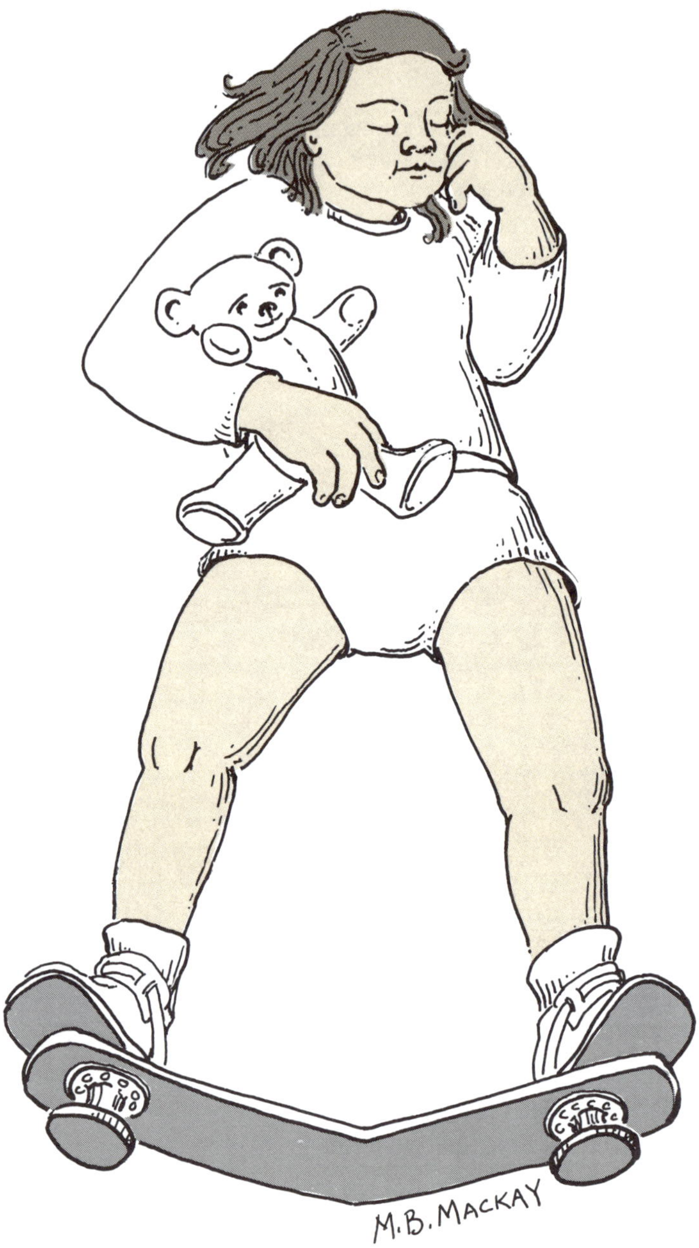

Figure 16.5
This boot splint is worn at night for at least one year to correct a clubfoot deformity.

deformity becomes progressively more resistant to correction. The orthopedic surgeon gently but firmly manipulates the newborn infant's clubfoot to obtain as much correction as possible (without undue force) and then applies a plaster cast.

The cast is changed every few days, for about a week, with more correction attempted each time. The baby does not have to be kept in the hospital during this time. Following that, there are weekly cast changes for about six weeks, and then cast changes every other week for six weeks.

If the casts have corrected the problem, the child is given straight-last shoes (no left or right foot distinction) to wear during the day. At night the child wears a boot splint (Fig. 16.5). The boot splint is easily applied by the parents, and causes no discomfort to the baby. This regimen continues for 12 to 18 months, and is the best way to prevent a recurrence of the deformity.

Surgical Treatment

Approximately 60 percent of clubfeet treated within the first few weeks of life will have responded to non-surgical treatment by the end of the first three months. The remaining 40 percent will require surgery, which involves dividing the tight joint capsules and lengthening the tight tendons. At the end of the operation, which takes about 90 minutes, a plaster cast is applied. The child usually goes home after a few days.

The cast is maintained for at least two months, with a cast change at one month. It is then replaced by a boot splint. Occasionally such operations prove ineffective, and a tendon transfer may be required. Very rarely the joints in the back part of the foot must be fused to correct a remaining deformity, but this cannot be carried out until growth is nearly complete.

With appropriate treatment, the child should enjoy a normal childhood and be able to participate in all sports. The foot and calf may be slightly smaller than the normal one, but overall the appearance is cosmetically acceptable.

Congenital Dislocation of the Hip

The term "congenital" means present at birth. The hip is a ball and socket joint.

A dislocation of the hip occurs when the ball is not properly located in the socket, i.e., it is "out of joint."

A relatively minor abnormality of any part of the hip joint can significantly disturb normal walking and can eventually lead to chronic arthritis (degeneration of the joint). A hip joint that has been abnormal in a patient's early years is destined to "wear out" in early or middle adult life. One-quarter of all arthritis of the hip in adults is the direct result of residual defects from congenital dislocation of the hip.

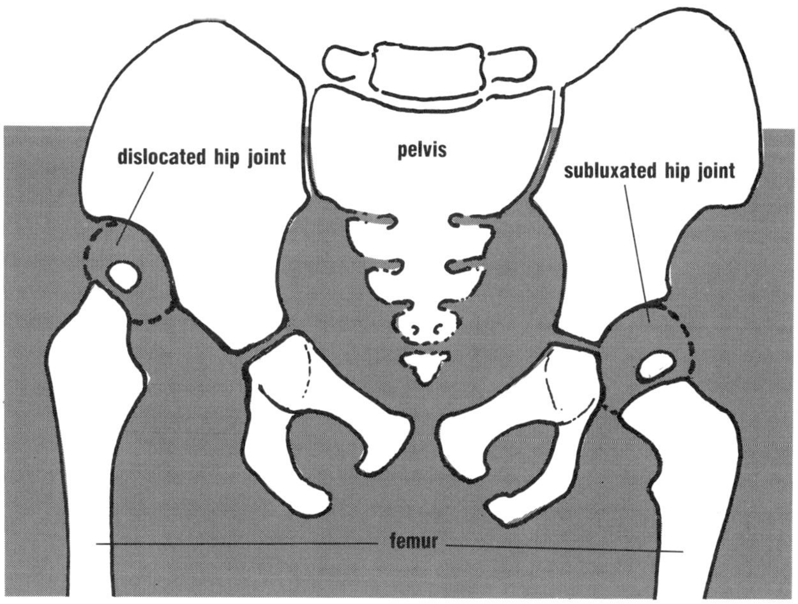

Figure 16.6
A front view of a completely dislocated right hip and subluxated (partially dislocated) left hip.

Diagnosis

In congenital dislocation of the hip, the hip joint is loose or unstable (subluxated) at birth because the joint capsule is loose. At birth, one child in 80 has an undue degree of looseness of the hip joint capsule, predisposing the hip to dislocation as the hip joints straighten from their previously flexed position before birth. In the first few weeks after birth the majority of loose hip joints tighten up spontaneously, but some (one in 650) remain unstable and, if untreated, are liable to dislocate. Girls are affected at least eight times as often as boys. In over 50 percent of cases, both hips are abnormal.

The longer the dislocation or subluxation goes untreated, the more severe — and the less reversible — any secondary abnormalities become. An untreated (or unsuccessfully treated) congenital dislocation causes a severe limp when the child begins walking. During childhood the condition is painless, but in adolescence or early adult life the hip becomes painful as the result of secondary chronic arthritis.

Unlike a congenital clubfoot, a congenital dislocation of the hip is not obvious to anyone at birth. During the first few weeks of life, a specific physical examination of the infant's hips is more accurate than X-ray examination, since much of an infant's hip joint is still formed of cartilage, which is not visible on X-rays. After the first few months, certain signs on examination and X-ray make the diagnosis less difficult (Fig. 16.6).

If the child reaches walking age with an untreated congenital dislocation of the hip, a severe limp will usually indicate the condition. If the dislocation is partial, however, a limp does not usually become apparent until several years later.

All newborn babies should be carefully examined on the first day of life, so that if treatment is needed, it can be started early, when it is simpler and the results much better than if treatment is started months or years later.

Non-Surgical Treatment

During the newborn period when the hips are usually only loose, rather than permanently dislocated, the only treatment required is maintaining the hip, or hips, in the flexed and spread position with either a pillow splint (Fig. 16.7) or a harness (Fig. 16.8).

If treatment is started between two to 18 months, traction is required for a few weeks before a gentle closed reduction of the hip is performed under general anesthetic by orthopedic manipulation. The hips are then immobilized in a cast

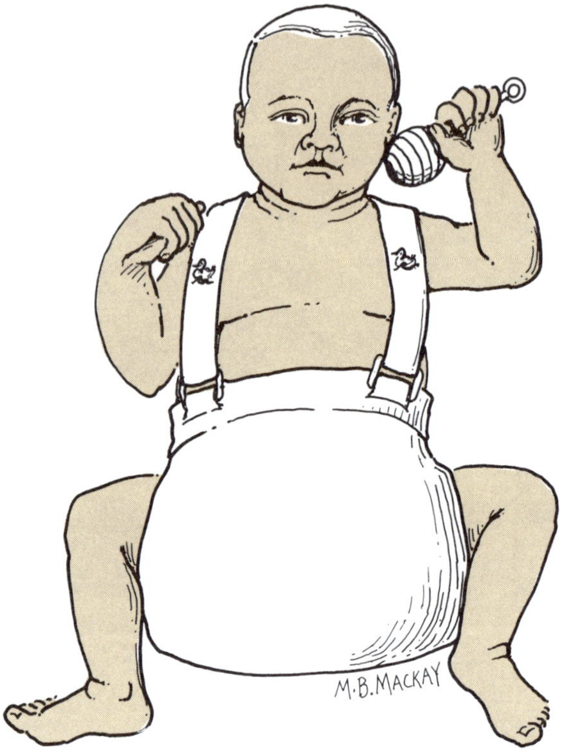

Figure 16.7
Pillow splint.

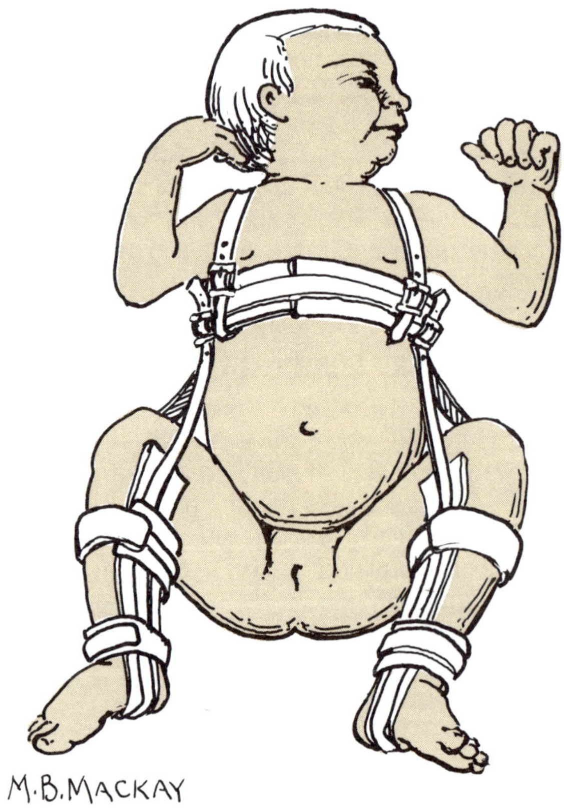

Figure 16.8
Hip harness.

which is changed every two months until the X-ray appearance of the hip(s) is virtually normal. This takes from four to 12 months, depending on the age of the child when treatment was begun.

Surgical Treatment

In approximately 20 percent of children treated under the age of 18 months, the dislocated or subluxated hip does not respond adequately to non-surgical treatment, in which case surgery is required. The hip joint is opened, tight muscles are released and the stretched joint capsule is repaired. The hip is then immobilized in a stable position for several months.

After 18 months, the secondary abnormalities of congenital dislocation are not only more severe but also less reversible. By this age the child is usually walking and has a limp that has been described as ''waddling like a duck.'' For children aged 18 months to five years, the most effective surgery involves dividing the pelvic bone to correct the abnormality of the socket (innominate ostertomy). After six weeks in a hip cast, the child can walk again.

A child with a well-treated congenital dislocation or subluxation of the hip should enjoy a normal childhood and be able to participate in all sports. Nevertheless, all children who have been treated for this condition must be assessed by an orthopedic surgeon at regular intervals in order to monitor the subsequent development of the treated hip(s).

Recent Advances

The screening of all newborn babies by special physical examination to detect congenital dislocation of the hip at birth is the most important advance in the diagnosis of this condition. It enables the orthopedic surgeon to treat the infant effectively, usually without surgery.

Scoliosis (Curvature of the Spine)

While scoliosis, or curvature of the spine, may be congenital (present at birth), 85 percent of all scoliosis is acquired during growth, usually during adolescence. The precise cause of this type of scoliosis is unknown.

The normal spine consists of 24 cylindrical-shaped bones connected in front by discs and behind by additional joints. The normal spine is held straight by a combination of muscles, ligaments and joint capsules. During the growing years it usually grows equally on the right and left sides, remaining straight.

Scoliosis occurs to some degree in one person out of every 200. It usually first becomes apparent between ages 10 to 15, and affects girls much more frequently than boys. Although this type of scoliosis is not inherited in any particular pattern, it does tend to run in families.

Scoliosis usually increases in severity, especially during the rapid growing years of adolescence, because of unequal growth on the two sides of the spine. Mild degrees of scoliosis show up to about 30 degrees of curvature on an X-ray, and do not produce a visible deformity. More severe degrees of the condition are obvious, especially when the patient is bending forward (Fig. 16.9).

Uncorrected scoliosis of over 40 degrees slowly increases in severity even when the child has finished growing, and does produce a visible deformity. It may lead to painful degenerative arthritis of the lower part of the spine in adult life.

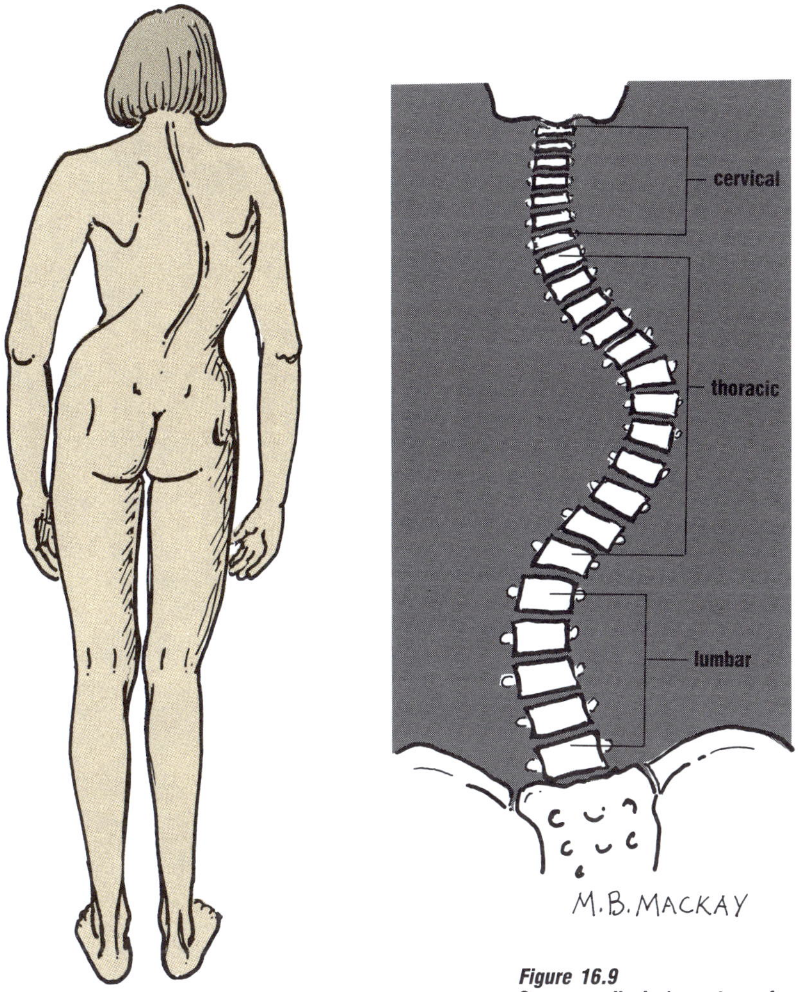

Figure 16.9
Severe scoliosis (curvature of the spine).

Diagnosis

Idiopathic (no apparent cause) scoliosis begins slowly, insidiously and painlessly. By the time the curvature has become readily detectable, it has already reached 30 degrees. Well-trained school nurses can help to make the diagnosis while the curvature is still mild.

Once the diagnosis of scoliosis has been made by physical examination, the orthopedic surgeon will carry out a complete musculoskeletal examination including lower limb length measurement and neurological assessment in order to exclude other causes of scoliosis, such as muscle disease or a congenital bony abnormality. X-ray examination, which should include thc full length of the spine in the standing position, reveals the true degree of curvature, which is always more severe than would be suggested by the external physical appearance.

Non-Surgical Treatment

The adolescent with idiopathic scoliosis should be seen by an orthopedic surgeon to determine the need for correction of

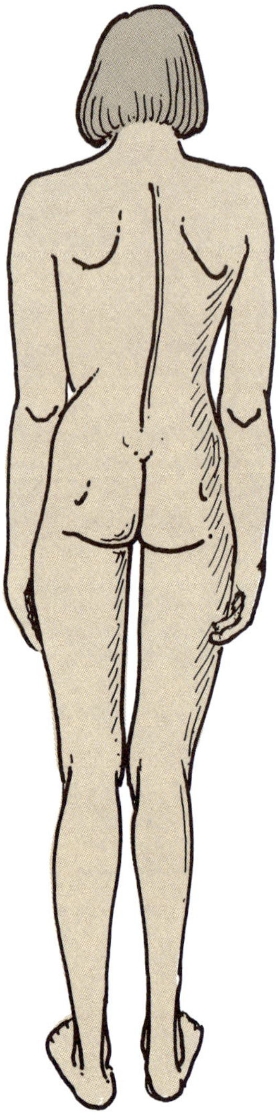

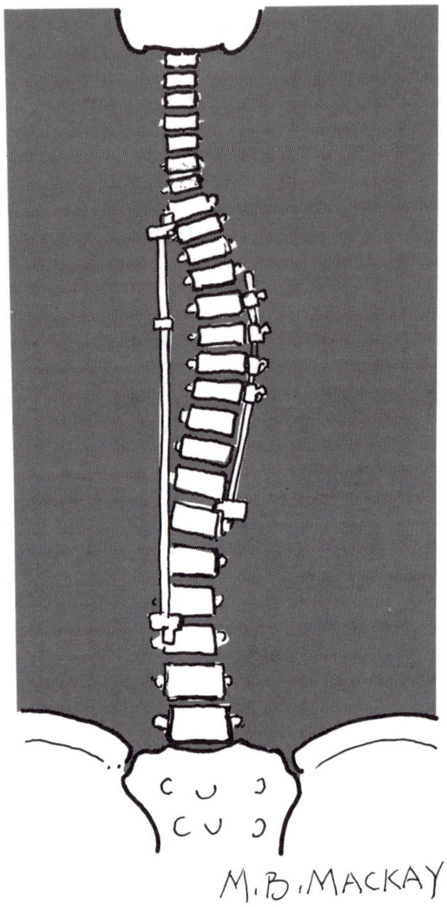

Figure 16.10
Spinal instrumentation rod.

the deformity, and should be assessed at regular intervals throughout the growing period. The aims of treatment are to prevent progression of mild scoliosis and to correct and maintain correction of more severe scoliosis.

For children with curves of 20 to 40 degrees and with two or more years of anticipated growth, a spinal brace can usually reduce the curve and prevent it from increasing. The patient is fitted for the brace in a special scoliosis clinic attended by orthopedic surgeons, physiotherapists and brace-makers (orthotists). The brace is worn until growth is complete and the curve has stabilized. It is easily worn night and day and is removed for washing only.

Surgical Treatment

For adolescents with a curvature of over 40 degrees that is already producing an obvious deformity, or which is likely to do so in the future, the most effective operation to date is the combination of mechanical correction with a rod, which straightens and stabilizes the spine and is left in place permanently, and spinal fusion (Fig. 16.10). The results of such surgery are generally excellent, provided that the curvature has not been allowed to progress to an extreme degree.

The patient usually remains in the hospital for 10 days after the surgery, in a cast and in bed. Once the child is allowed to walk, a back splint or brace is worn day and night, removed only for washing. On discharge from hospital, the child may go to school, but should not participate in sports for one year. The splint or brace is worn until X-rays show that the spinal fusion is complete, usually within three months. Upon successful completion of the treatment, the child gradually returns to a normal lifestyle.

Recent Advances

The most important recent advance in treating scoliosis is the screening programs of adolescents in schools, so that scoliosis can be detected and treated while the curvature is still mild.

Surgical instruments are always improving, allowing more perfect correction and better stability. It is sometimes possible to avoid using casts and braces, even immediately after surgery.

Chapter 17

Orthopedic Surgery Adult

Allan E. Gross
Latner Professor and Chairman
Division of Orthopedic Surgery
University of Toronto
Orthopedic Surgeon
Mount Sinai Hospital, Toronto

Jean Calder
Illustrator

Orthopedic surgery deals with disorders of the bones, joints and muscles. The term orthopedic actually means "straight child," but today orthopedic surgery is divided into pediatric and adult. Most orthopedic surgeons in community hospitals do both, with the major part of their practice being adult. In teaching centers, surgeons tend to do either pediatric or adult orthopedics.

Bones

The human skeleton is made up of long bones, flat bones and irregular bones. Although bones are rigid because they contain calcium, they are alive, with both a blood and nerve supply.

Bones have several functions. One of these is to protect vital organs, the way the rib cage protects the lungs and heart. Bones allow movement by forming joints and serving as levers for muscles. Bones are the storehouse for calcium and phosphorus and also contain marrow, which forms blood cells.

Surgery of Fractures

A break in a bone is called a fracture. Acute traumatic fractures occur as a result of a significant force, like a fall. Stress fractures occur from repeated minor forces such as excessive unaccustomed walking. Pathological fractures happen when a minor force is exerted on a bone weakened by disease, such as cancer.

Acute traumatic fractures can be open (compound) or closed. With an open fracture, a wound exposes the fracture to the air; a closed fracture has intact skin over it. Fractures are also classified by the pattern of the break, such as horizontal, oblique, spiral or comminuted (splintered, or broken into small pieces).

Fractures heal spontaneously. Bones are covered by a thin envelope of fibrous connective tissue (periosteum), whose bone-forming cells help in the repair process. Blood vessels around the fracture and within the bone will also contribute to this repair process. A collar of repair tissue (callus) forms around the two ends of the broken bone, bridging the break.

Fracture healing requires a good blood supply and a soft tissue envelope called the periosteum, both of which contain cells that aid in the healing process. The greater the force causing the fracture, the greater the disruption of the blood supply and soft tissue envelope, which thus retards healing.

Because of their anatomical site, certain bones have a poor blood supply and are therefore slow healers. Some fractures may heal in three weeks. Others may require up to six months, depending on the bone and the amount of soft tissue damage. The shin bone (tibia), requires several months, while the wrist (distal radius) will usually heal in four or five weeks. Fractures in growing bones heal much faster than those in adult bones.

A busy hospital emergency department handles about ten fractures every day, but at least 75 percent of these are minor, requiring little or no treatment. The other 25 percent are major, possibly even life-threatening. The eventual outcome of the treatment depends upon the bone fractured, the type of fracture, and the patient's general state of health.

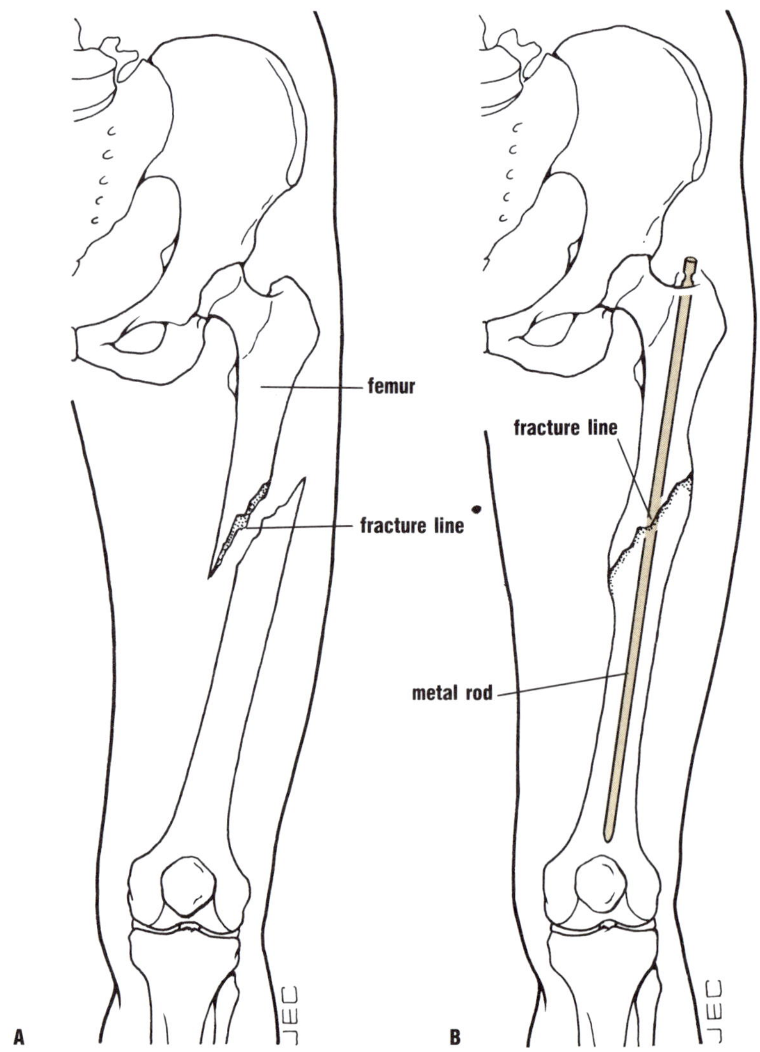

Figure 17.1
A fracture of the femur (thigh bone) of the left leg, before (A) and after it has been surgically fixed by a metal rod (B).

Diagnosis

There are three basic kinds of forces that may break a bone. Traction or pulling can result in a fracture when a joint is twisted and a ligament pulls off a piece of bone. Compression from a vertical force may cause a fracture, such as when a fall from a height produces a compression fracture of the spine. A bone may also be broken due to bending and twisting — the most common causes of limb fractures.

When a bone breaks, pain and swelling develop immediately because of soft tissue damage and bleeding. The break in the bone causes instability, so that the patient is unable to bear weight on that bone. The magnitude of the force determines the degree of displacement — how far the bone ends are separated and therefore the degree of soft tissue damage. In some fractures, the bone ends may be close to their normal anatomical position, causing less pain.

Non-Surgical Treatment

Some fractures may be undisplaced and stable, requiring only treatment for the symptoms. For example, an undisplaced fracture of a foot bone may require only a pressure bandage and the use of crutches for a few days. A cast may allow the patient to walk more easily, but is not necessary for healing.

If a fracture is badly displaced, it must be put back into its normal position, so that healing can occur. This is called "reduction" of the fracture. Reduction can usually be accomplished by simply manipulating the bones back into place (closed reduction), but sometimes surgery is required to reposition the bones (open reduction).

General or local anesthetic may be used in a closed reduction. Afterwards the fracture is held in position by a cast. Casts are used to decrease pain by protecting the fracture and, after a closed reduction, to hold the fragments in position until they heal.

A cast or plaster is a roll of soft bandage impregnated with a calcium salt. The soft roll of plaster is first immersed in water, then applied in layers to the fractured limb, where it hardens in a few minutes. The patient is usually asked to return the next day so that the cast can be checked to make sure it is not too tight, which would impair circulation, and for an X-ray, to see that the fracture is still in optimal position for healing.

The diagnosis of a badly displaced fracture is easily made by physical examination and X-rays. A less displaced fracture may be more difficult to diagnose on physical examination, and the X-rays may be more difficult to interpret. A bone scan is sometimes necessary to diagnose undisplaced fractures. A bone-seeking isotope is injected intravenously, which travels to areas of increased new bone formation, such as a fracture site. It shows up as a hot spot when the skeleton is scanned by the isotope detector.

Surgical Treatment

When an open reduction is necessary, the fracture is usually very unstable and must be held in place by metal pins, screws or a plate. This is called "internal fixation." In these cases a cast is not usually required to hold the bone in position.

Open reductions are done if a closed reduction is technically impossible or difficult to hold in plaster once achieved. Open reductions are also done if there are associated injuries to major blood vessels, nerves, tendons or visceral organs (like the bowel or the bladder) which must be repaired, and the fracture must be held rigid by a metal fixture at the same time to avoid further damage by sharp bone ends. Open reductions are usually necessary for multiple fractures because it is difficult to immobilize more than one limb in plaster and still have the patient walking and receiving good nursing care. Finally, fractures involving joints must be perfectly reduced, or arthritis will develop.

The most common metal devices used in open reductions are screws, plates held by screws, and rods placed within the canal of the bone (Fig. 17.1). The metallic devices may be left in forever if they do not irritate the surrounding tissues or cause changes in the adjacent bone. Most hardware is, however, removed one or two years after surgery.

Case Study: Fracture Surgery

It was toward the end of the first day of their skiing holiday that the accident happened. Marjorie and Hazel were on their last run when Hazel lost control on a tricky part of the hill. She took a fall and was grimacing with pain when Marjorie reached her.

The ski patrol responded quickly and Marjorie was soon moved to the nearby hospital. X-rays showed that her shin bone was broken just at the boot line. The surgeon said he could get the bone ends back into place, but she'd need a cast from groin to ankle — and she'd have to return home for further treatment. Marjorie wouldn't hear of letting her go home alone, or of staying on without her. Holiday hopes dashed.

At her local hospital, Hazel found out that the fracture had slipped out of place. The surgeon wanted to operate, but she really didn't like the idea. "Can't you just put it back in place and put another cast on?" The surgeon explained that it was possible, but she'd have to return in a week for more X-rays to check that the bone ends were still in place. To Hazel, that seemed a small price to pay.

But a week later the fracture had slipped again. Hazel was sure they were doing something wrong. Because Hazel was skeptical, the surgeon took extra care in explaining what was involved. She would be given a general anesthetic, and they'd put in a metal plate during surgery. She would be in the hospital for five or six days and would be on crutches for three months, then partial weight-bearing for three months, with physiotherapy to her knee and ankle. It was a long time, but she wouldn't be in a cast, which was some consolation.

Hazel found the physio hard work, even though the surgery itself hadn't bothered her very much. At her 18-month checkup, the surgeon asked Hazel if she was having any problems with the metal plate in her leg. "I know it's there, especially in the cold, but that's about all," she said. "Some people experience pain," said the surgeon, "but another worry in someone of your age would be what we call bone atrophy. If you don't stress bones, as you normally do in walking, their ability to remain strong is reduced. The metal plate is taking the stress at present. Now that the bone has healed, we should let it take the strain again."

This would entail the removal of the metal plate, and a further six weeks on crutches, to allow the holes left by the screws to fill in with bone. Once off crutches Hazel began to get more exercise, and one year later she was again enjoying herself on the slopes.

Complications

Some complications of fractures are common to all surgical procedures. (See chapter 4.) Some relate specifically to fractures and may occur up to two months after the fracture, or later.

The early complications are mainly injury to nearby tissues or organs. There may be damage to the adjacent skin and the surrounding muscle in an open fracture. If this damage is extensive, the fracture site may become infected. Skin and sometimes muscle grafts are used for coverage, usually put on seven to 10 days after the fracture has occurred. Tendons, blood vessels and nerves injured by the sharp bony ends must be repaired as soon as possible and prevented from further harm by fixing the fracture with a metal device.

The late complications are failure to heal, healing in a poor position and infection. When a fracture does not heal, it is called a non-union. This may be caused by poor positioning of bone ends (a poor reduction), persistent movement between the bone ends, infection or a poor blood supply. Soft tissue damage around the fracture interrupts the blood supply, and is worse in badly displaced fractures.

If a fracture does not heal in the expected period of time (up to six months for some bones), surgery is needed to put in a bone graft and a metal fixture. The bone graft is used to induce bone formation, and is taken from the patient's iliac crest near the hip. The graft consists of small bone chips, which are laid around the fracture site.

A fracture may heal in a poor position, causing a deformity. This is called a malunion. If significant, it is treated by surgery. The surgeon breaks the bone again and then places it in proper anatomical alignment, holding it with a metal fixture.

Chronic infection (osteomyelitis) is a very serious complication of fractures. It is usually associated with open fractures and is difficult to cure except by extensive surgery to remove the infected bone — often in several stages. Bone, skin and muscle grafts may also be necessary, because fractures that become infected are usually accompanied by extensive soft tissue damage. Antibiotics are used but are ineffective without surgery, because the poor blood supply to infected bone prevents antibiotics from getting to the fracture site. Surgery helps to improve the blood supply.

Recent Advances

If a non-union occurs, electrical stimulation of the fracture site may stimulate bone formation and healing in some cases. However, this technique is still very controversial.

Microvascular surgery has improved the treatment of bones that do not unite because of an extensive gap between the bone ends. A piece of living bone, with its blood supply intact, can be used to bridge the defect. (See chapter 15.) This provides a living bone graft, which promotes rapid healing.

Three common fractures exemplify the principles of fracture treatment, and the possible complications.

Fractures of the Distal Radius (Colles' Fracture)

The forearm bone that ends at the wrist is called the radius. A fracture of the end of the radius is the most common fracture seen in any emergency department (Fig. 17.2). It usually occurs in children and elderly women, and is caused by a fall on the outstretched hand.

The patient has a painful, swollen wrist and a characteristic deformity if the fracture is significantly displaced. An X-ray confirms the fracture and shows the degree of displacement. If there is no significant displacement, a cast is applied without manipulation.

If the bone ends are displaced, they are manually moved back into the correct anatomical position after the patient has

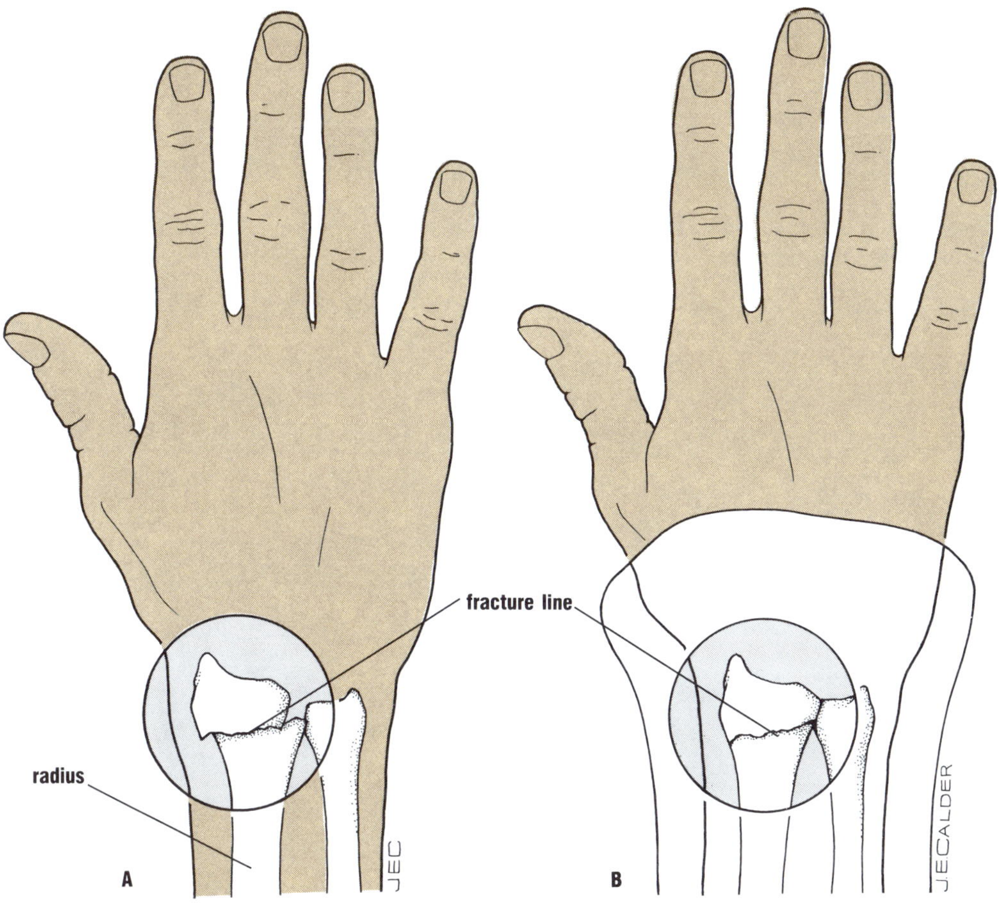

Figure 17.2
A fracture of the distal radius (Colles' fracture), before (A) and after it has been manipulated back into its normal position (B).

been given local or general anesthetic. A cast is applied from the base of the fingers to just below the elbow, and an X-ray is taken. If the position is acceptable, the patient is allowed to go home but returns the next day for another X-ray and an assessment of the circulation and nerve supply to the hand.

Patients are seen again at about 10 days for another X-ray and cast check, and at about five weeks for cast removal and another X-ray. While the wrist is in a cast, the patient must exercise the fingers, elbow and shoulder to prevent stiffening of the joints.

Since this fracture is caused by a minor injury, early complications are rare. However, troublesome late complications may occur. Because this fracture occurs most commonly in elderly females, the bone may be soft (osteoporotic). The fracture may heal in mal-union, causing a deformity at the wrist. This complication, although quite common, does not usually interfere with function or cause pain, and it only rarely requires surgery. If the deformity is severe in a younger patient, the bone may have to be surgically refractured and fixed with metal.

Another complication that may occur early or late is compression of the median nerve that passes through a fibrous tunnel next to the fracture. This causes numbness and weakness in the hand and is called carpal tunnel syndrome. If the nerve compression is severe, surgery may be necessary to release the fibrous tunnel, allowing more space for the nerve. (See chapter 18, page 237.)

Fractures of the Hip

Fractures of the hip occur in the elderly, particularly in women, because their

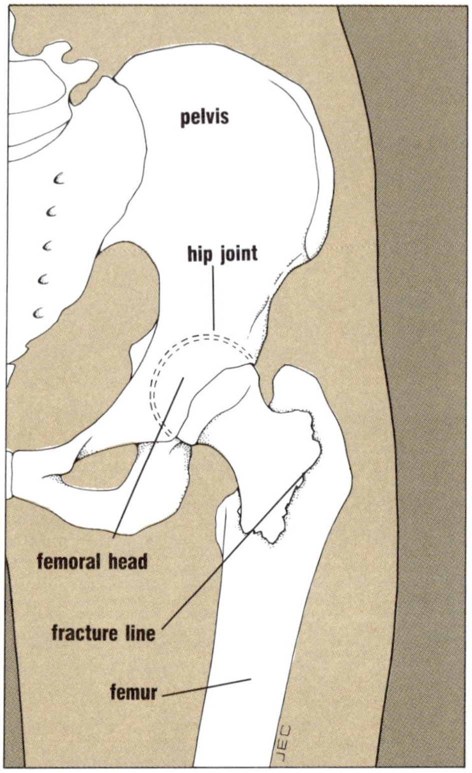

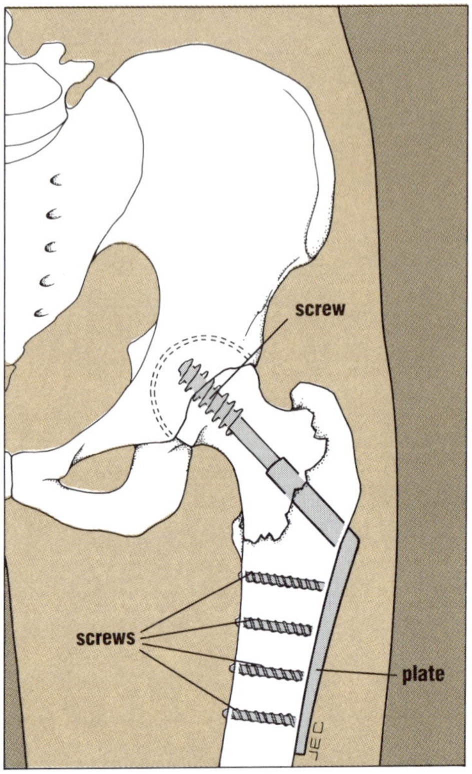

Figure 17.3
A fracture of the left hip, seen from the front, before (A) and after the fracture has been surgically stabilized with screws and a plate (B).

bones are weakened by post-menopausal osteoporosis. Most of these fractures occur in the home after a simple fall. In some cases, the bone may break during a minor twisting force before the fall.

This fracture has greater socio-economic implications than any other: up to 25 percent of the patients in an adult orthopedic ward will have fractured hips, and will need several months of rehabilitation, often ending in transfer to a nursing home.

Fractures of the hip are usually operated on and fixed with metal (Fig. 17.3). This allows the patient to walk, thus avoiding all the complications of bed rest in the elderly, such as blood clots in the leg veins that may spread to the lungs, swelling of the extremities, pressure sores, urinary infections, stiffness of the joints, and osteoporosis due to lack of activity. The patient is allowed out of bed the day after surgery, usually with a walker.

A patient who was active and completely independent before the fracture will most likely return to his or her former capabilities. If the patient was somewhat frail, the fracture might be "the straw that breaks the camel's back," and the patient may require permanent assistance for walking and self-care.

In about 25 percent of fractures that occur within the neck of the femur, the blood supply may be interrupted and the femoral head dies, causing osteoarthritis of the hip joint. The more displaced the fracture, the more likely this is to happen. A surgeon may insert an artificial hip in an elderly patient with a badly displaced femoral neck fracture, but would fix the fracture in a younger, more active patient.

The mortality rate in elderly patients who suffer this fracture is at least 10 percent at six months, but this is due more to failure of other organs than specific complications at the fracture site. The fracture may precipitate a downhill course for some patients, and it is important for the patient's family to understand the seriousness of the situation.

Fractures of the Tibia

Fractures of the shin bone (tibia) occur most commonly in the young adult. This fracture is often caused by motor vehicle accidents, especially those involving motorcycles. Fractures of the tibia used to be commonly caused by skiing injuries, but with the new high ski boots, the force of a fall is now transferred to the knee.

Fractures of the tibia are often open, because the bone is close to the skin. If the fracture is closed, relatively undisplaced and stable, a cast is applied from the toes to the groin, and the patient is kept in the hospital for only a day or two. During this time the patient is observed for circulatory problems and is taught how to walk with crutches.

If the fracture is displaced and mildly unstable, it is put back into its correct anatomical position while the patient is under general anesthetic, and a cast is applied (Fig. 17.4).

If the fracture cannot be manipulated back into place, or if it is so unstable that it cannot be held in a cast, then an open reduction is carried out, and the fracture is held in place with a metal plate or a nail placed in the canal of the bone. In this case, a cast is not necessary, and the patient is allowed to walk with crutches but without bearing weight.

The wound of an open fracture must be cleaned with the patient under anesthetic. If the wound is small and relatively clean, it can be closed by sutures when the fracture is treated, but if it is extensive and relatively dirty, it is cleaned, dead skin and muscle are removed, and the wound is left open. Under these circumstances the fracture

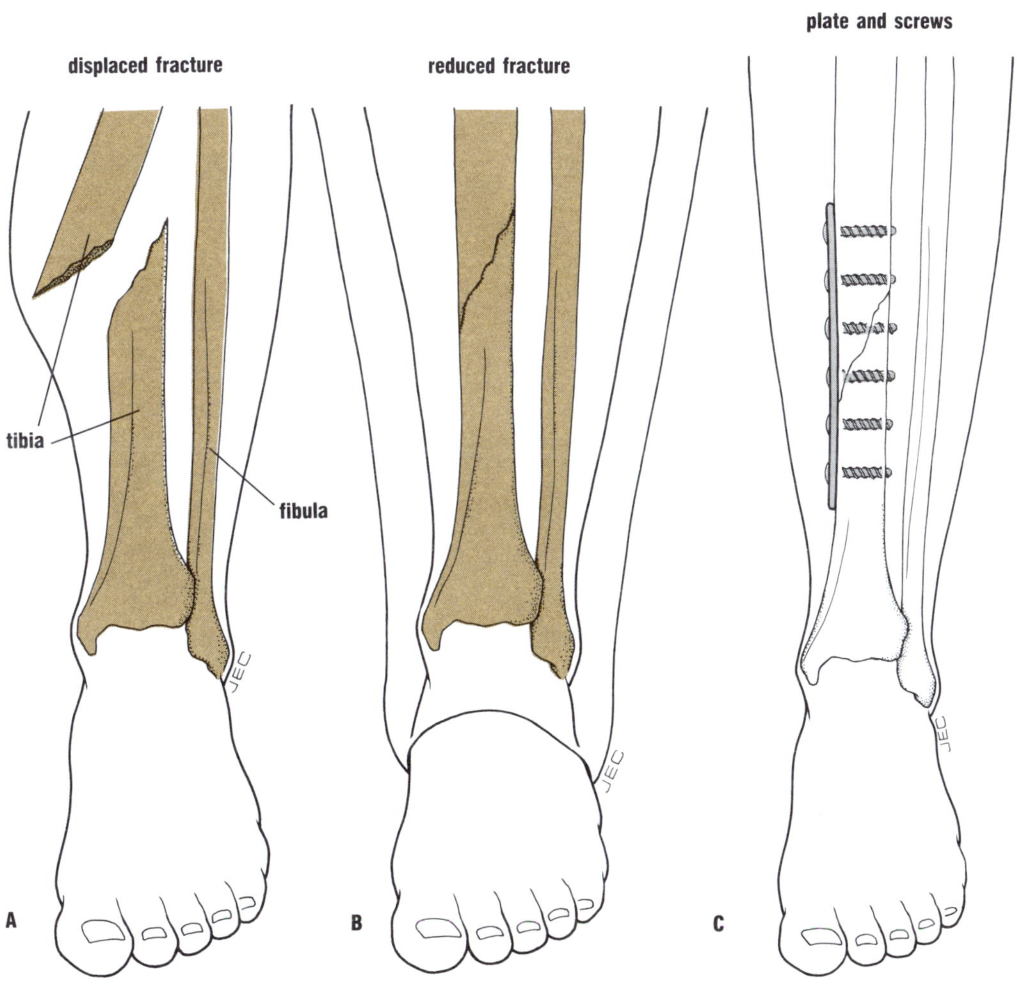

Figure 17.4
Fracture of the tibia (shin bone), before (A) and after a closed reduction (B), and after an open reduction (C), where the fracture is stabilized with a plate and screws.

Case Study: Knee Surgery

Stan was looking forward to his squash game with one of the guys from his department. Although he hadn't been going to the club as long as his colleague, he enjoyed the game and the friendly competition.

His opponent placed a tricky shot, and Stan, his foot placed firmly on the floor, twisted to return the ball. A sharp pain shot through his knee, causing him to drop his racquet. "You okay?" asked his opponent. Stan, a bit breathless, walked to the side and back a few times, then decided he was all right. They finished the game, even though Stan's knee still felt sore. The next day his knee was swollen and painful, but seemed to be on the mend.

He didn't play squash for about a week while his knee felt sore. But the club tournament was coming up. He decided his knee felt a bit better, so he let himself be persuaded to try a game. In the very first game his knee locked. He sat out a game, then tried again, but this time his knee gave way and he fell.

He saw his family doctor the next day. "You may have damaged a ligament or meniscus, Stan," Dr. St. Clair said after examining him. "I'd lay off the sports, wear a tensor bandage, use ice when the knee is swollen, and have physiotherapy." He also arranged for Stan to see an orthopedic surgeon.

is usually unstable and difficult to manage in a cast, so an external fixation device may be used. This allows rigid fixation of the fracture without putting hardware into the wound, which can become infected. Small diameter pins are placed in the bone above and below the fracture and attached to an outrigger on the outside of the leg, to stabilize the pins. The patient is then able to ambulate with crutches.

While the external fixator is in place, the soft tissues may be repaired with skin and muscle grafts as soon as the wound appears to be clean and healing. The surgeon may elect to use the external fixator until the fracture heals, or to remove the external fixator and fix the fracture with a metal plate when the wound appears to be healing without infection.

The early complications are injuries to skin, nerves and blood vessels. Damage to nerves is usually dealt with later by either a nerve repair or a tendon transfer. Damage to blood vessels is dealt with immediately; otherwise, the limb tissue will die and have to be amputated.

The plastic surgeon becomes involved if there is extensive soft tissue damage. Simple skin grafts are usually all that is necessary. If the damage to the skin and surrounding muscles is extensive, a combined muscle and skin graft may have to be carried out, usually by transferring tissue from another part of the same leg. Grafts are carried out when the wound appears to be healing without infection (any time from one to four weeks).

The tibia has a poor blood supply, so even undisplaced stable fractures may take up to six months to heal. More displaced fractures have greater soft tissue damage and a more precarious blood supply. Some of these fractures may not heal even after several months, and further surgery then becomes necessary. This surgery involves rigid fixation of the fracture with metal, and a bone graft taken from the patient's iliac crest near the hip. If the fracture has already been fixed with metal, just the bone graft is inserted. If the device is not effectively holding the fracture, it is removed and a new one is applied.

Surgery of the Knee

The knee joint is the "prince" of joints. It is pampered with tape and braces, and revered by those who love to flaunt their knee incisions like duelling scars. This status is often underlined by the fact that many highly paid athletes have abruptly had their careers ended by injuries to this joint.

Two societal trends have increased the need for knee surgery. One is the fitness craze. The other is our extended lifespan. The elderly now expect to maintain their quality of life to a greater age. Both of these trends depend on mobility.

We move our bodies by means of our joints. A joint consists of bones that meet, a capsule that surrounds the bone ends, holding them together, and cartilage to line the bone ends as they move against each other. The joint is moved by the muscles. The knee joint is a complex hinge that not only permits bending (flexion) and straightening (extension), but can also rotate about 10 degrees inward and outward.

There are three bones in the knee joint: the lower end of the thigh bone (femur), the upper part of the shin bone (tibia), and the knee cap (patella). Where the bone ends meet to form the joint, they are covered by cartilage — a smooth, slippery, ice-like substance that allows friction-free movement between the bones (Fig. 17.5).

The ends of the bones forming any joint are held together by strong connective tissue, called the capsule. Where the joint is most stressed, the capsule is reinforced by strong strips of connective tissue called ligaments. The knee has four ligaments — one on each side and two within the joint itself (Fig. 17.6). The menisci are on top of, and attached to, the cartilage of the tibia.

The knee is also stabilized by muscles. The two major groups of muscles around the knee are the quadriceps and the ham-

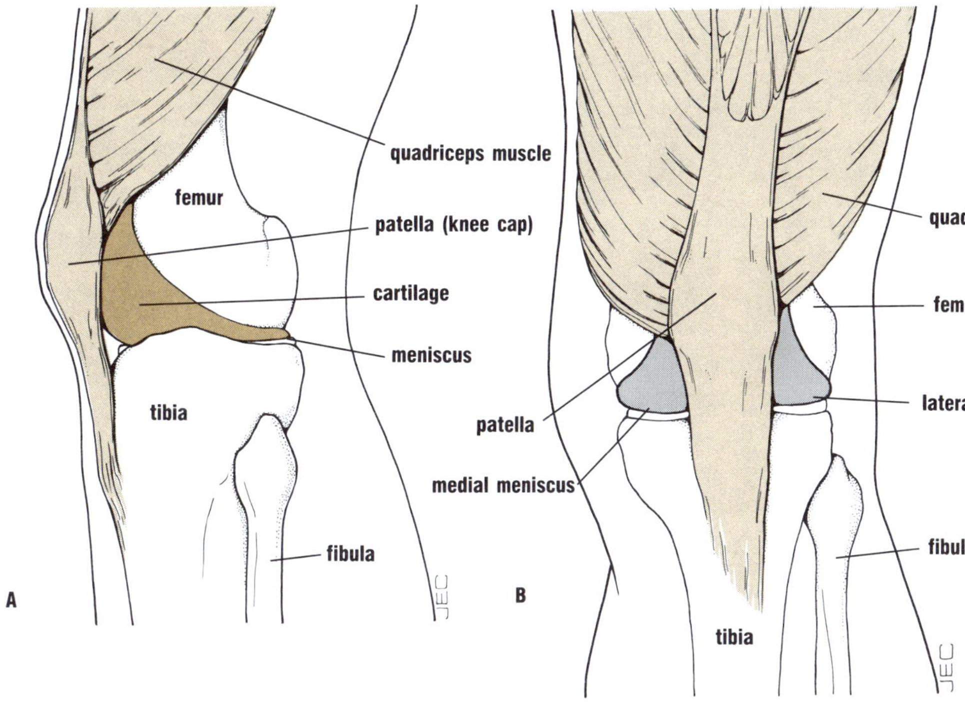

Figure 17.5
The left knee joint from the side (A) and front (B), showing the bones and muscles.

strings. The quadriceps are in front of the thigh bone (femur) and insert into the shin bone (tibia). They extend or straighten the knee. The kneecap (patella) serves as a fulcrum for the quadriceps muscle, increasing its efficiency in straightening the knee. The hamstrings are behind the thigh bone and also insert into the shin bone. They bend the knee.

Menisci act like shock absorbers between the two bones forming the joint. They are unique to the knee, which is subjected to high impact forces during activities such as jumping and running. The menisci consist of fibrocartilage, a firm, rubbery substance. The knee has an inner meniscus (medial) and an outer (lateral) one. When you hear that an athlete has torn a cartilage, they really mean a torn meniscus, not the cartilage that lines the joint (Fig. 17.7). The menisci are on top of, and attached to, the cartilege of the tibia.

Diagnosis

The symptoms of a torn meniscus depend on the pattern of the tear. Sometimes the tear produces a mobile frag-

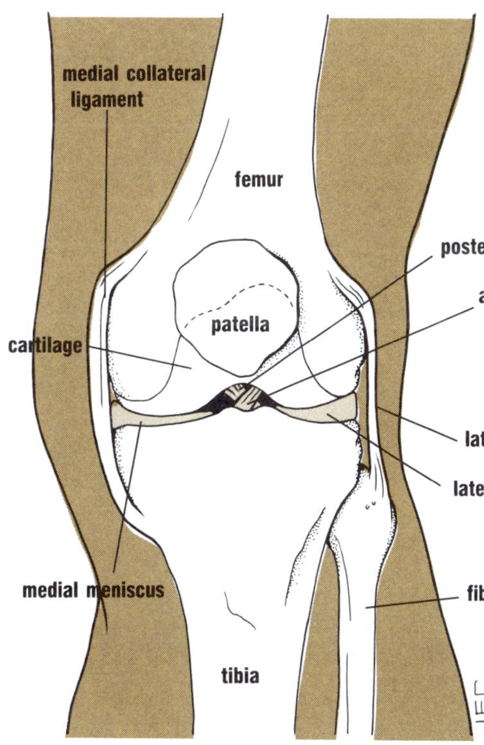

Figure 17.6
A front view of the left knee, showing the four major ligaments and the menisci.

Figure 17.7
The knee menisci and ligaments shown from above, before (A) and after a "bucket handle" tear to the medial (inner) meniscus (B).

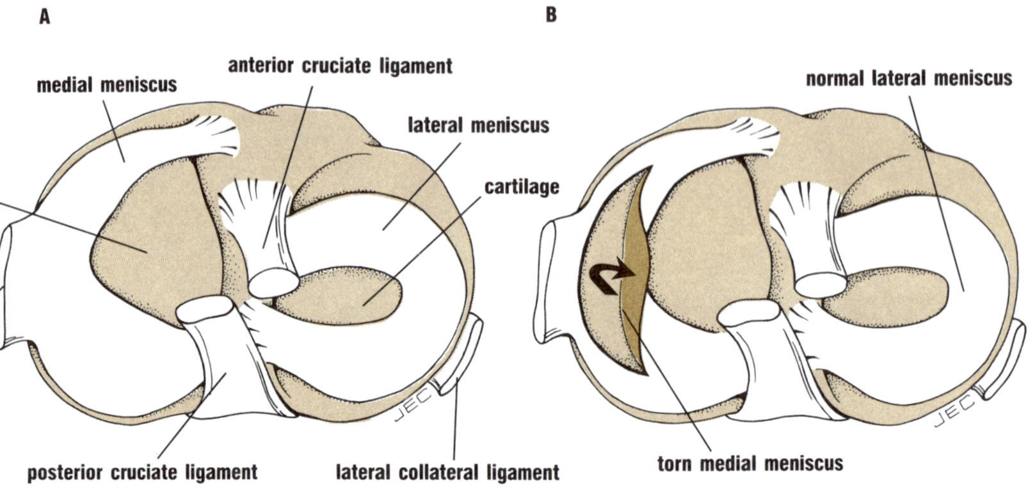

The orthopedist suspected that Stan had torn a meniscus rather than a ligament. He increased the physiotherapy. Stan was back on the squash court in a few weeks. But his knee still locked or gave way, and was painfully swollen. Two months later he saw the orthopedist again. This time Dr. Bertrand recommended a procedure called arthroscopy.

Stan was pleased that he was in and out of the hospital the same day. After the surgery, his knee still felt a bit sore and swollen. The surgeon had removed the torn part of a meniscus. Stan's knee had three puncture wounds covered by Bandaids. Dr. Bertrand had used absorbable sutures, so Stan wouldn't have to have them removed. He could return to work the next day. Dr. Bertrand said he wouldn't feel like running for about two weeks, but started Stan on physiotherapy two days after surgery and told him it would continue for about a month. After that Stan could get back to playing squash where he gradually regained his former ability.

ment, which can get caught between the femur and the tibia, causing the knee to catch and give way. This is usually followed by pain and swelling. Between these episodes, there may be no symptoms.

When the pattern of the tear is in the shape of a bucket handle, the "handle" is pushed into the middle of the joint, causing the knee to lock so it cannot be straightened. When this happens, walking is impossible.

The menisci can be torn during twisting of the knee, most often during sports, but also during less vigorous activities, such as squatting. The inner meniscus is more vulnerable to damage than the outer one.

Diagnosing a torn meniscus can be difficult, because the history given by the patient and the physical findings are often vague. For a more precise diagnosis, an instrument called an arthroscope is inserted into the joint through a small puncture wound, so that the surgeon can see inside the knee. This procedure is called diagnostic arthroscopy.

Non-Surgical Treatment

Most meniscal tears will not heal spontaneously, but small, simple tears may become symptom-free after three or four weeks of restricted activities, and need no further treatment.

Surgical Treatment

If a tear continues to cause symptoms such as pain, swelling, locking or giving way, then surgery is carried out, usually by arthroscopy. The surgeon looks through the arthroscope, inserts instruments through small puncture wounds and removes the torn portions of the meniscus.

If arthroscopic surgery is not possible, the surgeon will make an incision about an inch long and will remove the damaged part of the meniscus. This operation is called an arthrotomy. Arthroscopic surgery tends to be less painful postoperatively and results in a shorter convalescence than arthrotomy.

After arthroscopy the knee is supported by a pressure bandage. The patient returns to daily activities in about two days and sports within a month. After an arthrotomy the patient has to wear a large groin-to-ankle pressure bandage for two weeks and use crutches for weightbearing. Sports are out of the question for at least six weeks.

Physiotherapy, consisting of muscle-strengthening exercises, is usually required for about one month after arthroscopic surgery and two months after an arthrotomy. Patients eventually return to their normal lifestyle, including sports.

Recent Advances

Surgeons now feel that if possible, only the damaged part of the meniscus should be removed, rather than the entire meniscus, which was the common practice ten years ago. Entire removal causes wear and tear on the cartilage after many years, so surgeons now leave as much meniscus as possible.

Recent research suggests that certain patterns of tears can be repaired. The repair can be done by arthrotomy or through the arthroscope.

Torn Ligaments

Ligaments are strong, leather-like fibers of connective tissue that enclose a joint. They can be stretched (sprained), or partially or completely torn.

A patient can tear one or more ligaments, or ligaments and menisci simultaneously. The degree of damage depends on the direction and magnitude of the injuring force. The most common combination is an injury to the medial collateral and the anterior cruciate ligaments, often seen in football after a player is hit from the side (Figs. 17.8 and 17.9). The high incidence of knee injuries from this mechanism led to the abolishment of the "crack-back" block in American football. Most ligament tears are caused by severe forces, but the anterior cruciate ligament may be damaged by more moderate forces, such as landing from a jump. An isolated tear of the anterior cruciate ligament is the most common ligament injury.

A ligament tear causes a hemorrhage, producing a swollen, painful joint that will not bear weight. A chronic tear causes symptoms only during vigorous activities such as sports, usually in the form of giving way. Over a period of time, this can damage the menisci and cartilage, leading eventually to degenerative wear and tear osteoarthritis.

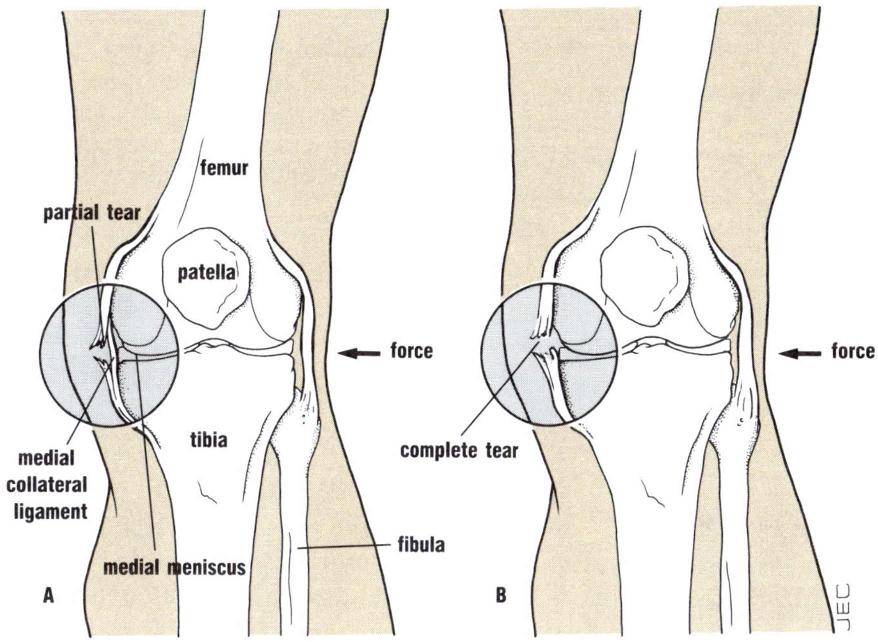

Figure 17.8
Front view of the left knee, showing a partial tear (A) and complete tear (B) of the medial collateral ligament.

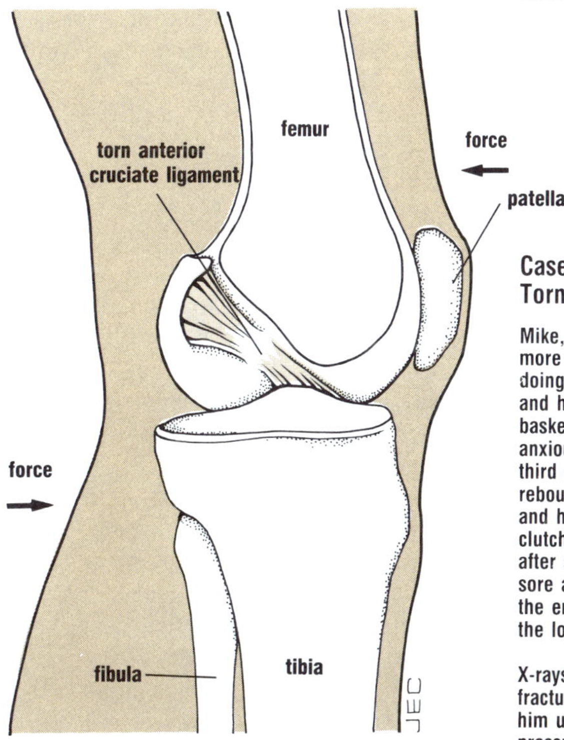

Figure 17.9
Side view of the left knee, showing a complete tear of the anterior cruciate ligament.

Case Study: Torn Ligaments

Mike, aged 21, was a sophomore at university. He was doing well. He liked his courses and he had just made the basketball team. He was anxious to show his stuff. In his third game, he went up for a rebound, landed on one foot — and his knee gave way. He fell, clutching his knee. The coach, after seeing that his knee was sore and swollen, sent him to the emergency department of the local hospital.

X-rays showed that Mike hadn't fractured a bone, which cheered him up a bit. They gave him a pressure bandage and crutches. He saw the doctor at the university health service the next day, and was sent for physiotherapy. After about three weeks, his knee felt much better.

Mike's coach kept him out of the game until he seemed recovered. After six weeks, having worked hard at physiotherapy so that he could get back on the team, Mike played his first game. All went well until his first sudden turn, when his knee gave way. The same thing happened when he stopped suddenly. He couldn't continue the game. Frustrated and disappointed, he returned to the doctor at the university health service, to be given an appointment to see an orthopedic surgeon. The orthopedist examined Mike's knee and told him that he'd torn the anterior cruciate ligament. The choices of treatment were a brace, or surgery.

Mike thought over the orthopedist's alternatives carefully. He wasn't crazy about the idea of surgery, but the prospect of a brace was even less appealing. "If you were older and winding down your sports, I'd recommend a brace," the surgeon said. Mike agreed. It was too early to put an end to any chance of playing competitively.

During the operation, the surgeon used Mike's own tissue, from the fascia of his thigh — connective tissue with physical characteristics of a ligament. Mike was in a cast for five weeks, on crutches for 12 weeks and in physio for three months. He was out of basketball — and all other sports — for nine months.
After the physiotherapy he gradually returned to sports, but his surgeon said that although he had an 80 percent chance of achieving a reasonable level in sports again, he only had a 50/50 chance of getting to the pro level.

Diagnosis

After a significant ligament injury, the patient's knee becomes very swollen, and weightbearing is difficult or impossible. Ligament sprains can be diagnosed by physical examination, but more extensive injuries require examination under anesthetic and arthroscopy. If torn ligaments are not diagnosed and treated in the acute situation, they become chronic, leading to recurrent instability. This is particularly true for the anterior cruciate ligament.

Non-Surgical Treatment

Within two weeks of the injury, a simple sprain or partial tear are treated in a plaster cast (groin to toes) for four to six weeks. This is followed by approximately six weeks of physiotherapy and a return to sports in three to six months. Non-surgical treatment of a chronic tear depends on the patient's age and needs. The low demand or unathletic person may be content to decrease activities so that the knee never gives way. More athletic individuals may be able to cope by wearing a brace to stabilize the knee during sports.

Surgical Treatment

An acute complete tear of one or more ligaments usually requires surgery. The torn ligaments are sewn up and the patient spends four to six weeks in a cast. Sometimes it is impossible to repair the ligament, because it is too shredded or has a poor blood supply. This applies particularly to chronic tears. Under these circumstances a new ligament must be constructed using the patient's own tissues (tendons or connective tissue), or by using synthetic materials.

After surgery for a torn ligament, the leg is in a cast from groin to toes, with the knee bent, for about five weeks. When the cast is removed, the patient gradually straightens the knee over several weeks during a course of physiotherapy. Once the knee is straightened, the patient begins to take weight on the leg with the help of crutches. The patient starts full weight-bearing about three months after surgery, but physiotherapy continues for four to six months, followed by a return to sports in nine months to a year.

A highly competitive athlete performing at an international level may or may not reach former performance levels after a major ligament repair. For example, it's unlikely that a running half-back in football could return to his pre-injury performance. On the other hand, Steve Podborski was able to win the World Cup men's downhill skiing title after reconstruction of his anterior cruciate ligament, because skiing places less demand on this ligament, due to the smooth snow surface. Recreational athletes usually return to their preoperative potential, but this cannot be guaranteed.

Recent Advances

New synthetic materials such as carbon fiber and polypropylene braid have been developed to replace ligaments. The early results have been encouraging but are still very preliminary.

The Arthritic Knee

Arthritis is a general term meaning inflammation of a joint. Osteoarthritis is degenerative wear and tear of the cartilage. This wear and tear is part of the normal aging process, but osteoarthritis accelerates this process, usually due to some precipitating factor like an injury or a deformity.

Any irregularity of the joint lining eventually leads to wear and tear of the cartilage. A torn meniscus, for example, can no longer serve as a shock absorber, causing increased localized pressure and damage to the joint. Bowleg deformity causes an unequal weight distribution; all

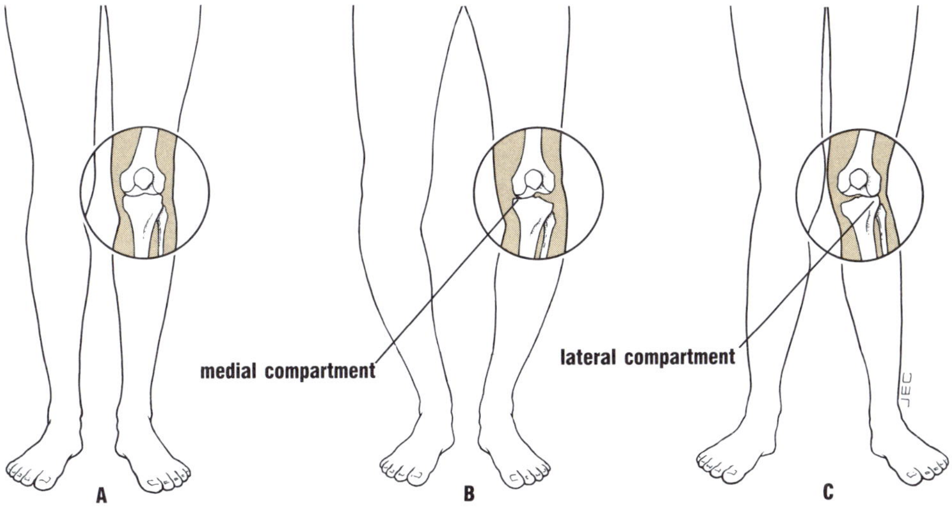

Figure 17.10
Knee alignment. Knees in neutral alignment (A) are straight, and the body weight is taken equally on both the lateral and medial compartments. Knees in a varus alignment are bowlegged (B), leading to all the weight being taken on the inside, causing wear and tear arthritis (osteoarthritis) of the medial compartment. Knees in valgus alignment are knock-kneed (C), so the body weight is taken on the outside, causing wear and tear arthritis of the lateral compartment.

the pressure is taken on the inside compartment of the knee, leading to wear and tear of the cartilage. Other causes of osteoarthritis are infection and fractures of the joint surface. In some cases there is no apparent cause.

The knee has three compartments: the inside (medial), the outside (lateral), and the patellofemoral. Osteoarthritis can affect all compartments (congruous osteoarthritis) or just one or two (incongruous osteoarthritis). The process may start in one half of the joint, if there is a malalignment like bowlegs or knock-knees (Fig. 17.10).

Osteoarthritis of the patellofemoral compartment causes pain under the kneecap. The pain may be increased by squatting, kneeling, using stairs, and sitting for a long period with knees bent. Osteoarthritis of the medial or lateral compartments causes pain, limited movement, swelling and progressive disability. Osteoarthritis most commonly starts by affecting primarily one compartment.

Rheumatoid arthritis is much less common than osteoarthritis. It is an inflammation of the joint lining (synovium) which eventually invades and destroys the cartilage in all compartments.

Diagnosis

The diagnosis is based on the patient's history, physical examination and X-rays. Occasionally diagnostic arthroscopy is helpful in estimating the degree of the disease. Certain blood tests can diagnose some types of arthritis, mainly rheumatoid.

Non-Surgical Treatment

The initial treatment of arthritis consists of restricted activities, weight loss, physiotherapy, walking aids such as a cane and anti-inflammatory drugs. Injecting cortisone into the joint can decrease symptoms, but is not effective after multiple injections. Cortisone relieves symptoms by lessening inflammation — but it also decreases the normal repair process.

Surgical Treatment

There are two types of surgery for the arthritic knee — realignment and replacement.

Realignment

If the disease is confined to the inside medial compartment, a bowleg deformity is often the cause of the wear and tear. A realignment operation transfers the weight to the relatively healthy outside lateral compartment of the knee. The bowleg is transformed to a slight knock-kneed position by an operation called a

Case Study: The Arthritic Knee

Frances, a 65-year-old homemaker, had always led a busy life.

She had had rheumatoid arthritis of several joints for a few years, but her major problem was her left knee. She'd been through all the regular treatments — medication, physiotherapy and even cortisone injections — but the knee remained a problem. Otherwise, her rheumatologist was pleased with the control of her disease. She was conscientious about taking her medication, and was careful not to overdo things.

But Frances had had to use a cane for the past few months. She said it made her feel like an old lady. She'd even had to ask for help with her grocery shopping. The family was worried that she was becoming frail.

Frances's rheumatologist said arthritis had destroyed the knee, and wanted to send her to an orthopedic surgeon. The orthopedist recommended knee replacement surgery, which sounded very drastic. He explained that because her knee joint had been destroyed by rheumatoid arthritis, and because she led a relatively sedentary life, knee replacement was the most appropriate surgery.

Figure 17.11
To correct a bowlegged deformity of the left knee, which is causing wear and tear arthritis of the medial compartment (A), a wedge of bone is removed (osteotomy), and the gap is stapled closed (B). This will realign the knee so it is straight, and transfer the body weight to the healthy lateral compartment.

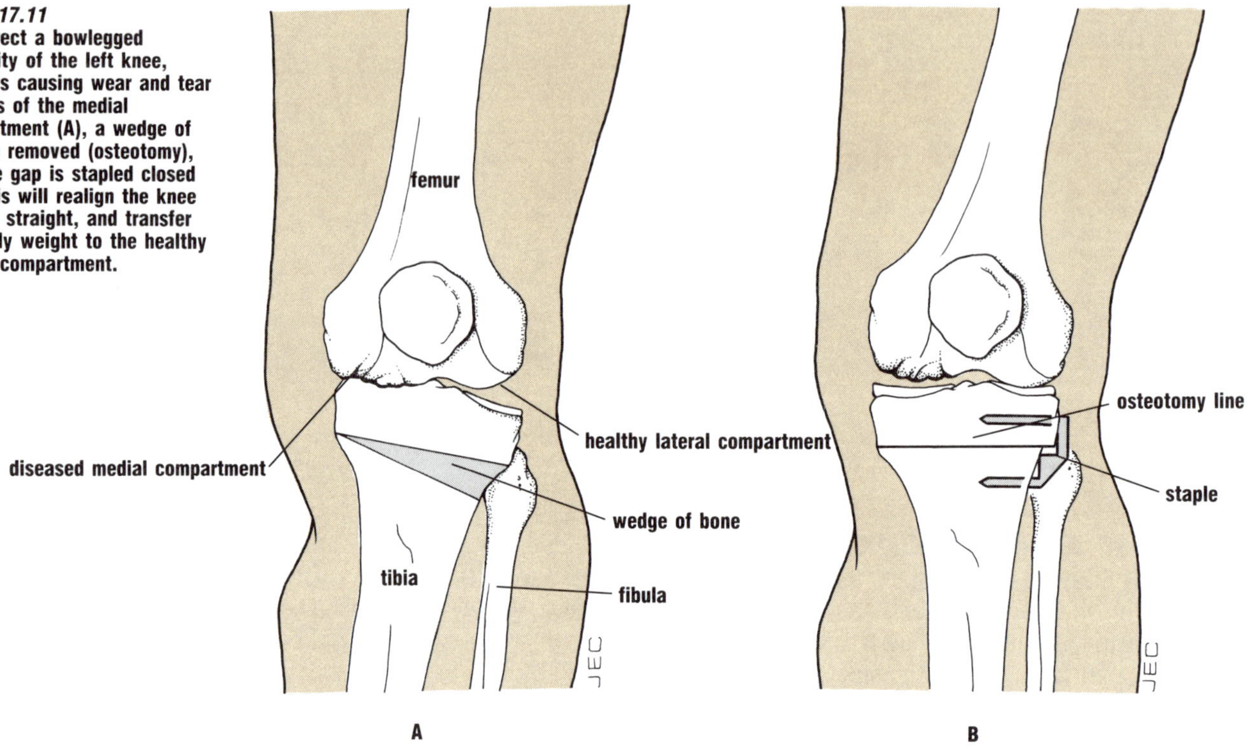

After discussion with her family and her rheumatologist, Frances opted for replacement surgery. Since in all other respects she was healthy and could expect a normal lifespan, she wanted to spend her last years as independently as possible.

The operation lasted for two hours, and Frances was hospitalized for ten days. A device called a continuous passive motion machine was used to get her knee moving — right in the recovery room. She was allowed partial weightbearing immediately, using a brace and crutches, and she progressed to full weightbearing in two weeks.

When her knee could bend to 90 degrees and the wound was clean and dry, Frances faced the next big decision. Should she go home or to a convalescent hospital? She opted for the convalescent hospital where she would receive care and treatment. She would be there for about six weeks.

high tibial osteotomy. A wedge of bone is removed from the upper segment of the tibia and the bone is usually maintained in its new position by staples until it heals. If this operation is done before the cartilage is completely worn out, the developing arthritic changes in the affected half of the joint are arrested (Fig. 17.11).

If the disease is confined to the lateral compartment, there is often an associated knock-knee deformity. This is much less common than bowleg deformity. In this case a realignment is achieved by removing a wedge from either the upper end of the tibia or the lower end of the femur, depending on the degree of deformity (Fig. 17.12).

The knee is wrapped in a well-padded plaster splint, which is left on for about five days, when knee flexion and extension is started. Weightbearing depends on the degree of stability of the bone fixation after realignment, but may be started as early as a few days or delayed for a few weeks. Crutches are used for approximately six weeks and a cane for four to six weeks. If the surgeon prefers that weightbearing be delayed, then crutches may be used during that time.

Postoperative procedures vary according to the surgeon. Recently, immediate knee movement in the recovery room has been made possible by the use of a continuous passive motion machine, which flexes and extends the knee. Some surgeons, however, delay mobilization for up to four weeks.

Complications

An early complication of realignment is foot drop. The peroneal nerve, which controls the muscles that hold up the foot, may be damaged by the surgery. Peroneal nerve injury is usually due to pressure during surgery rather than laceration of the nerve. The damage is not usually severe, and the patient will likely recover within a few months, during which time a ''drop-foot'' brace is worn to hold up the foot during walking. This small brace is attached to the shoe and extends to just above the ankle.

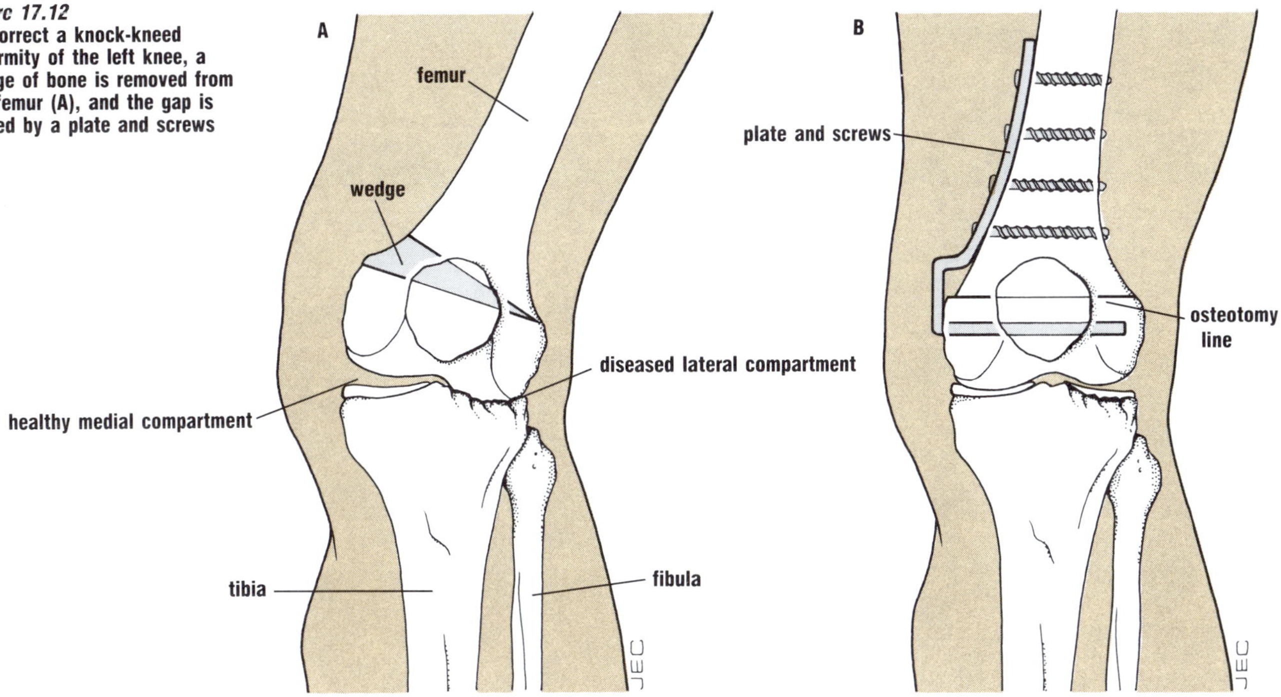

Figure 17.12
To correct a knock-kneed deformity of the left knee, a wedge of bone is removed from the femur (A), and the gap is closed by a plate and screws (B).

If the nerve injury is severe, surgical repair may be carried out. If repair is impossible because of the degree of damage, tendon transfers may be necessary.

The major late complication of realignment surgery is undercorrection of the deformity. If this occurs, further surgery may be necessary. It may be possible to do another realignment, but if not, then the insertion of an artificial knee is considered.

If successful, realignment surgery allows the patient to return to unrestricted activities — even the most vigorous sports — since the surgery involves no artificial components that could wear or loosen. If treated early enough, osteoarthritis can be relieved by realignment surgery, rather than replacement surgery. This may provide relief for the patient's lifetime, or at least delay the necessity for knee joint replacement for many years.

Replacement

If left too long, incongruous arthritis can become congruous, affecting all three compartments so that realignment is impossible. If a patient's entire knee is diseased, an artificial knee may be inserted. This is called total knee replacement. The artificial knee consists of plastic and metal components, which are attached to the bone ends with special cement. This combination of metal and plastic resembles the smoothness of cartilage on cartilage (Fig. 17.13).

An artificial knee provides a pain-free, stable joint with good motion and no deformity. The weak link in this operation is the use of cement to bond the artificial components to the bone ends. With heavy demands and over time, the bone-cement junction will break down and the components will loosen. This procedure is therefore reserved for "low-demand" patients who have a relatively sedentary lifestyle. A "high-demand" patient is advised to wait until a later age when his or her knee demands will not be as great. In general, the accepted minimum age for knee replacement surgery is 55, but exceptions are made for the very low-demand, younger patient with crippling arthritis.

After surgery, the leg is enclosed in

It was three months before Frances could walk without the aid of a cane, but when she did, her knee was relatively pain-free. Frances could do her own shopping, housework and gardening. The orthopedist said she'd have to see him at three, six and 12 months after the operation, and then annually.

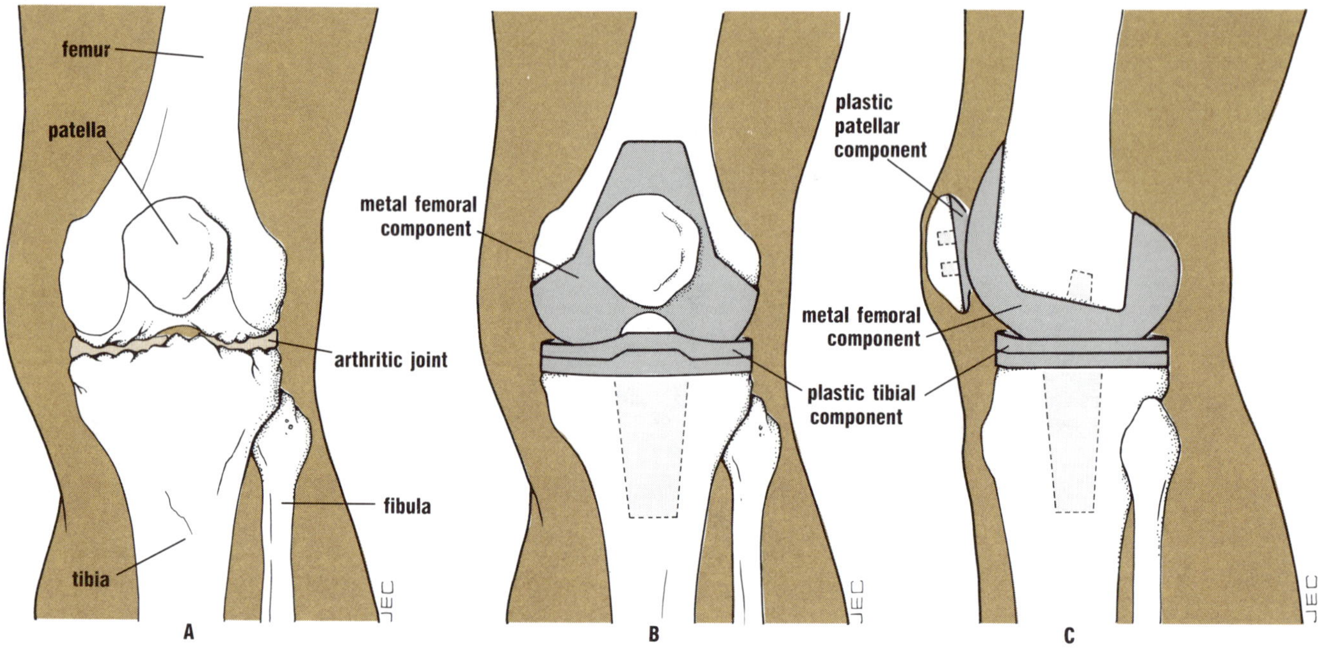

Figure 17.13
An arthritic left knee (A) in which both major weight-bearing compartments (medial and lateral) are diseased, making realignment impossible. The correction involves a knee replacement, shown here from the front (B) and side (C).

a well-padded dressing, usually with a splint. Knee motion is started at three to five days. Some surgeons prefer mobilizing the knee on a continuous passive motion machine starting in the recovery room. After one or two days the patient is allowed to walk and bear partial to full weight. Crutches are used for several days, and a cane is used for two or three months.

Complications

Infection, a rare complication, may become apparent a few days after surgery. If the infection extends deep into the bone, the artificial knee components will have to be removed. A superficial infection is therefore treated immediately with intravenous antibiotics and surgical drainage if necessary, to prevent the infection from spreading into the bone.

Infection is a very serious complication after knee replacement, because an artificial knee can be reinserted successfully in only half of the cases. Infection can occur up to a year or two after the surgery — or even longer if the infection is carried in the bloodstream from another source, such as a dental abscess. To avoid late infections, patients are given antibiotics when they have dental work, genito-urinary examinations, or infections of any kind. By using contemporary surgical techniques and preventive antibiotics, the infection rate can be kept below 3 percent.

After replacement surgery, the knee may become stiff if physiotherapy is not carried out in an organized program. If the knee does not regain a functional range of motion in a month, it may have to be manipulated under general anesthesia. This occurs in 5 to 10 percent of cases.

The most serious and common complication of knee replacement is loosening of the components. This occurs where the artificial components are cemented to the bone. In a low-demand patient, significant loosening occurs in about 10 percent of cases after five years. A new knee can be inserted, but the results are usually not nearly as good as the original. For this reason, research is attempting to find ways of fixing these implants without using cement.

Replacement surgery does not mean a return to a vigorous lifestyle. Activities such as running or jumping are discouraged. Obesity and occupations involving a lot of walking or heavy lifting must be avoided. If excessive demands are placed on an artificial knee, early loosening may occur, necessitating difficult and not always rewarding revision surgery.

Recent Advances

A new technique allows insertion of an artificial knee without the use of bone cement. Metal spheres or fibers cover the surface of the components inserted against the bone. These spheres or fibers create a porous surface that the bone can grow into. About six weeks after the surgery, the bony ingrowth is sufficient to fix the component firmly to the bone without using cement. Theoretically, this should decrease the rate of loosening, because the bony ingrowth should provide a permanent bond. Results so far have been encouraging, but are still preliminary.

The Arthritic Hip

The hip is a ball and socket joint of two bones — the femur and the pelvis. The head of the femur is the ball, and the acetabulum (a part of the pelvis) is the socket. The surfaces of the ball and socket are covered by cartilage (Fig. 17.14).

The joint is enclosed in a thick, leathery tissue called the capsule. In some places the capsule thickens to form ligaments. The whole joint is surrounded by muscles.

The ball and socket configuration allows movement in every direction. Ligament injuries, so common in the knee, are not a problem for the hip.

Problems of the hip are rarely described in the sports pages, because it is less vulnerable to injury than the knee. However, hip problems can be far more disabling than knee problems. Arthritis of the hip is a common cause of disability in North America and Europe.

Case Study: The Arthritic Hip

Joyce was in her mid-60s. For about three years she had been experiencing stiffness in her hip. Then it began to pain her. The family doctor took X-rays and discovered that she had arthritis. Joyce was told it was common in people her age, and she was given medication to ease the pain. But her hip seemed to get worse, and didn't improve after physiotherapy. Now she could only get around with the assistance of a cane.

When she found that she was unable to endure any kind of mild exercise, such as walking the dog, she decided to meet with her doctor to see what could be done. Her doctor explained that the next option was surgery, and an appointment was made with an orthopedic surgeon.

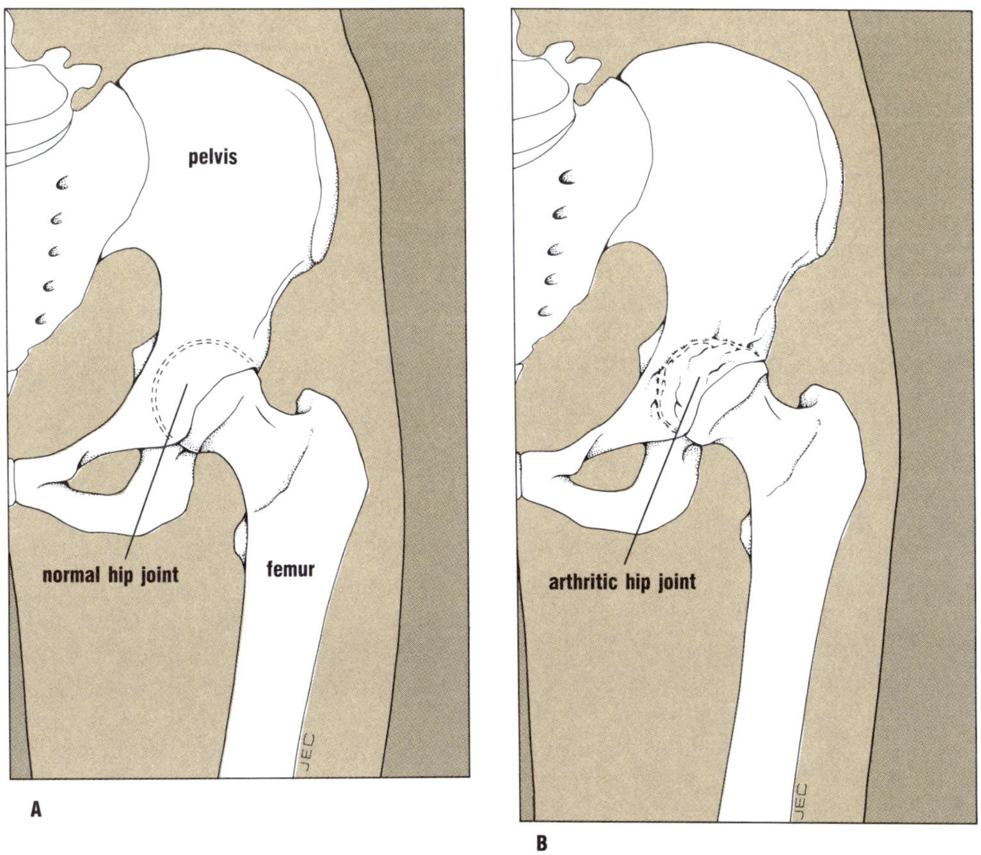

Figure 17.14
A normal (A) and arthritic (B) left hip joint, seen from the front, showing the ball (femoral head) and socket (acetabulum) hip joint.

Dr. Wendell asked Joyce a lot of questions about her daily life. He wanted to know if she could tie her own shoes, do her housework, go shopping, how far she could walk. She had expected things to be far more technical, but she appreciated the chance to talk about what mattered most to her. Dr. Wendell was very matter-of-fact. "Things seem to have been getting worse for quite a while. I notice that you've been taking painkillers. Do they help? Not anymore? I think, then, given the fact that you're otherwise well, you just want to be able to do light exercise, and you're not overweight, we should book you for hip replacement surgery."

He explained carefully what was involved, said she'd probably have to wait a couple of months for a hospital bed, but in that time she should watch her weight and not take aspirin for pain, and refrain from smoking.

In two month's time Joyce was scheduled for surgery. The operation lasted about two hours. The next day Dr. Wendell saw her to discuss the things she'd have to be careful about. She mustn't cross her legs, sit in low chairs or do any real bending. She could take showers, but no baths for the first while. All of these precautions were to lessen the chance of dislocating the new hip joint.

Diagnosis

Arthritis simply means inflammation of a joint. There are many different types of arthritis of the hip, but by far the most common is degenerative or "wear and tear" arthritis. It is the cartilage lining the joint that wears out. Osteoarthritis, as this is called, may develop for no apparent reason (idiopathic osteoarthritis), or there may be an identifiable cause, most commonly congenital deformity or injury.

Rheumatoid arthritis is another type, fortunately less common than osteoarthritis, because it is more serious and affects many joints. In rheumatoid arthritis the joint envelope is the source of the problem. It becomes inflamed, eventually invading and destroying the cartilage. Medication may control the inflammation, but eventually the joint may be completely destroyed, and surgery is necessary. Although rheumatoid arthritis is potentially far more crippling than osteoarthritis, less than 10 percent of people with rheumatoid arthritis become crippled by it. The disease is more common in women.

In arthritis of the hip, pain occurs during walking and is relieved by rest. The pain is felt around the hip, groin and thigh, interfering with such activities as walking, sitting, putting on shoes, and getting into a bathtub.

The majority of patients with disabling arthritis of the hip are elderly, but rheumatoid arthritis and arthritis caused by injury or congenital maldevelopment may also occur in young patients. Hip replacement, now a safe and effective operation, has had a great impact on the treatment of arthritis of the hip.

Arthritis of the hip is diagnosed by the history, physical examination and X-rays. No invasive diagnostic tests are necessary. The extent of the patient's disability must be documented (for example, the patient might be asked how many blocks he or she can walk) because hip replacement is not performed until a certain level of disability is reached.

Non-Surgical Treatment

Restriction of activities, rest, weight loss, physiotherapy and anti-inflammatory medications may help. A cane in the hand opposite the hip serves as a strut to keep the pelvis parallel to the ground, eliminating the need to limp. Arthritis of the hip can cause shortening of the leg, which will also cause a limp. This can be corrected by a lift inserted into the shoe.

Patients with rheumatoid arthritis are initially treated with anti-inflammatory medication, but may eventually require stronger drugs to suppress the inflammation. These medications are prescribed by rheumatologists, who specialize in the non-surgical treatment of joint disease.

Surgical Treatment

There are three surgical alternatives for the arthritic hip: realignment osteotomy, fusion and replacement. Replacement is by far the most common surgical approach. The choice of operation depends on whether the entire joint has been destroyed (congruous arthritis) or only part of the joint (incongruous arthritis), and whether the patient is low demand or high demand.

A lightweight patient over age 60 and with a sedentary occupation is considered low demand. A younger, obese patient with a physically demanding occupation or an interest in sports is considered high demand. Since artificial hips perform much better for a longer period of time in low-demand patients, alternatives to hip replacement must be found for high-demand patients.

Realignment

In incongruous arthritis, where a significant portion of the cartilage is still healthy, it may be possible to realign the joint so that the weight is taken on the healthy cartilage. Either the ball (head of the femur) or the socket (acetabulum) must be repositioned by an operation

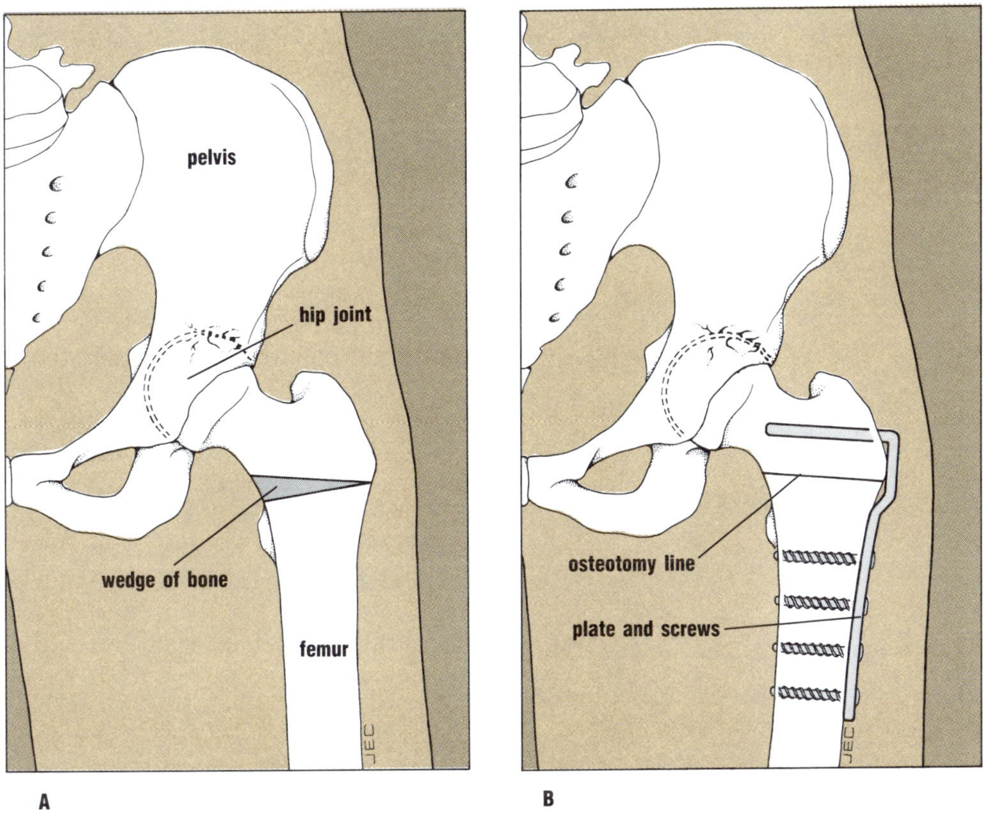

Figure 17.15
With incongruous arthritis of the hip (A), part of the joint is arthritic, while the rest is normal. To realign the hip, a piece of bone is removed from the femur, and a plate and screws are inserted to close the gap, transferring the weight to the healthier part of the joint (B).

called an osteotomy (cutting of a bone). Either the pelvis or the femur may be operated on, and a metal device holds the bone in its new position until it heals. If done early, this type of surgery may eliminate the need for hip replacement, or at least delay it for many years (Fig. 17.15).

Fusion

If the hip cartilage is completely worn, so that realignment is impossible, and the patient is too young for hip replacement, the hip can be fused to stop all movement, stiffening the joint in a functional position. This produces an immobile but strong, pain-free joint, although it causes a slight limp. Childbearing and sexual function are not inhibited.

Realignment or fusion allows the patient to take part in even the most vigorous activities without fear of wearing or loosening a synthetic joint. Hip replacement can still be done if necessary when the patient is older. Both realignment and fusion operations require the use of crutches for three to six months.

Replacement

The hip was the first joint to be replaced successfully by synthetic materials. In the late 1950s the concept of total hip joint replacement was developed, and this revolutionary operation, which dramatically improved the quality of life for people with arthritis of the hip, was being performed around the world in less than ten years. It is now one of the most common and successful orthopedic operations performed. In North America, in 1988, more than 100,000 synthetic hip joints were inserted.

An incision 10 to 12 inches long is made over the thigh and hip. The surgery takes up to three hours, and blood transfusions are usually required. The head of the femur is replaced by a metal ball attached

Joyce was practicing with her walker the next day. The pain bothered her, but as the nurse said, she could expect to have pain where the incision had been made. She was taking painkillers which eased the pain and helped her get going on the walker. Dr. Wendell had told her she'd be in hospital for about 10 days. At that point they'd decide whether she could go home, or if she'd be better in a rehabilitation hospital. Joyce made good progress, and was allowed to return home.

Dr. Wendell saw her again at four weeks, when she was down to using one cane and looking forward to getting rid of that. She had very little pain now, and was really beginning to believe that the surgery would give her a chance at a more active life.

At three months, Joyce felt strong enough to walk without the cane. Dr. Wendell checked the hip. The replacement seemed to be holding up well, so the cane could go. One further checkup was scheduled in six months, and after that Dr. Wendell would need to see her only on an annual basis.

to a stem that is anchored to the patient's thigh bone by bone cement. The acetabulum is replaced by a plastic socket that is anchored to the pelvis by cement, which grouts into the rough surface of the bone (Fig. 17.16).

The routine after total hip replacement varies slightly depending on the surgeon, but the major components are the same. After the operation, patients are in bed for one to five days, with their legs kept apart by a pillow to prevent the ball from dislocating from the socket. The patient is then allowed to walk with crutches or a walker. Most surgeons allow weight bearing within a day or two. The crutches or walker are used for one to four weeks, then two canes for two weeks, then one cane in the opposite hand for up to three months after the operation, when the patient should be able to walk unaided. The average length of hospital stay is two weeks, during which time physiotherapy is given, consisting of instructions for walking with crutches and canes, muscle strengthening, and gentle hip stretching. The need for rehabilitation and physiotherapy is minimal after this operation.

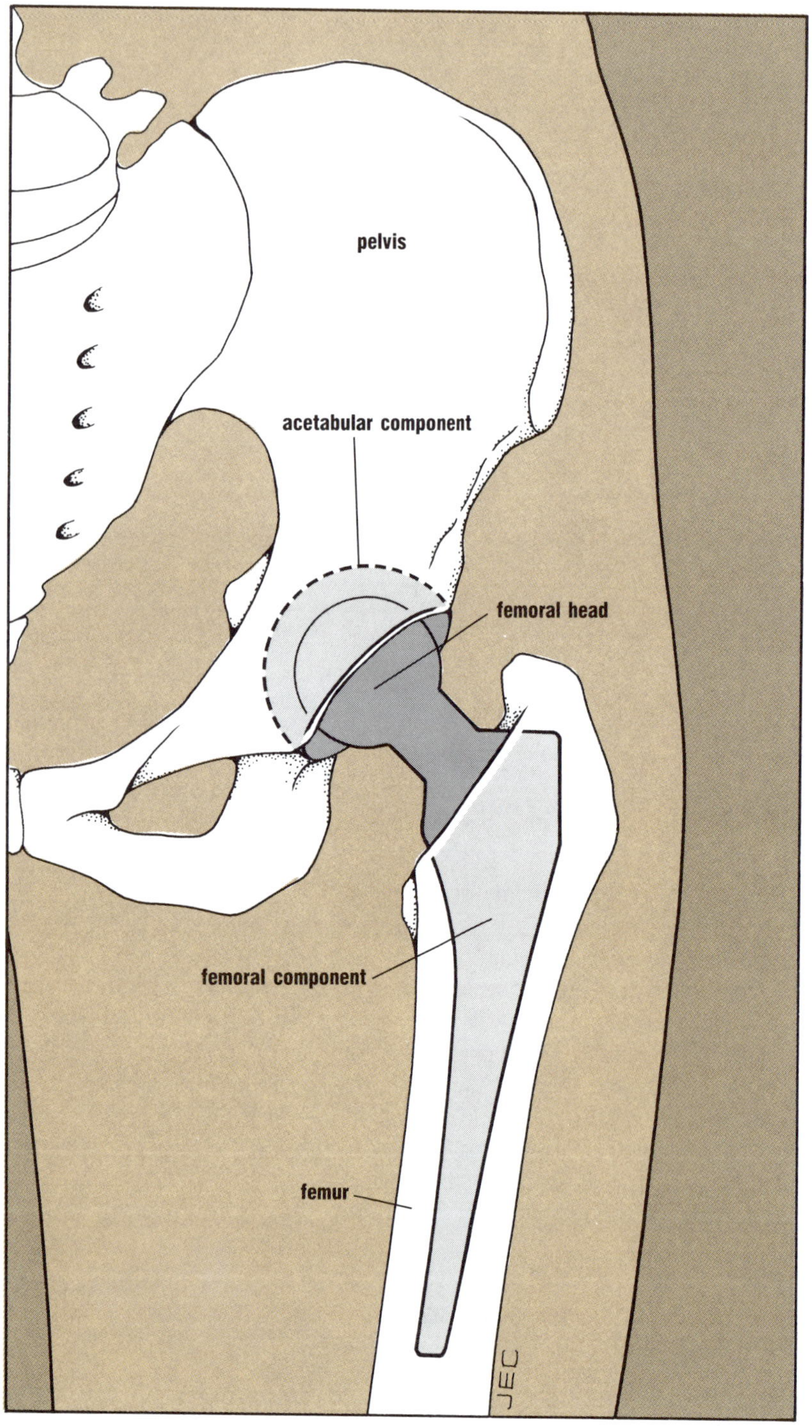

Figure 17.16
In total hip replacement, a prosthesis is inserted, involving an acetabular component (socket), femoral head (ball) and femoral component.

Complications

Complications can occur after any operation (See chapter 4), but thrombophlebitis and pulmonary embolism occur more commonly after hip replacement than other surgical procedures. Thrombophlebitis is the formation of a blood clot in a vein. Pulmonary embolism occurs when a piece of a blood clot breaks off and travels to the lung. The veins that develop thrombophlebitis are usually in the leg that is operated on, but it may occur in the other leg.

Following hip surgery, the surgeon may take certain measures to prevent thrombophlebitis. An elastic bandage or stocking may be used to prevent swelling and improve blood flow in the veins. The foot of the bed may be elevated slightly to improve the return of blood from the legs. The patient may be given certain medications to inhibit blood clotting. Probably the most important factor is physical activity, including deep breathing, coughing, calf pumping (moving the feet up and down) and early walking, all of which improve the return of blood from the leg veins.

Reports on the incidence of thrombophlebitis after hip surgery range from 5 to 50 percent. The incidence of pulmonary embolism after hip surgery is probably 5 to 10 percent, and death due to pulmonary embolism less than 1 percent. If thrombophlebitis does occur, the treatment is medication that prevents further clots from forming. These medications are given for three to six months.

Dislocation of the metal ball from the plastic socket may occur at any time, even several years after surgery, but it usually happens within the first three months. The dislocated ball must be placed back in the socket as quickly as possible, sometimes under general anesthetic. If it is stable, the patient is nursed in bed with the legs spread wide apart for three to six weeks. If the joint is unstable, the surgeon studies the X-rays to see if either the ball or the socket are in a position that might encourage them to dislocate. If so, the surgeon will operate to reposition the component.

The two most common nerves to be injured during hip surgery are the femoral (which controls the muscle that straightens the knee) and the sciatic (which controls the muscles that bend the knee and move the foot). These nerve injuries are usually due to pressure at the time of surgery. They resolve without treatment within a few days to a few months. Another common nerve injury is caused by the patient lying with the foot turned out, causing pressure on a nerve as it winds around the outside of the calf. This interferes with the ability to elevate the foot at the ankle. This usually clears up within three months, but during this time a special ankle brace must be used.

A very serious complication is infection, which can occur from a few days to several years after surgery. Usually infection occurs within the first few months, often within the first few weeks, due to contamination by airborne bacteria at surgery. When it occurs several months or years later it is due to infection elsewhere; the bacteria reach the hip via the bloodstream. Infection due to contamination at the time of surgery is far more difficult to eradicate because it may be deep in the bone where the circulation is poor, so that antibiotics cannot reach it.

When total hip replacements were introduced in the 1960s, the infection rate in most centers was over 5 percent. Today's rate is more acceptable: about 1 percent. The surgery is now done more quickly, and in most centers antibiotics are given intravenously on the day of surgery and continued for about 48 hours, followed by five more days by mouth. If the patient has any other infection, it must be eradicated before hip replacement. Many hospitals use special operating rooms, where the air is changed 300 times per hour, and flows in one direction (either vertical or horizontal). The surgeons may also wear special protective suits and helmets.

If there is significant infection, the wound is drained as soon as possible. This may cure the infection if it is done within a few days of surgery, but is unlikely to work for an infection that appears later. If the infection persists, the ball and socket and all the cement must be removed. At that point there are three alternatives. A new hip may be inserted, using cement impregnated with antibiotics, or insertion of the new hip might be delayed for about three months, during which time the patient would receive antibiotics. The third alternative, usually chosen only if the first two fail, is to permanently remove all components and cement, leaving the patient with a loose (flail) joint. This is called an excision arthroplasty. The patient's leg will be short and weak, but mobile and pain free. Walking is possible with a leg brace or using at least one cane.

Infections occurring years after surgery are carried by the blood from another site of infection. Any implant is susceptible to bacteria present in the blood. To protect the artificial hip, patients who have infections elsewhere, or are undergoing dental work, surgery, or examination of other organs, must take antibiotics. If not on antibiotics and infection does spread via the blood to the hip, cure is often possible by surgical drainage and antibiotics.

If the hip components loosen at the bone cement junction, pain develops and the operation must be done again. The results will not be as good the second time, because when the first artificial hip is removed, along with the cement, the surfaces left on the pelvis and femur are smooth, lacking the rough lattice necessary for good cementing. Since bone is lost due to the surgery and from abrasion by the loose cement, larger artificial components must be used. Loosening occurs more often and in a shorter period of time after the second operation.

The incidence of loosening ranges from 10 to 50 percent at ten years. The incidence of loosening in high-demand patients is 50 percent at five years. Improved cementing techniques have lowered these figures recently, but not to the point where this type of surgery can be recommended for high demand patients. It has taken orthopedic surgeons about ten years to realize this, because long-term results have only just become available.

In low-demand patients (light, elderly, unathletic) the implants work well for at least 15 years, perhaps longer. The high-demand patient can expect a good result for only about five years, which is why realignment or fusion are considered as alternatives. Patients with cemented hips are advised not to gain weight, not to do heavy lifting, and to avoid any activities that produce impact, such as running. For example, golfing using a cart is allowed, but tennis is not. Optimally the patient should be at least 50 before hip replacement is performed but exceptions are made for severely crippled patients.

Recent Advances

Research is concentrating on fixing the ball and socket to their respective bones without cement. One approach involves press-fitting the components, so that they fit tightly in the bone without moving. This is technically difficult and often minute movements do occur, causing slight pain. This, however, may be a reasonable trade-off.

The other approach is to use a porous metal coating on the surface of the components that lie within the bone. Over six to 12 weeks, bone grows into the pores of this coating, stabilizing the component. The results of this approach are gratifying to date, but it is too early to determine long-term results.

Chapter 18

Neurosurgery

Alan R. Hudson

James Wallace McCutcheon Chair
Surgeon-in-Chief
Toronto Hospital Corporation and Toronto General Hospital

Megan Welsh
Illustrator

Neurosurgery is surgery of the central and peripheral nervous systems. The central nervous system consists of the brain and the spinal cord; the peripheral nervous system consists of the nerves that originate in the central nervous system and finish in the extremities, the trunk and the face.

The Brain

The brain is contained within the skull and is attached to the spinal cord. Within the brain are a series of chambers (ventricles) that are connected by narrow passageways. Cerebrospinal fluid (CSF) flows through the ventricles and passageways, eventually reaching the surface of the brain, where it acts as a water-cushion around the brain and spinal cord. The fluid is eventually absorbed into large veins on the inner surface of the skull.

The brain is nourished by four major blood vessels, two on each side (Fig. 18.2). Those supplying the front part of the brain are called the carotid arteries; those supplying the back part of the brain are called the vertebral arteries. These blood vessels break up into branches, distributing blood throughout the brain.

Brain cells are extremely sensitive to the supply of oxygen and glucose carried in the blood. If this supply is interrupted for more than a few minutes, the brain cells will be rapidly damaged and ulti-

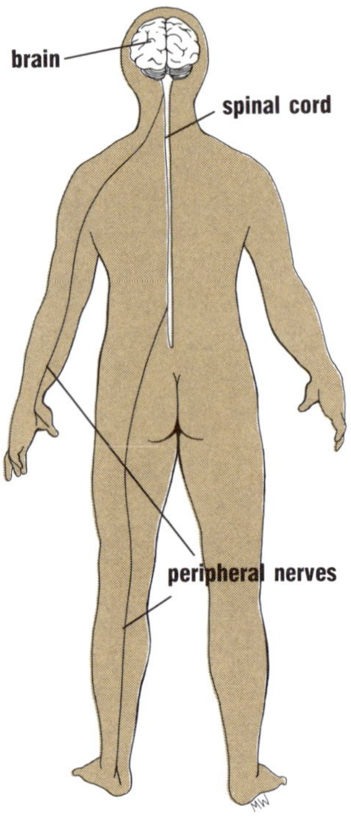

Figure 18.1
Central nervous system.

mately killed. Many of the conditions seen by neurosurgeons result from damage to the brain's blood vessels, which knocks out function in that part of the brain, causing a stroke.

The brain is an extraordinarily sophisticated computer. Information is conveyed to and from the brain by nerves, which reach every corner of the body. The nervous system in the body can be thought of as an electrical circuit. The main distribution cable enclosed within the spine is called the spinal cord and is attached to the brain. The impulses that travel to and from the brain are like small electrical currents, which arrive at transformer stations and cause minute amounts of chemical substances to be released. These initiate the next set of electrical impulses in the appropriate adjacent circuits.

Interruption of any specific part of this complex network will give a reasonably predictable result, no matter what the cause of the interruption. For example, the motor control center in the front part of the brain may be affected by a head injury, tumor or stroke. Although these conditions are quite different, they produce the same result — weakness or paralysis in the area controlled by that part of the brain.

The first task confronting the neurosurgeon is to decide where the diseased part (lesion) is. For example, if a patient has a paralyzed and unfeeling hand, the surgeon must decide if the problem is in a peripheral nerve leading to the hand, in the spinal cord, or in a particular part of the brain. Disease or injury at one of these three sites can cause the problem.

Having established where the lesion is, the neurosurgeon must next determine what the lesion is. A tumor, injury or stroke affecting the nervous system at a particular point will each cause the same abnormality, so special tests will be required to reach a diagnosis, in order to indicate the correct treatment.

The brain eventually replaces damaged tissue with scar tissue, rather than with normal, functioning brain. Likewise, the spinal cord repairs itself with scar tissue, but the peripheral nerves do have the capacity to repair by reproducing functioning nerves. Thus it is vitally important that the diagnosis of neurological abnormality be made as soon as possible. Occasionally, neurosurgical operations are matters of extreme urgency; in rare cases, even minutes can make the difference between success and failure. In many instances the situation is "semi-urgent" — transportation to a neurosurgical center, diagnosis and treatment are required within one or two days.

Neurosurgery may be needed at any age. Operations have even been performed on the unborn child, although this is rare. Occasionally, an operation may be required at birth, or within the first few days of life. Children or adults may require an operation because the normal circulation of the cerebral spinal fluid is obstructed — a condition known as hydrocephalus. Surgery may be required for a brain tumor, stroke or infection. In rare cases, operations are performed to control chronic pain or persistent tremor in patients who do not respond to medication.

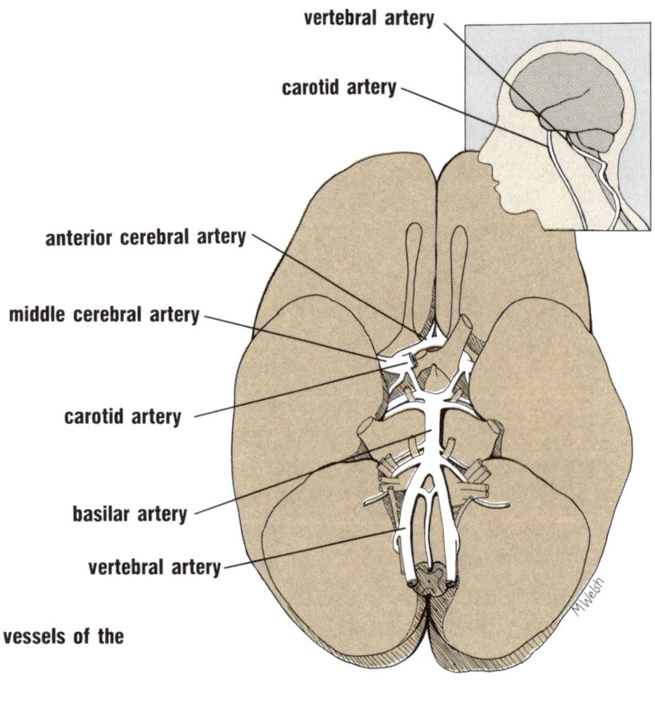

Figure 18.2
Major blood vessels of the brain.

Some operations on the brain, spinal cord and peripheral nerves are extremely simple; some are very intricate. Some of the procedures can be completed at low risk to the patient; others carry a significant risk, but a risk that is lower than the one the patient would face if the condition were left untreated.

Brain Function

Certain functions are located in certain areas of the brain (Fig. 18.3).

Level of Consciousness

The area of the brain primarily responsible for maintaining level of consciousness is located in the upper brain stem. When this area is functioning normally we are alert and respond to our environment. If the area is impaired slightly, the patient may appear drowsy, but will respond to a shouted question or command. If the area is impaired more significantly, the patient will respond only if a painful stimulus is applied to some part of the body. Severe impairment results in no response to a stimulus. The patient is then described as being unconscious, or "comatose."

Motor Power

The right side of the brain is responsible for the motor (muscle) movement of the left side of the body and vice versa — the circuits previously described cross from one side of the brain to supply the opposite side of the body. Interruption of the circuits conveying impulses for motor control from the brain, result in weakness or paralysis of the opposite side of the body. The terms "hemiparesis" or "hemiplegia" are sometimes used to describe this state.

Sensation

The central computing station related to sensation is located in the brain on the opposite side of the body from which that information is being gathered. Disturbance of function in that part of the brain will therefore result in failure to appreciate sensory stimuli on the opposite side of the body. This abnormality may occur alone, but more frequently occurs with abnormalities of motor control, because the areas of the brain controlling these two functions are located side by side.

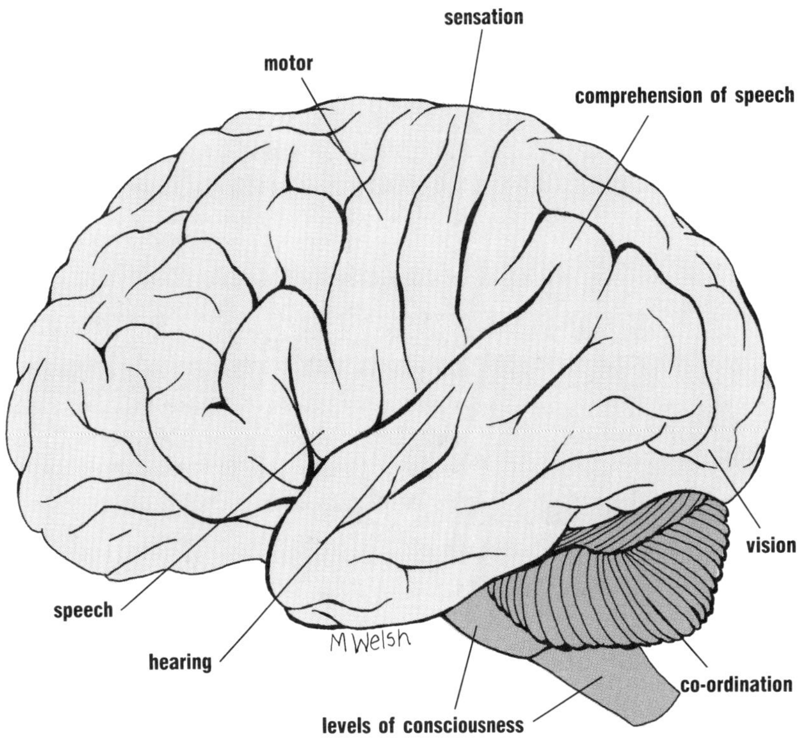

Figure 18.3
Brain function.

Expression and Comprehension

The computing station for these vital functions is situated in the left brain in most patients, although in some left-handed patients it is on the right side. Lack of function in this area causes the frustrating inability to express one's thoughts adequately. If this situation is severe, the term "aphasia" is used. Lesser grades of severity are called "dysphasia." The site for comprehension of speech or writing is immediately adjacent to the site controlling expression of thought, so these patients are frequently unable to understand either spoken or written communication, despite being neither blind nor deaf. In relatively minor forms of this condition, the term dyslexia is used.

Brain Disorders

The majority of patients suffering from conditions that require neurosurgery will have alterations in consciousness, motor weakness, sensory disturbance, or difficulty in comprehension or expression. They may also experience seizures, resulting from a sudden abnormal electrical impulse and short-circuiting in one part of the brain. For example, if the computer center responsible for the arm is suddenly the site of such firing of electrical impulses, the opposite arm will suddenly jerk and move, frequently in a rhythmical manner. This is called a focal seizure. The neurosurgeon can determine from the patient's or family's description of the seizure which part of the brain is involved. If the electrical firing and short-circuiting is more generalized, ''grand mal'' seizure will result. In this situation patients may cry out and then fall unconscious, while their limbs jerk. They may bite their tongues or wet themselves. Both focal and generalized seizures are symptoms of underlying abnormality, not diseases in themselves.

Diagnostic Tests

Diagnosis of a neurological disorder is determined from three sources: the patient's history, a physical examination, and special tests.

After a preliminary diagnosis has been made by the family doctor, the patient is usually referred to a neurologist, a specialist in neurological disorders who is concerned with diagnosis and non-surgical treatment. If surgery is indicated the patient is referred by the neurologist to the neurosurgeon. If the problem is obviously surgical to begin with the patient may bypass the neurologist.

In taking the history, the neurosurgeon is particularly interested not only in the specific symptoms, such as headache, weakness or seizure, but also the overall pattern of the illness over time. Did the symptoms come on abruptly and subsequently slowly improve? For example, a patient who suffers a small hemorrhage into the fluid surrounding the brain may suddenly experience a very severe headache that improves over the next few days. A patient harboring a rapidly growing brain tumor may have a gradual onset of symptoms, with steady and relentless deterioration.

Certain symptoms are intermittent with periods of absolute or relative normality. For example, a patient may suffer loss of motor power in an arm or a leg for 30 minutes and then have complete restoration of function. These attacks may suggest temporary interruptions of the blood supply to that part of the brain, which may be caused by hardening and narrowing of the main arteries supplying the brain (arteriosclerosis).

During the physical examination, the surgeon will be looking for information to confirm the impression formed from the history. The surgeon will look for signs that suggest the patient's intracranial pressure may be raised, such as looking into the eye with an ophthalmoscope to see whether the optic nerve head is swollen. The surgeon will also look for evidence of localized weakness, numbness or lack of coordination, which may indicate which part of the brain is affected.

Absolute diagnostic precision is required, however, before a neurological disorder can be treated. The surgeon will select from the wide variety of diagnostic tests available — those that will provide the most information at the least risk to the patient.

Computerized Axial Tomogram (CAT scan)

This is a sophisticated X-ray test, usually abbreviated as CAT or CT scan. A brain scan presents a series of pictures depicting slices from the top to the bottom of the brain. Thus, the location of a brain tumor, blood clot or abscess can be accurately defined. The risk to the patient from this test is extremely low, but the cost of installing and running such machinery is high.

Magnetic Resonance Imaging (MRI)

The magnetic resonance image is similar to the CAT scan in that images are depicted as slices of the organ being studied. The main difference is that instead of X-rays, magnetic fields are used to generate the images. In certain circumstances magnetic resonance images provide greater detail than CAT scan pictures.

MRI machines are expensive and require specially constructed rooms. Exciting advances are being made in this technique, however, and when MRI reaches its full potential, other tests will likely become obsolete. Spectroscopy is a new technique that uses MRI to study the chemical composition of brain tissue.

Angiography

An angiogram is an X-ray of the blood vessels. The four main blood vessels to the brain may be partially or completely blocked. Branches of these blood vessels at the base of the brain may dilate, forming balloon-like structures called aneurysms, which may break and cause bleeding around the brain (subarachnoid hemorrhage). Branches of these arteries within the brain may also rupture, causing an intracerebral hemorrhage, or arteries within the brain may have an abnormal structure from birth (arteriovenous malformation). A cerebral angiogram will reveal all of these conditions.

The test is usually conducted by sliding a small tube (catheter) through an accessible artery in the patient's groin. Usually a local anesthetic is used, but a restless patient may require a general anesthetic. A catheter is then threaded through other major blood vessels in the abdomen and chest and then into the four vessels supplying the brain. Contrast material is injected and a rapid sequence of X-ray films is taken, tracking the passage of the fluid through the blood vessels.

There is a small but definite risk of stroke from a cerebral angiogram. However, large centers perform several such tests every day, so that the neuroradiologist is particularly skilled. In many instances, life-threatening conditions cannot be diagnosed without an angiogram. In these situations the patient is advised to accept the small risk for the sake of acquiring the necessary information.

Isotope Brain Scan

Radioactive isotopes, "visible" to a counting machine are injected. These isotopes will accumulate in abnormal areas of the brain. Isotope brain scans are safe and are far more widely available than CAT scanning. Unfortunately, they are not as precise as CAT scanning or angiography.

Lumbar Puncture

Samples of cerebral spinal fluid (CSF) can reflect abnormalities within or near the brain. Sampling is particularly useful in diagnosing infections around the brain (meningitis) and in confirming that there is bleeding around the brain (subarachnoid hemorrhage). The test is performed by inserting a needle through an anesthetized area of skin over the lower spine (Fig. 18.4). The needle is passed between the bones of the spine into the water-cushion around the spinal cord, and samples of the cerebral spinal fluid are withdrawn for analysis.

Figure 18.4
Lumbar puncture.

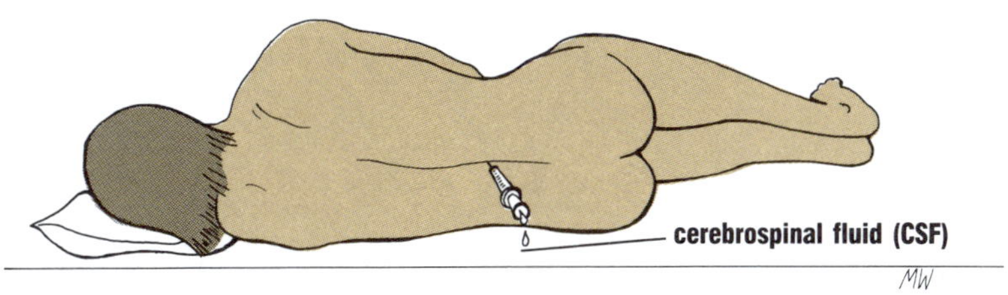

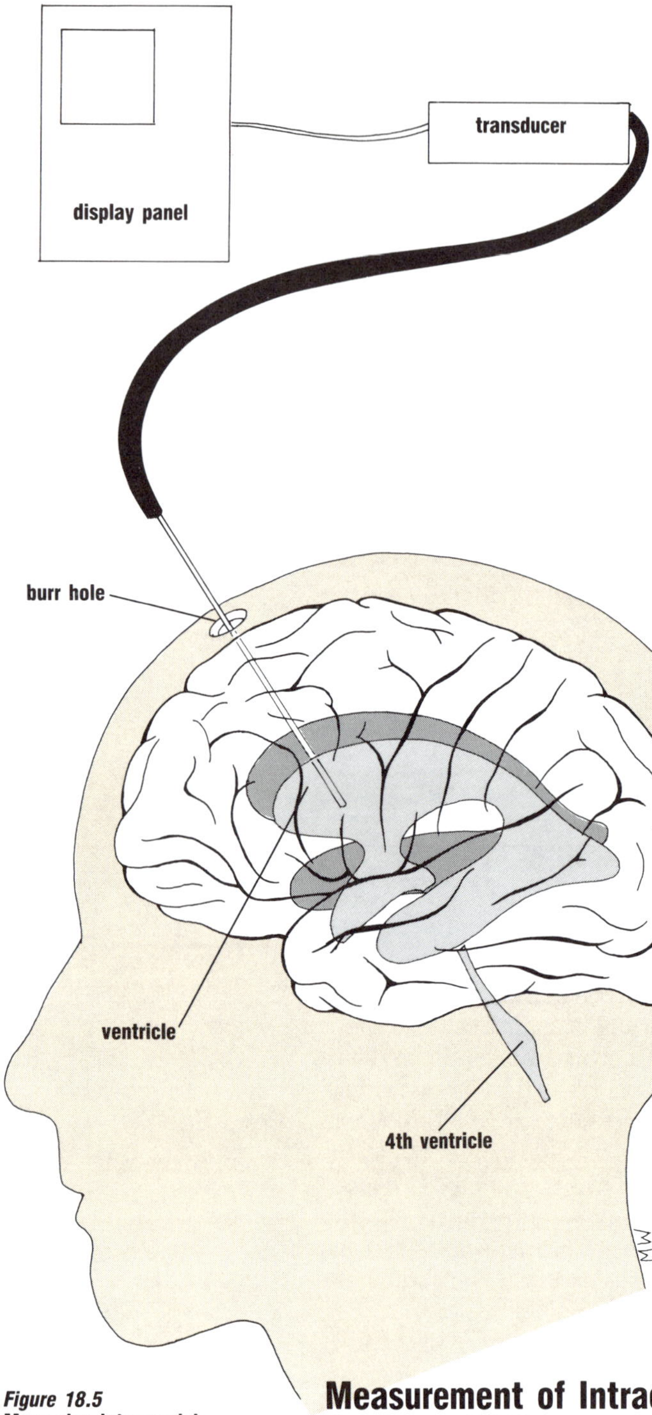

Figure 18.5
Measuring intracranial pressure. A tube is inserted into the ventricle, which contains cerebrospinal fluid (CSF).

Measurement of Intracranial Pressure (ICP)

The brain is contained within a fixed space — the skull. If anything is added to this confined space, such as a brain tumor or blood clot, or if part of the brain swells, the pressure inside the skull will be raised, affecting brain function.

A direct measurement of intracranial pressure is performed only in an intensive care unit. A tube is inserted through a burr hole into the skull, under local anesthetic (Fig. 18.5). The test can detect rising intracranial pressure at an early stage, before irreversible damage results. There are certain risks from the technique, the major one being the introduction of infection via the tube, which is usually left in place for two or three days, since intracranial pressure must be recorded over a period of time. An alternative technique measures the pressure immediately inside the skull via a sensor that is screwed into the burr hole.

Sensory-Evoked Potentials

This is a new technique now being evaluated in the intensive care unit. In this technique, a peripheral nerve is stimulated with a small electrical current, causing a nerve impulse to travel up the nerve, through the spinal cord to the brain. The passage of these little currents can be measured at both the spinal cord and brain surface. Any interruption of this circuit will change or stop the currents, pinpointing damage.

Ultrasound

Ultrasound is also being used to study the blood vessels in the neck and the main blood vessels of the brain. This technique transmits and receives sound signals, which are then analyzed to provide an image of the structure being studied. At the moment these tests are used primarily for the initial screening for diagnosis, but may eventually take the place of some angiographic tests.

Positive Emission Tomography (PET)

PET can provide a map of the functioning brain. The patient inhales an isotope which then links with a normal molecule in the brain. A color-coded map of the brain is produced, showing the distribution of the particular isotope under study. This extremely expensive device has already yielded considerable information about normal brain function and the abnormalities associated with brain tumors and stroke. Researchers also hope to find new information on the abnormalities underlying mental disease.

Electroencephalogram (EEG)

The EEG used to be a commonly performed screening test but the test is now primarily performed in patients suffering from seizure disorders. The frequency and amplitude of the "brain waves" (formed by the millions of electrical currents flowing through the brain) are altered when a seizure occurs and the EEG may help characterize the specific nature of the seizure disorder.

Non-Surgical Treatment

Antibiotics

If the patient has an infection of the nervous system, high doses of antibiotics are the main treatment. Antibiotics will also be used to treat any other infections such as infections in the lung (pneumonia) or urinary tract (cystitis). Infection following neurosurgery is extremely serious so some surgeons give patients antibiotics before the operation, to prevent infection. The disadvantage is that should an infection occur after antibiotic therapy, the organisms will be resistant to the antibiotics already present in the patient's body.

Anticonvulsant Medication

These drugs are widely used to treat or prevent seizures. Frequently the patient will be required to take anticonvulsant medication for several months after the operation. The patient and the patient's family must clearly understand the instructions and the importance of taking these drugs as prescribed.

Steroids

Cortisone is frequently used before, during and after brain operations, to prevent or treat brain swelling, which may complicate the underlying condition of the operation. Steroids are particularly useful in controlling the swelling that occurs around brain tumors, but they are far less successful in controlling the swelling following head injury.

Nutrition

All patients undergoing brain operations will have intravenous lines usually attached to plastic tubes in arm veins, occasionally leg veins, and rarely neck veins. Patients with depressed levels of consciousness may have to be artificially fed for a prolonged period, which is impossible by conventional intravenous feeding. In this circumstance, a nasogastric tube is passed through the nose, down the esophagus and into the stomach so that the patient may be fed intermittently. The family will hear the nursing staff refer to "D feeds," and will notice plastic bags containing fluids with the appearance and consistency of milkshakes, which are allowed to drip by gravity down the tube into the stomach.

Ventilatory Support

Patients with a depressed level of consciousness may not breathe deeply or cough adequately, which may cause portions of the lung to collapse. Unconscious patients may inhale material from their mouths or any vomited material, causing acute inflammation in the lung as well as blocking off some of the air tubes. They may breathe very shallowly or irregularly because the brain centers con-

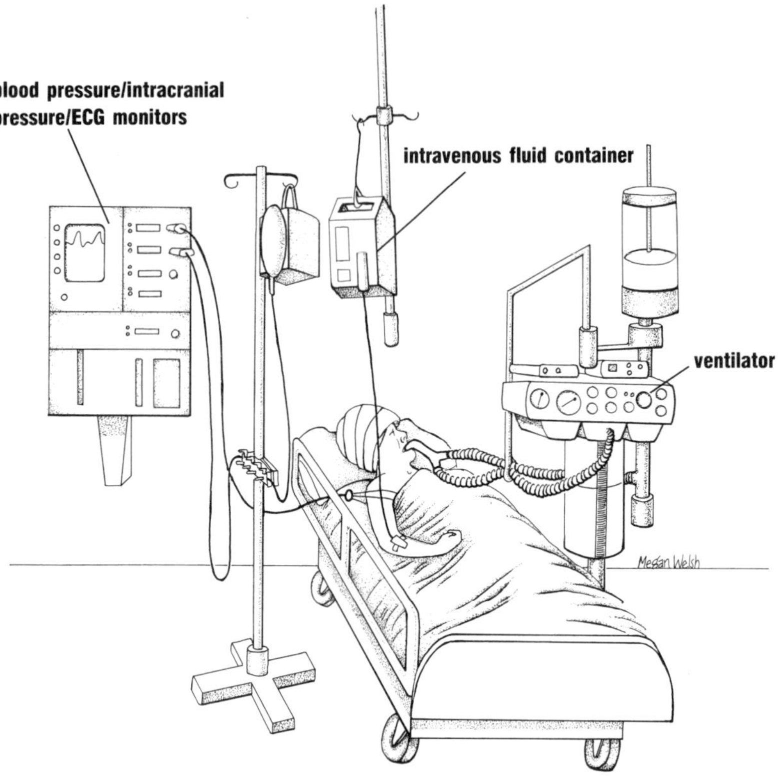

Figure 18.6
Life-support systems.

trolling respiration are damaged. Patients may have both chest and head injuries. In all of these situations, artificial ventilation is required to ensure that the blood receives a full supply of oxygen, which is transported to the brain and will help speed recovery (Fig. 18.6). A tube is passed into the windpipe and a small balloon is inflated around this tube to ensure a tight seal. The tube is then hooked up to a ventilator machine set to control the volume, frequency and pressure of each cycle of breathing. Patients who are lightly unconscious may resist mechanical ventilation, so they are given medication in order to let the machine take over their breathing.

Various life support systems (ventilation, intravenous fluids, etc.) support the patient while the underlying condition is dealt with or while awaiting improvement following head injury. Unfortunately, instances occur in which the function of the brain stem is permanently lost. In this situation, even though mechanical ventilation keeps the heart working, the patient is dead. The initiation and control of normal breathing is a brain function, so a dead patient will not breathe spontaneously. The contraction of the heart is not initiated by the brain; the heartbeat is an isolated phenomenon peculiar to the heart. However, if the patient is dead and the ventilator is turned off, the blood will no longer be oxygenated because the dead patient does not breathe. Then the heart will slowly fade and eventually cease beating.

The determination of death is always made extremely carefully, by more than one physician. If the dead patient is to be an organ donor, it is essential that the organs donated be retrieved in the best possible condition. In this situation, the dead patient will be kept on the ventilator so that the organs to be donated can be fed with oxygenated blood until the recipients can be prepared to receive them. The organs are then surgically removed, and at that stage the ventilator is turned off.

Surgical Access to the Brain

Craniotomy means opening the skull to gain access to the brain. Most craniotomies are conducted under general anesthetic but, on occasion, local anesthesia is appropriate. The hair has to be shaved from the area of the incision, but not necessarily from the whole head.

By the time the patient comes to surgery, the surgeon should know the exact location of the lesion and be fairly confident about what the lesion is likely to be. The approach to the lesion is planned to give the surgeon maximum visibility, and to disturb the surrounding brain, particularly vital centers, as little as possible.

If the incisions are made in the forehead, they are usually placed within frown creases to minimize any postoperative cosmetic defect. In most intracranial

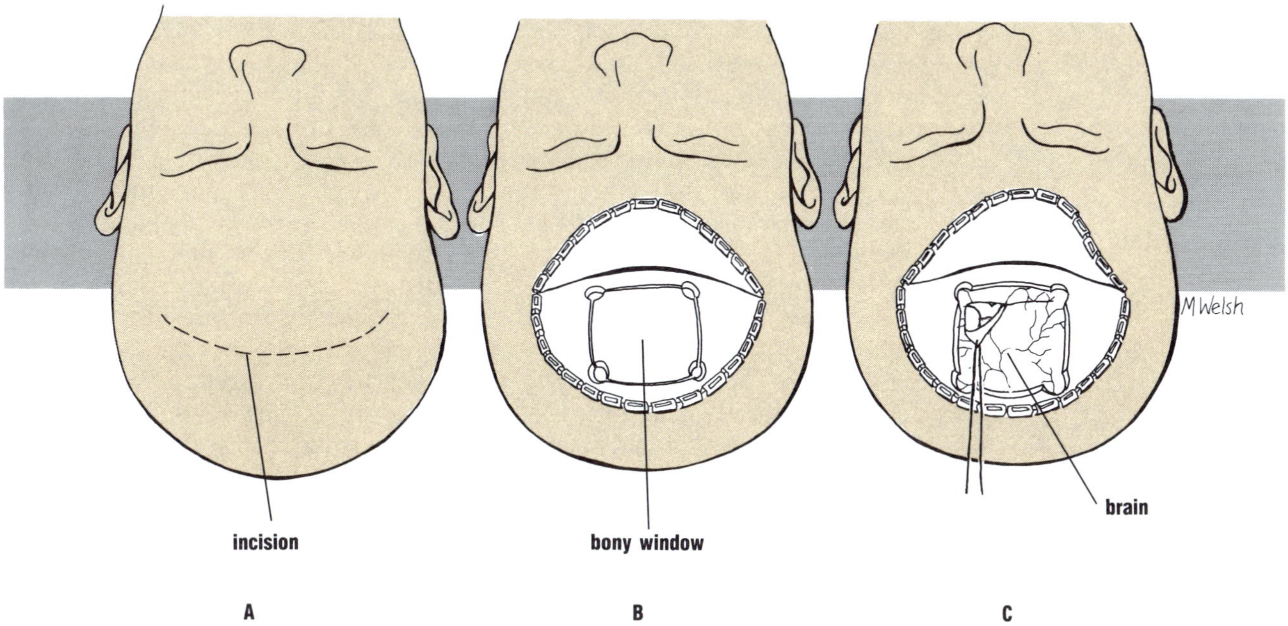

Figure 18.7
Craniotomy. An incision is made in the scalp (A), and a bony window is cut out of the skull (B) to gain access to the brain (C).

operations, a series of pins are inserted into the bone of the skull and held in an apparatus attached to the operating table, to hold the skull firmly in place at the best angle for direct access. After the operation, the patient will find small puncture wounds through the scalp at points distant from the operation site; these puncture wounds are caused by the pins.

In most cases, a hinged bony ''window'' is opened in the skull to give access to the brain (Fig. 18.7). If the lesion is within the skull but outside the brain, the surgeon will gently separate the adjacent brain with metal spatulas, which may be held by the surgeon's assistant or may be fixed to the frame that is supporting the fixation pins. This must be done with extreme care to avoid damaging the brain. The expert neuroanesthetist aids the surgeon at this stage by giving an intravenous drug which will shrink the brain slightly, and by controlling the patient's breathing so that the veins in the brain are not distended (engorged with blood).

If the lesion is within the brain, the surgeon must cut down to the lesion. The surgeon may choose to chart a course by first passing a probe into the abnormality and taking a small sample, or by applying an ultrasound device to the surface of the brain. By using an ultrasound device the lesion will be visible on a nearby television screen.

Blood vessels are first sealed off with heat before being cut. As each bleeding point appears, the vessels are sealed. The bleeding must be completely controlled to give the surgeon a clear view of the structures to be operated on and to prevent postoperative oozing from the blood vessels.

The surgeon uses many specially-made and delicate instruments during surgery. Throughout the operation the brain and surrounding tissues are kept moist with a saline solution, so that the surrounding brain is kept in as perfect a condition as is possible.

Once the surgery is completed, the surgeon will lower the bone flap into place and then close the skin incision with sutures or staples. Frequently, a padded head dressing resembling a football helmet is applied.

There are three groups of complications from craniotomy. The first includes those complications that may result from any major operation under general anesthetic. (See chapter 4.) The second group relates to craniotomy itself and includes postoperative blood clot formation, brain swelling, infection, and epilepsy. The third group includes risks and complications peculiar to the specific site of operation. For example, removal of a tumor attached to the eighth cranial nerve (hearing) may be complicated by injury to the seventh cranial nerve (supplying the muscles of facial expression on half of the face).

Both the patient and family should be aware of these general and specific risks before surgery. No operation is risk-free, nor is success guaranteed. The surgeon will advise the patient and family as to what can be accomplished by craniotomy and what the risk will be.

In addition to standard craniotomy instruments, a wide variety of precision instruments have been designed for use at various depths of the brain. New devices combine ultra-high-speed fragmentation of tissue with suction, so that very little physical pushing and pulling of tissues is required. Tumor tissues may be sucked out with precision, within millimeters of normal structures.

Lasers are also being used more frequently in brain surgery, for either cutting or vaporizing tissues. Once again, the advantage is that very little movement of tissue occurs, and the surgeon can operate with delicacy and precision. Because the high-speed fragmentation suction apparatus and the laser apparatus are extremely expensive, most operating rooms are forced to choose one instrument or the other.

The combination of advances in anesthesia, instrument design and other new devices has significantly shortened the duration of most neurosurgical procedures. Many complex and dangerous procedures may be accomplished within three or four hours. However, in unusual circumstances, the operations may be very prolonged, due to the need for special caution or special testing; a long operation does not in itself indicate that the surgery is going badly.

Head Injury

Patients who sustain a head injury may be admitted for observation at a hospital. In some circumstances, the physician may allow the observation to be conducted at home rather than in hospital. In that situation the family must be fully instructed as to what the signs of complications are, so that they can return the patient to the hospital immediately should such signs develop.

Concussion is a significant brain injury. Patients are strongly advised not to allow children to engage in athletic activities in which the express intent is that of creating a head injury (e.g., boxing). If a player suffers a concussion during a football or hockey game, that player must be removed from the game and should not be allowed to participate in body contact sports for at least three months following the injury.

Skull fractures range from cracks in the bone to complex patterns of bony fragmentation. Some of the bone fragments may be depressed and driven into the brain substance.

Patients suffering from severe head injuries will be admitted to a hospital. In emergency situations, holes may be made in the skull to allow rapid removal of blood clots that may develop between the skull and the brain. If these blood clots continue to expand, the patient could suffer irreparable brain damage. Patients suffering from head injuries which are initially very serious, or in whom serious complications may develop, are usually transferred to neurosurgical centers. In some instances, an operation is required to remove blood clots or to remove swollen and lacerated parts of the brain. In many instances, however, the damage is characterized by diffuse bruising and hemorrhages within the brain. The situation may be complicated by brain swelling. These patients may require prolonged nonoperative management in a neurosurgical unit while complications of the original injury are treated and the patient is supported in the hope that recovery will occur. Intracranial pressure monitoring and ventilatory support may be used.

A patient in a neurological center may eventually be discharged, either to his or her home, to the original referring hospital, to a rehabilitation facility, or to a chronic care facility. The patient's ability to re-enter society is determined by the degree of intellectual or physical impairment resulting from the injury. A prognosis of the eventual outcome can usually be expressed in very broad terms about a week after the injury.

In general, the long-term complications following head injury are related to the severity of the original injury. Patients who suffer moderate head injury may have symptoms of headache, dizziness, difficulty in comprehending abstract thought, impaired judgment and difficulty with complex mathematical problems. Families of patients with these symptoms should be supportive in the hope that the symptoms will resolve over three or four months. The family should consult with the family doctor during this phase of rehabilitation, so that they can reasonably establish what is anticipated of the patient at that stage.

A patient suffering from severe head injuries may experience more profound and possibly permanent impairment of intellectual ability. Psychometric tests can help to measure the degree of intellectual impairment so that the family will know whether the injured patient can ever return to previous employment, other gainful employment or whether he or she will require custodial care. This is also true for children and whether or not they will be able to continue in a regular school environment. Patients may have to be retrained in simple tasks such as dressing and routine toilet needs.

Some patients survive a very severe head injury but regain little ability to interact with their loved ones and their environment. Such patients usually require heavy nursing care and are best managed in appropriate chronic care settings.

Although technical advances are constantly being made, the key to overall advancement in the management of head-injured patients will be prevention. The most significant recent advances have been legal ones — regulating the use of seat belts, crash helmets and speed limits. A stricter attitude toward drinking and driving is a positive but partial response to this enormous problem.

Brain Tumor

Tumors within the skull may be situated within the brain itself or may arise from adjacent structures, such as the brain coating (meninges), and press on the brain. Malignant brain tumors may be primary (arise from the tissues within the skull) or secondary (grow within the brain as the result of spread from malignancies occurring in other parts of the body).

Diagnosis

Brain tumors may occur at any age. The patient may have symptoms of raised intracranial pressure such as vomiting, headache or seizures. The patient may also show evidence of loss of function in the part of the brain harboring the tumor. This may mean increasing weakness or lack of coordination in a leg or other body part.

Surgical Treatment

Benign brain tumors can be totally removed, resulting in cure. Occasionally, small portions of benign brain tumor may be left behind because their removal might constitute too great a danger to the patient. In that situation, a benign tumor may regrow, necessitating another operation.

Unfortunately, it is virtually impossible to remove a malignant brain tumor in its entirety. After initial surgery,

Case Study: Brain Tumor

Bonnie was worried. Twice now, Malcolm had complained about "writer's cramp" in his right hand. Like all writers, he complained about physical discomforts when he was working, but this was different. They used a computer at home, and for the past two evenings Malcolm had got up restlessly when he had a real flow going, asking her to keyboard while he dictated. Usually he was restless only if the writing wasn't going well. Now he paced while he dictated, and complained about a pins and needles sensation in his right arm.

After a few minutes he resumed his work at the keyboard. Bonnie left the room, but rushed back when she heard Malcolm cry out. He was staring wide-eyed at his right hand, which jerked and flailed as if it had a life of its own. "That does it. We're going to the hospital *now!*"

Upon the completion of initial tests and a physical examination, the family physician on duty requested the assistance of the neurology resident. Once the resident had asked Malcolm about the kind of symptoms he'd been having, the next step was for Malcolm to have a CAT scan.

The resident soon came in with the results. She mentioned the word "tumor," which led Bonnie to question whether Malcolm had cancer. "From the appearance and the location, we don't think so," the resident replied. "But it must be removed, because it's pressing on the brain and causing the symptoms. During the operation we'll find out for sure."

Malcolm was booked for surgery the following day. Once he was bedded down for the night, Bonnie peppered the resident with questions. Although it seemed that her worst fear — cancer —wouldn't be realized, there were possible complications from the operation that would be horrific for Malcolm, such as loss of one of his senses, particularly sight.

The operation lasted for three and one-half hours. The resident saw Bonnie immediately after surgery, to report the removal of a benign tumor, which the neurosurgeon removed with little damage to the brain.

For the next 48 hours Bonnie anxiously watched Malcolm's every movement. He recognized her when he came round from the anesthetic — one hurdle jumped. He heard her speak to him — a further hurdle. She couldn't yet be sure if he understood, because he was still groggy. Later he gestured for a glass of water — with his right hand. Another hurdle.

On the third day after the operation, Bonnie was at the hospital when the resident came in to see Malcolm. All this evidence so far was good — Malcolm's senses had returned, his blood pressure was good, and all other physical signs were normal. The resident carefully reviewed with both of them what they should watch for, and warned them again that the specific risks of this operation were the formation of a blood clot, swelling of the brain, infection or epilepsy. "I can't overstate how important it is to follow instructions exactly and to report any symptoms immediately, however minor they seem."

patients are repeatedly re-examined and checked with CAT scans, so the surgeon can judge the rate and extent of tumor regrowth.

The operation to approach a brain tumor is called craniotomy. (See page 226.) Instead of a craniotomy the tumor is sometimes reached using a specialized neurological procedure called stereotactic surgery. This technique allows deep areas of the brain to be reached by passing probes through a single hole in the skull. The depth and direction of the probing is carefully predetermined by CAT scans and magnetic resonance imaging (MRI), and the probe is directed by an apparatus fixed to the patient's skull. This technique is used in obtaining biopsies from certain deep tumors, and in placing radioactive seeds to irradiate specific brain tumors. Stereotactic surgery is also used to sever deep circuits to treat certain movement disorders, and to place electrodes for management of some chronic pain states. The technique was once widely used to treat patients with Parkinson's disease (these patients are now usually treated with drug therapy). The main complication of stereotactic surgery is a hemorrhage occurring deep in the brain. On rare occasions this may require a craniotomy to stop the bleeding.

As soon as the tumor is located, a small portion is taken to the laboratory in the operating room and the tissue is frozen. Very thin slices are then taken from this block of tissue and are examined under the microscope by a neuropathologist, who can then tell the surgeon the nature of the tumor and the degree of malignancy. The surgeon will usually make every effort to remove as much of the tumor as possible. If the tumor is malignant, however, this procedure is not curative.

The other two mainstays of treatment for malignant brain tumors are radiation and chemotherapy. The benefits and risk of these two forms of treatment are discussed with the patient and the family after surgery.

Recent Advances

Because surgery, radiation therapy and chemotherapy are all treatments, not cures, researchers are constantly striving to find new methods of treating malignant brain tumors. For example, lasers are being studied as a way of destroying malignant brain tumor cells. Surgeons are also studying the effect of local radiation from implanted radioactive seeds (brachytherapy) and the effect of heat on malignant brain tumors (hyperthermia).

Cerebral Vascular Disease (Stroke)

A stroke is the sudden occurrence of neurological disability as a result of blood vessel disease in the brain (cerebral vascular disease). There are many types of cerebral vascular disease that may cause a stroke. A sudden hemorrhage may occur when a brain blood vessel, weakened by high blood pressure, breaks. The blood vessel may have an abnormal outpouching (aneurysm) or abnormal cluster of vessels (arteriovenous malformation) that may break, causing bleeding into the fluid surrounding the brain. The blood vessel may be blocked from the build-up of fatty deposits (atherosclerosis), so that an area of the brain is deprived of its blood supply. Another common cause of stroke is the lodging of a portion of a blood clot (embolus) which is washed up in the bloodstream. The clot gets stuck at a narrow point in the vessel and suddenly shuts off the blood supply to that part of the brain.

Diagnosis

The diagnosis of the site and nature of the stroke is made by information from the patient's history, physical examination and special tests. For example, the history and physical examination may show weakness affecting the right arm, leg and face, with an inability to compre hend speech or speak fluently. A CAT scan and angiogram may show a blockage of the left middle cerebral artery.

Non-Surgical Treatment

The most important elements are control of high blood pressure, taking aspirin and cessation of smoking. Aspirin is used for a variety of purposes, including pain control. However, the regular taking of aspirin also helps prevent the buildup of blood clots within diseased cerebral vessels. Physical therapy will aid the return of integrated and coordinated function of the weakened limbs.

Surgical Treatment

In certain situations, an operation can be done to treat the stroke, or prevent future stroke. For example, the main problem in a stroke victim may be narrowing and ulceration of a carotid artery in the patient's neck. Small pieces of cholesterol and blood clot can break off from these ulcers and be washed up into the blood vessels of the brain, where they may block the vessels, causing small or large strokes. The narrowing of the carotid artery itself may even become so extreme that the amount of blood flowing to the brain on that side is diminished. If the surgeon feels that the patient is likely to have future strokes, despite the best medical therapy, then they may advise the patient to accept the risk of a surgical unblocking of the carotid artery (carotid endarterectomy). In this common operation, the carotid artery is opened, and the narrowed, ulcerated segment is removed (Fig. 18.8).

Research is now being done to determine exactly which patients will do better with medical treatment and which patients will do better with medical treatment and endarterectomy. Neither treatment, however, can totally guarantee freedom from future stroke.

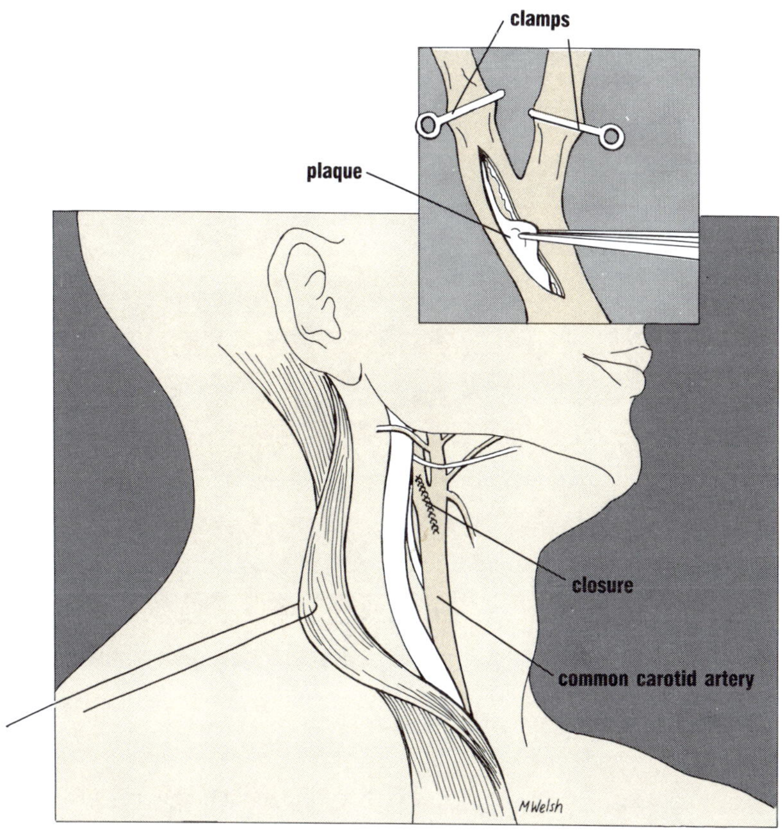

Figure 18.8
Carotid endarterectomy. The artery is temporarily clamped while plaque is removed from the inside of the artery. The artery is then closed.

Complications

Carotid endarterectomy may be complicated by the occurrence of a stroke during the operation itself, although the surgeon and the anesthetist will take every precaution to lessen this possibility. Rarely, a blood clot may develop in the neck a few hours after surgery. If this becomes severe, an emergency operation is required to remove it to prevent the clot from exerting pressure on the windpipe.

Aneurysm

An abnormal ballooning of a blood vessel on the brain (aneurysm) may burst and cause a hemorrhage. This is one of the most serious cases of bleeding into the cerebrospinal fluid (subarachnoid hemorrhage). Hemorrhage is likely to lead to neurological damage and possibly death, so the surgeon may advise an

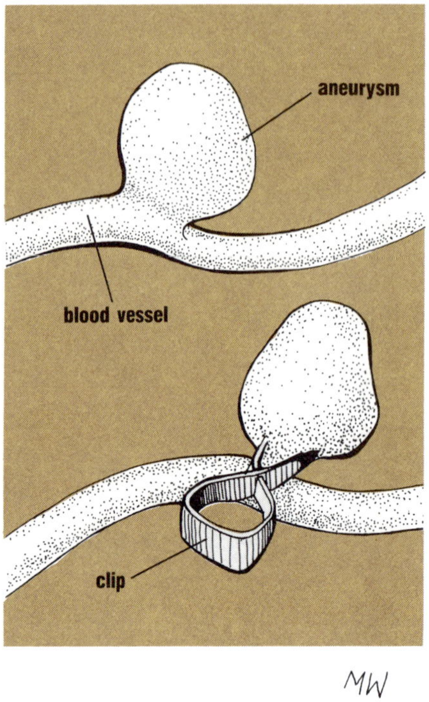

Figure 18.9
An aneurysm can be treated by placing a clip across the neck of the balloon.

operation to place a clip across the neck of the aneurysm so that blood can no longer enter the ballooned part of the artery (Fig. 18.9). This is done via a craniotomy. (See page 226.) The clip remains permanently in place.

Subarachnoid hemorrhage may be complicated by severe brain damage due to the initial hemorrhage, or the surgery itself may cause brain damage. In rare instances the clips may partially close off the parent blood vessel.

The most important recent advance in treating subarachnoid hemorrhage has been the education of the public and the medical profession about the significance of the first abrupt headache which indicates that the aneurysm has leaked. Generally the outcome of surgery is related to the patient's level of consciousness at the time of the operation. If the diagnosis is made promptly following the first hemorrhage and the patient is quickly transferred to a neurosurgical center, the overall outcome will be improved. In addition, the great strides made in surgical instrument design, aneurysm clip design and operating microscopes have given rise to cautious optimism in dealing with these extremely difficult problems.

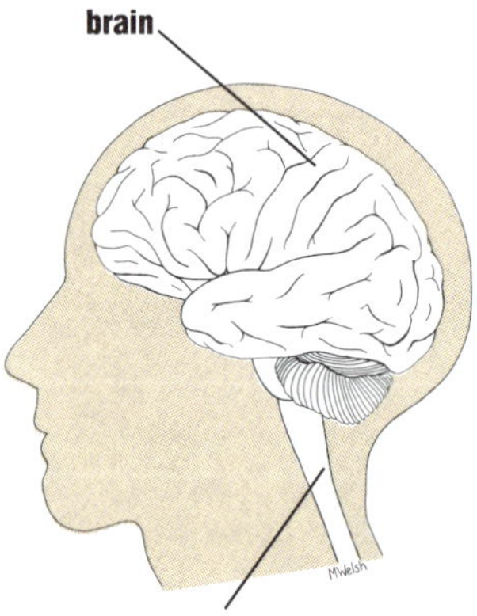

Figure 18.10
Brain and brainstem.

Spinal Cord

The spinal cord leads down from the brain and is totally enclosed by the bones that make up the spine (Fig. 18.10). Its function is very similar to a telephone cable, with individual wires conveying messages to and from the brain. An interruption at any level of the spine will prevent sensory messages from reaching the brain, and motor messages from reaching the muscles. Complete interruption results in total paralysis of the muscles below the level of the interruption. Injury to the spinal cord in the neck will affect the arms and legs and, in its most severe form will result in paralysis of all four limbs (quadriplegia). Injury affecting the spinal cord below the neck results in paralysis of the legs, but arm function is maintained (paraplegia). The spinal cord also conveys the messages that control bladder, bowel and sexual function, so spinal cord disease frequently affects these functions as well.

The manifestations of spinal cord disease depend on the location of the abnormality in the spinal cord, whether the abnormality is caused by an injury to the spinal cord, pressure on the cord from a tumor, or compression from an abscess. When the cord is compressed, the spinal canal must be surgically enlarged. This operation (laminectomy) is described under degenerative disc disease (page 234), but it is also done for tumors or infections.

Traumatic fracture dislocations, tumors and, more rarely, infections may cause the spinal column to become structurally weak and unstable. If the spine is unstable, the cord may be further damaged by abnormal movement of the vertebrae. To prevent this, the spine may be held in line by externally applied splints or internally implanted devices. Cervical traction, a device similar to old-fashioned ice tongs, can be applied to the outside of the skull. Traction is then applied using weights suspended over pulleys. This is frequently the initial method of stabilizing the cervical spine and realigning broken bones in the neck that have been displaced after injury.

Another external device, the halo, allows the patient greater mobility, while maintaining the cervical spine in a straight line. A metal ring is attached to the skull at several points by pins screwed into the bone. A close-fitting plastic vest is applied to the chest, and the metal ring around the skull and the plastic vest are joined by external bars, thus maintaining the cervical spine in correct alignment (Fig. 18.11). At first glance, this apparatus appears to be most uncomfortable, but patients prefer the relatively minor inconvenience to spending 12 weeks in traction in bed.

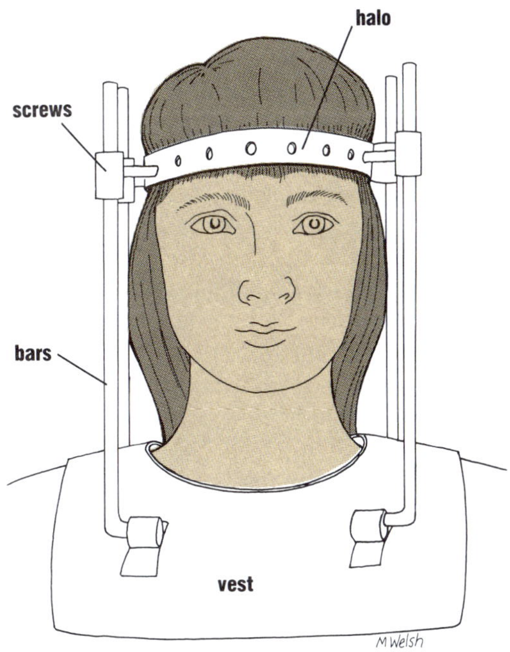

Figure 18.11
Halo spinal-support device.

The internal fixation of spinal bones is usually performed by a team of surgeons. Orthopedists have developed an ingenious series of rods, wires and springs that enable them to splint abnormal areas of the spine, and thus prevent further spinal cord damage. These internal fixation devices may be applied to either the back or the front of the spine; occasionally both types are required.

Operations on the spine may be performed from behind or from in front. In the case of the neck, the operations are fairly straightforward from either direction, but in the case of the back, the surgeon may have to gain access to the front of the spine through the chest or abdominal cavity.

Diagnostic Tests

While ordinary X-rays of the spine may be very useful in determining both the level and nature of the abnormality, the myelogram is the most frequently ordered test in diagnosing spinal cord problems. CAT scanning may also help; frequently the myelogram and CAT scan are combined in a single test.

For a myelogram, the patient is placed face down on a table and local anesthetic is injected into the lower spine. A needle is inserted into the space containing the cerebrospinal fluid, and the radiologist injects a contrast fluid that can be seen on an X-ray machine. The table is tilted up and down, causing the fluid to flow in the space immediately around the spinal cord. The radiologist can watch its progress on a screen or can take X-ray pictures for future examination. If an abnormality is pressing against the spinal cord, or if there is an abnormality within the substance of the spinal cord, the flow of the dye will be blocked or deflected, enabling the radiologist to pinpoint the exact site of the problem.

For CAT scanning and magnetic resonance imaging (MRI), a series of slices are produced on a screen by scanning the appropriate level of the spine. With greater refinement of technique, CAT scanning will decrease the need for some myelograms. When MRI techniques are fully developed and available, myelography will be used infrequently.

Case Study: Degenerative Disc Disease

A construction worker for the past 15 years, Gordon was proud of his skill and his lack of fear for dangerous work. But a few months ago he'd "put his back out" lifting something, and it had been getting steadily worse. He'd had X-rays and a myelogram. The doctors said he could have surgery, but he'd drawn the line there. Even the thought of surgery bothered him, but when they'd talked about the things that could go wrong, he didn't want to hear any more. But now, his wife would point out that surgery would help to remedy his condition.

On this particular evening he had arrived home and was playing with his children. He bent down to pick up his two-year-old. An agonizing spasm of pain shot through his back, and his wife came rushing in to find him unable to straighten up.

Gordon still didn't think surgery was a good idea, but he agreed to see the surgeon. "There's no doubt we can relieve the pain with an operation — but that doesn't mean you can carry on just as you have been doing. You won't by any means be an invalid, but you will have to take it more easily."

Gordon refused again to have surgery, to Marie's consternation. A social worker was assigned to help the family look at alternatives if Gordon couldn't do the work he was used to. But two months later, after a further agonizing bout of pain, he finally consented to the operation.

Rehabilitation

In patients with significantly impaired spinal cord functions, rehabilitation is liable to last many months. In the initial phase, the patient is wholly dependent on the attending doctors and nurses. This stage may last several weeks. In the intermediate period, the patient gradually assumes more responsibility, and in the final phase, the patient becomes almost totally responsible for his or her well-being, learning to maximize his or her residual function.

Family and friends play a vital role during all three of these phases. While the occurrence of permanent spinal disability may come as an enormous shock to both the patient and the family, physicians and nurses do have considerable experience in handling both the physical and emotional aspects of such a tragedy. At times, the relative will know more about the prognosis than the patient. It is essential that the family discuss the situation with the attending surgeon, so that the psychological aspects are handled harmoniously and to the patient's ultimate advantage. This involves a delicate balance, which is neither overly pessimistic nor unreasonably optimistic. To offer false hope does little to help a situation. On the other hand, constantly bemoaning the misfortune of the patient will hardly improve the patient's spirits. Such an illness is akin to a long-distance race and not a sprint. The family must summon up their energy for a long period of adjustment and support.

Degenerative Disc Disease

The spine consists of individual vertebrae that are separated from one another by discs, which act as shock absorbers. The discs are made of fibrous tissue and cartilage surrounding a core of much softer tissue. As a disc degenerates, the softer central material starts to push out through the firmer covering. This bulge may, in turn, press on either a branch of the spinal cord (nerve root), or the spinal cord itself (Fig. 18.12). If the condition worsens, the soft portion may eventually break right through the covering and apply even greater pressure and irritation to the nerve root or spinal cord.

If the disc is in the neck, this results in neck pain, muscle spasm and pain in the arm, frequently into individual fingers. Specific movements of the neck may aggravate the pressure on a nerve root and the arm pain. Weakness of the muscle supplied by a particular nerve root will result from prolonged pressure. Tingling and eventually loss of sensation may occur in the area of skin supplied by that particular nerve root.

When the degenerative disc occurs in the lower back, low back pain and muscle spasm develops (lumbago). Pressure on the nerve roots in this area can cause pain along the sciatic nerve down the back of the thigh and through the calf into the foot (sciatica).

Non-Surgical Treatment

Most patients suffering from degenerative disc disease are treated by non-surgical methods. Various forms of physiotherapy, bracing or prolonged bed rest may bring relief. Oral medications may dull the pain and lessen the muscle spasm. The patient has a significant role to play in this treatment, which frequently involves an exercise program, weight reduction and, possibly, a change of job. In a few cases, pain, weakness or loss of sensation persist. These cases are usually referred to a specialist, and at this time a myelogram is usually performed.

Sometimes an enzyme called chymopapain is injected into the center of the disc to shrink it. This material has been used almost exclusively in the low back for the treatment of low back pain and sciatica. However, despite many years of study, the benefits of this form of treatment are still being debated, and not all surgeons recommend it.

Surgical Treatment

If the diseased disc is in the neck, the surgical treatment is an anterior cervical discectomy. An incision is made along the line of a natural crease in the front of the neck, so that the final scar will not be very obvious. The soft tissues of the neck are gently separated, revealing the front of the spine. The disc is then cut out, releasing the pressure on the nerve root or spinal cord. In many instances, the surgeon will replace the disc with a bone graft, fusing that segment of the neck. Fortunately the cervical spine is similar to a bicycle chain with numerous joints, so that fusion of a single level does not usually impair neck movement once the patient has fully recovered from the operation.

If the diseased disc is in the back, a lumbar laminectomy and discectomy is performed from behind. The surgeon evaluates the evidence obtained from the patient's history, physical examination, X-rays and myelogram, so that he or she knows exactly where to perform the operation. The procedure involves cutting the skin and retracting the muscles from the area immediately above the spine. The laminae (the bony part of the spine covering the nerve root) are partially removed, under the operating microscope. The nerve root, which is stretched over the underlying disc, is then moved aside, and the disc is removed. In the lower back area, bone grafts are usually not employed; the disc is subsequently replaced by scar tissue.

Patients usually leave hospital within three or four days of the operation. The return to work depends on the patient's occupation. Patients at desk jobs are usually back at work within three to four weeks of surgery. Patients who have had uncomplicated anterior cervical discectomies usually have unrestricted activities three months after surgery. However, appropriate exercise programs, weight control and job modification must be respected.

Figure 18.12
Degenerated disc.

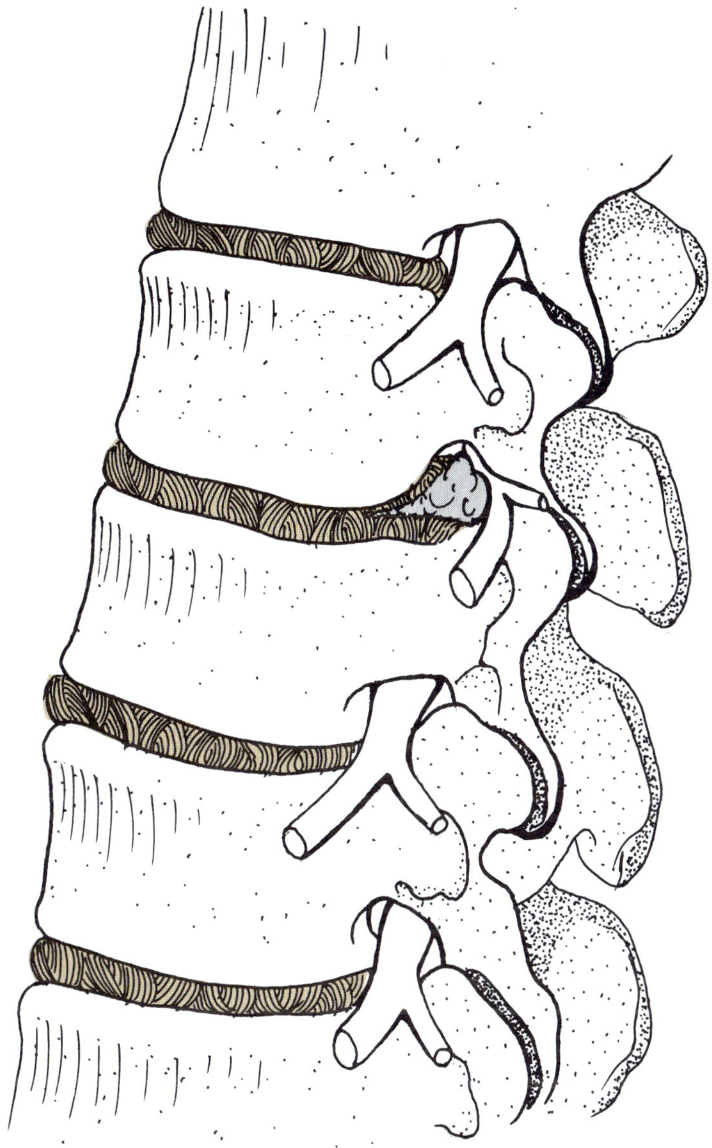

Complications

Every spinal operation has risks. The structures most likely to be damaged are the spinal cord and nerve roots.

The most significant risk of cervical disc surgery is spinal cord injury, with

After a month of recovery, Gordon was transferred to a new job at his construction firm that enabled him to combine desk work with on-site inspection. He was pleased by what a difference it made not to be worried about the threat of sudden searing back pain. The doctors had warned him repeatedly that he must avoid straining his back, and he'd been perhaps over-careful at first. Surgery, while it hadn't been the nightmare he'd envisioned, was still not his favorite way to spend time — he didn't want to do anything that would put him back in hospital.

Three months after surgery, Gordon could pick up his toddler again without collapsing. The surgeon was generally pleased with Gordon's condition. Together with the physiotherapist, he designed a program of exercises that actually had Gordon feeling fitter than he had been before he put his back out. The surgeon was pleased with that, too.

subsequent permanent quadriplegia. Other risks include postoperative blood clot formation and infection. In the lumbar area, the most significant risk is failure of treatment, necessitating a second and possibly a third operation.

The key to a good outcome in both cervical and lumbar disc surgery is careful patient selection and meticulous operative technique. The surgeon will advise the patient what the operation entails and what the risks are. The final decision for or against surgery is the patient's, not the surgeon's. Degenerative disc disease is a common problem; in carefully selected cases, the results of surgery are very good.

Peripheral Nerve

A peripheral nerve carries motor messages to a specific group of muscles and also conveys sensory messages from specific areas of skin. Lack of function of a specific peripheral nerve will therefore cause weakness and loss of sensation. The majority of cases can be diagnosed by a careful physical examination of motor power and sensation.

The nerve may be injured by a sharp object, such as being totally or partially severed by a piece of glass from a car windshield. In many instances, however, the nerve is stretched and damaged without being severed. A peripheral nerve may also be trapped where it runs through an anatomical tunnel. More rarely a peripheral nerve may be affected by a tumor.

Electromyographic (EMG) and nerve conduction tests can help diagnose nerve damage. A small electrode is inserted into a muscle and the electrical activity at rest, on action and on response to stimulation of the nerve is recorded. The nerve is then stimulated some distance away from the muscle, and the time taken for that stimulus to reach the muscle is recorded.

Trauma

The timing of surgery is extremely important in peripheral nerve injury cases. If the nerve is sharply severed (as in pushing an arm through a window), the best results are obtained if the nerve is sutured on the day of injury. If the nerve has also been crushed and pulled (as in a chainsaw injury), it is often better to postpone surgery for two to three weeks. This allows the exact extent of the damage to become obvious, so that the surgeon knows how much of the damaged nerve needs to be removed before it is sewn together again. When the injured nerve is simply stretched, the surgeon will usually wait about three months before operating, because the nerve may recover during the three-month period, thus avoiding an operation altogether.

Most operations on peripheral nerves are conducted under general anesthetic. The surgeon may remove surrounding scar tissue, part of a nerve, or the entire nerve. If the gap created by removing part of the nerve is small enough, the surgeon will sew the two ends of the nerve together. If the gap is too large, a nerve graft is placed between the two ends of the injured nerve. Usually the grafting material is obtained from sensory nerves in the leg.

It is extremely important that the patient follow whatever instructions are given for immobilization of the limb. If it is moved prematurely, the very fine nerve sutures will break, and the cut nerve ends will pull apart. A cast may be required for three to six weeks; the patient will then undergo a physiotherapy program to remobilize joints and prevent stiffness.

The recovery period lasts up to two years. During this time the patient must be very careful not to burn or injure the numb areas, or to allow paralyzed joints to stiffen. As the nerve regenerates, the patient may experience quite uncomfortable pins and needles and other strange feelings in the previously anesthetized area. The unpleasant feelings are usually easily controlled with mild painkillers.

Patients are usually reassessed eighteen months after the operation. Results are sometimes less than perfect, but sufficient to allow the patient to continue his or her occupation and social activities. By this point, the final degree of recovery can usually be determined. Reconstructive operations, joint fusions and tendon transfers may be performed at this stage, depending on the results of the nerve surgery.

Entrapment Syndrome

Peripheral nerves may be trapped in narrow tunnels. The most common cause of tingling in the fingertips is the carpal tunnel syndrome (see also page 201). In this situation, the median nerve is trapped in a tunnel immediately in front of the wrist. Patients complain of numbness and tingling in the thumb, index and middle finger. These symptoms are often worse at night. The symptoms may be aggravated by certain day-to-day tasks, such as driving a car, peeling potatoes, or knitting. Nerve conduction studies and electromyograms (EMG) are very useful in confirming the diagnosis of carpal tunnel syndrome. In mild cases, the patient may be treated with wrist splints applied at night, and other simple measures. The majority of patients will require an operation to relieve the symptoms and prevent further damage to the median nerve. The purpose of the operation is to cut a ligament, releasing the tight tunnel. This can usually be accomplished under local anesthetic during a day visit.

Another common site of nerve entrapment is at the elbow joint. In this situation, the ulnar nerve is caught in a tunnel behind the elbow joint. This can cause clumsiness in the hand and numbness in the small finger and half of the ring finger. If patients do not respond to simple conservative measures, the nerve is usually moved from its position behind the elbow joint to a new site in front of the elbow joint, stopping the pressure that occurs on the nerve every time the patient flexes the elbow.

Tumors

Peripheral nerves may be affected by tumors growing within or adjacent to them. Simple benign tumors, called schwannomas, can usually be removed from the nerve without damage. Another kind of benign tumor, the neurofibroma, may also be simply removed, but in many instances the nerve trunk must be cut, creating motor and sensory loss. A malignant nerve tumor poses grave danger to the patient's life and requires very radical surgery.

Complications

Peripheral nerve operations may occasionally be complicated by a worsening of the neurological condition. Wound infections are treated with appropriate antibiotics and the limb is rested. All patients suffering from nerve injury will experience discomfort while the nerve is healing, but a few patients experience extremely severe pain (causalgia). This is more common in patients with partial nerve injury and, if medications fail, further surgery may be necessary.

Chapter 19

Transplant Surgery

Michael A. Robinette
Assistant Professor of Surgery
University of Toronto
Urologic Surgeon
Toronto General Hospital

Marlene Herbst
Illustrator

Transplants make headlines. Everyone has seen pictures of smiling organ recipients as they leave hospital, or anxious relatives waiting for a donor to be found. But many don't realize that the waiting would be greatly reduced if more people considered organ donation. One donor can provide many organs, depending on the cause of death and the state of the donor's health during life.

The surgical techniques for organ transplantation were developed at the turn of the century. However, because the body reacts to a transplant as if it is an invading bacteria or virus, rejection usually resulted, and almost all transplant attempts (except those from identical twins) failed. In the 1960s, drugs were discovered to be highly effective in combating rejection. This marked the beginning of a new era in transplantation. Research during the following two decades led to a better understanding of the rejection process, and transplant physicians gained considerable experience with various anti-rejection drugs.

In the 1970s, the drug cyclosporine was invented, and its clinical introduction in the early 1980s caused a dramatic improvement in transplant survival.

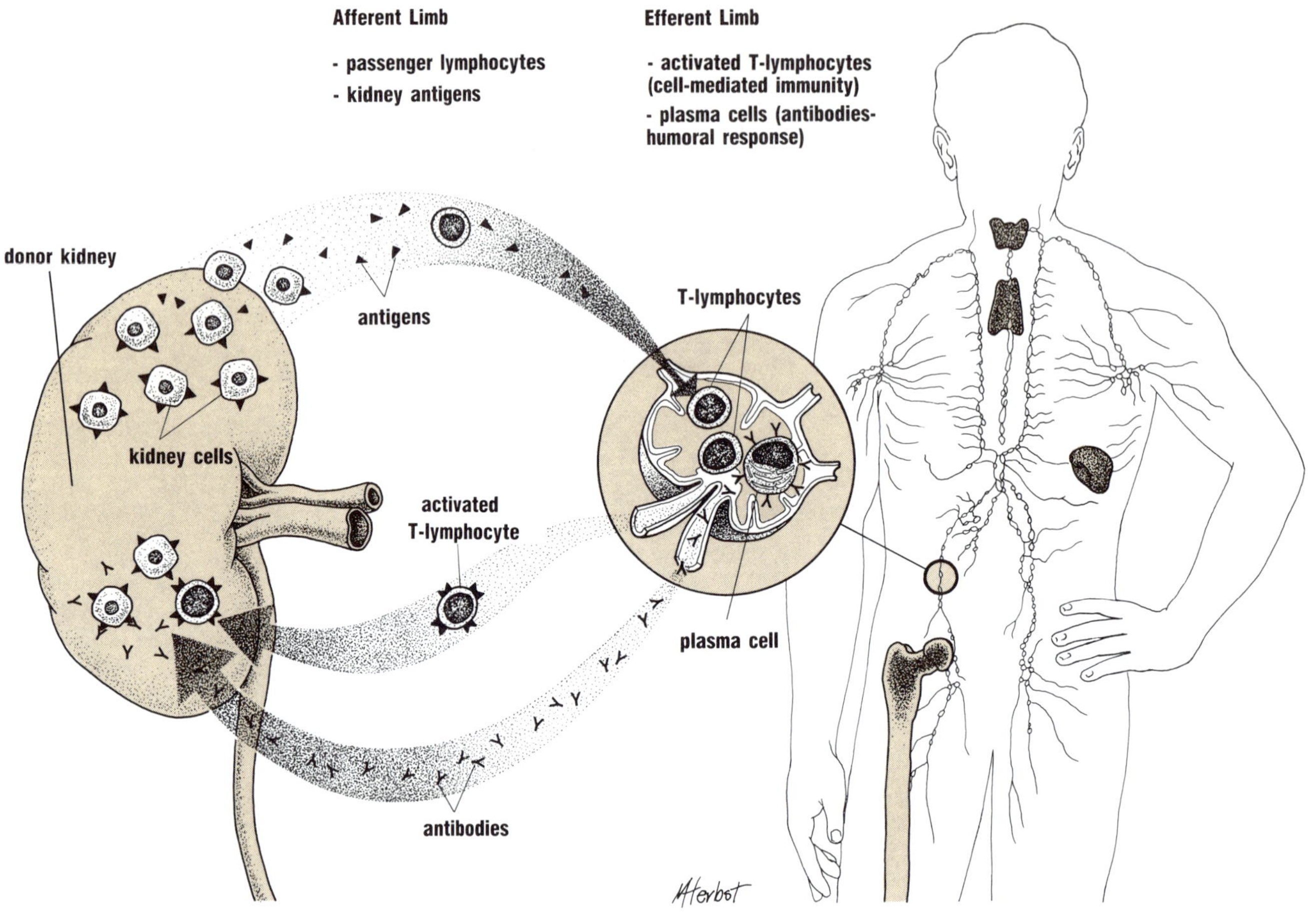

Figure 19.1
Immune rejection response.

Transplant failure from acute rejection or for technical reasons usually occurs in the first couple of months. Transplant success is therefore often measured by the percentage of grafts still functioning at the end of one year. Chronic rejection claims approximately 5 percent of transplants each year thereafter. Since the introduction of cyclosporine, one-year graft survival for kidneys has increased from 65 to 80 percent. For liver and heart transplants, the improvement has been even more impressive: from 35 to 75 percent. Lung, heart/lung and pancreas transplant results are also more successful. Corneal transplants have the best graft survival rate (95 percent) because the cornea is a membrane with no blood vessels and thus is not prone to rejection.

Organ Rejection

The cells of the transplanted organ have proteins called antigens on their surface that differ from those of the recipient. The recipient's immune rejection response is therefore "turned on" by the presence of these foreign antigens (Fig. 19.1).

For a transplant to succeed, the immune mechanism in the recipient's body must be "turned off," so that it will not reject the donated organ. This technique is called immunosuppression.

Attempting to match the donor and recipient's tissue type as closely as possible will also decrease the immune response. A perfect match is achieved if a transplant is exchanged between identical twins. The next best match is between siblings, followed by other close relatives. The tissue types of donor and potential recipient are determined by a blood test.

Immunosuppressive Drugs

Drugs that decrease the immune response inhibit the rejection process. In the early 1960s, investigators discovered that the combination of steroids and azothiaprine was a powerful inhibitor of rejection, and that acute rejection could even be reversed with large doses of steroids. However, these drugs decrease the body's ability to combat other foreign substances, such as infections. Steroids can also interfere with wound healing, increase the likelihood of bruising, stimulate cataract formation and contribute to the development of diabetes and bone problems. Azothiaprine is toxic to the liver and causes bone marrow suppression, which may eventually lead to increased risk of bleeding and infection. However, in spite of these risks both steroids and azothiaprine remain the cornerstone of immunosuppressive therapy.

Anti-lymphocyte globulin is another medication that is effective in both the prevention and treatment of acute rejection. Newer, more specific monoclonal antibodies have been developed to produce more selective immunosuppression and fewer side effects.

Cyclosporine is an antibiotic-like product of a fungus with a selective immunosuppressive effect. It does not affect other blood cells, so there is less chance of developing infection or bleeding complications. Furthermore, wound healing is not impaired. Cyclosporine is, however, toxic to the kidneys in high doses.

Organ Donation

Kidneys and other organs are donated from people who die as a result of head injuries from motor accidents, gunshot wounds or other physical trauma, ruptured vascular aneurysms, or conditions that irreversibly damage brain tissue (drowning, suffocating or drug overdose). Although the brain is not functioning and there is no chance of recovery, the vital organs are temporarily maintained by mechanical ventilation, intravenous fluids and special drugs. Brain-dead organ donors can be supported in this artificial manner for only a few hours, which allows time to prepare for organ donation.

Once the heart stops and circulation ceases, the lack of oxygen and nutrients rapidly damages the vital organs, and they are no longer usable for transplants. For this reason, people dying outside of hospitals cannot donate organs, except their corneas, which can be removed from the donor up to 12 hours after the heart has stopped beating. Other contraindications to organ donation include diseases such as cancer or infections affecting the organ to be donated, which could be transmitted to the recipient. As a result, only 1 to 2 percent of all deaths are suitable for organ donation. Age limitations depend on the organ being donated. Kidneys can be transplanted from donors aged one to 65. For liver and lung donations, the upper age limit is 50, and for heart donors it is 45.

If a potential donor is rapidly approaching death, a tremendous effort and close collaboration of many people, especially nurses and physicians, is necessary to ensure that organs are properly retrieved and transported to the recipients. The donor must be carefully monitored and maintained, using special medication and equipment. Once specialists determine that brain death has occurred, consent for organ donation is obtained from the relatives. Regional coordinators working for organ retrieval programs identify the most appropriate recipient for the avail-

Case Study: Organ Donation

Claudette had always wondered what it would be like to watch at the bedside of someone you loved who was close to death. Her heart had gone out to mothers she'd read about in the paper, waiting to see if their children were going to make it. Now here she was herself, watching over her 19-year-old-son, massively injured in a head-on car accident. He'd had surgery to stop the hemorrhaging inside his skull, but the doctors told her that the next 48 hours would be critical. Looking down on him, with all the tubes and wires attached to his body, she could hardly believe it had all come to this.

Claudette was joined by her husband, Andrew, a nurse and Dr. Khan. Dr. Khan began to say that their son did not appear to be progressing, and it looked very much that he was going to die.

As Dr. Khan left the room, the nurse followed him out into the corridor. "Doctor, do you think Michel would be a suitable organ donor?" The doctor slowly turned. "I hadn't thought about it. It seems awfully callous to go in and suggest that to them now." The nurse shook her head. "You know, I've seen lots of parents like this. They stand around waiting for the end, wondering what it's all been for. Sometimes it really helps them to know that something good came out of it all, even if not for them."

They left Claudette and Andrew alone with Michel for a while after they had suggested organ donation. It was not an easy decision to make, but Claudette and Andrew both agreed that they should allow Michel's organs to be donated.

* * *

Melanie had never known waiting could be this hard. When they had been waiting for their baby to be born, there was excitement. When they had been waiting to find out if her kidney problem could be solved, there was hope. Now, there was nothing but waiting — for a kidney donor. Caroline had endured seven years of operations, diets, dialysis — and waiting. The doctors had told her parents three months ago that the only chance now was a kidney transplant, but at the time, she wasn't very high on the priority list. Now, each day took her a little closer to death, and Melanie felt she was almost dying herself — of frustration.

She rarely left the hospital now, afraid that a call might come when she was on her way home. She and her husband, Alan, made sure that one of them was always within reach of the phone, and one was at the hospital with Caroline. Until last week, they'd brought Caroline in to the hospital three times a week for dialysis, but this week her condition had deteriorated so badly that she had been kept in.

There was a bustle outside the door, and the surgeon came in. "What is it — any news?" Melanie asked breathlessly. "I don't want to give you any false hopes, but there's a possibility we may have a donor."

This time the waiting wasn't nearly so long. It had been three hours before they could find out whether the donor kidney would go to Caroline. While they waited, Melanie had thought about that other mother who was losing her son.

able organ according to matching tests and clinical status (status 6 is the most urgent in "need" of a transplant). The recipient transplant physician is notified and preparations for the transplant surgery are initiated. Teams of surgeons, nurses and technicians work together, carefully removing the vital organs in a way that prevents tissue damage. The organs are flushed with a special cold solution that prevents blood from clotting and rapidly induces cooling (hypothermia), and are individually stored in sterile containers surrounded by ice. In this cold condition, the organs' metabolic requirements are lowered, allowing time to prepare the recipient for the transplant and to transport the organ to the recipient's center. The length of time for this is limited and is different for each organ. Following removal of the organs, the donor's body is sutured and sent to the funeral home. Organ donation does not interfere with funeral arrangements.

Organs are distributed to recipients using a complex network of regional transplant centers, based on blood group, tissue type, medical need and a roster that ensures that each center gets its "turn" for donated organs. When a suitable recipient is not found locally, a computer search among a collaborative network of organ retrieval programs identifies another recipient elsewhere in North America. On rare occasions the search is expanded to include Europe, South America and even the Far East.

Each organ donor provides a gift of life to several patients. Two patients receive the kidneys and may no longer require dialysis. Sight can be restored to two blind people as a result of the cornea transplants, and the recipients of the liver, heart, lung, pancreas and joints can be given new lives. Skin and bone are also donated for grafts.

There are still significant medical barriers to the donation process. Confusion about the correct steps to follow, insufficient guidelines and coordination, a lack of familiarity with the donation process, and concerns about the time demands of becoming involved are frequently expressed by doctors, nurses, residents and interns. Legal questions, financial issues (affecting the hospital budget rather than the individual doctor's fee) and personal feelings are other obstacles. Many physicians are still inhibited about requesting the consent of a grieving family, despite recognizing the potential benefits of organ donation to the family in their grieving process.

In order to facilitate organ donation, hospitals are being encouraged to create an organ donation committee to establish policies and assign individuals to act as organ donor coordinators. Education of health-care professionals concerning donor identification and management is being introduced in medical and nursing schools and will continue as postgraduate hospital lectures. In order to lessen the chance of missing potential donors, the concept of "recorded consideration" is being implemented in several centers. Under this system, each "brain-dead" patient about to have life-support systems withdrawn has to be considered as a potential donor and, when appropriate, consent should be requested from the next-of-kin.

Kidney Transplants

Although the first human kidney (renal) transplant was performed in Europe in 1936, the first successful identical twin transplant occurred in Boston in 1954. Four years later, kidney transplants donated from relatives were successfully performed in Paris and Boston. These patients are the longest-surviving kidney recipients in the world. Techniques to prevent rejection allowed kidney transplant programs to expand rapidly. By 1970 4,000 transplants had been performed worldwide; by 1988 the number exceeded 200,000.

The most common cause of chronic kidney failure is glomerulonephritis, a condition that results in progressive

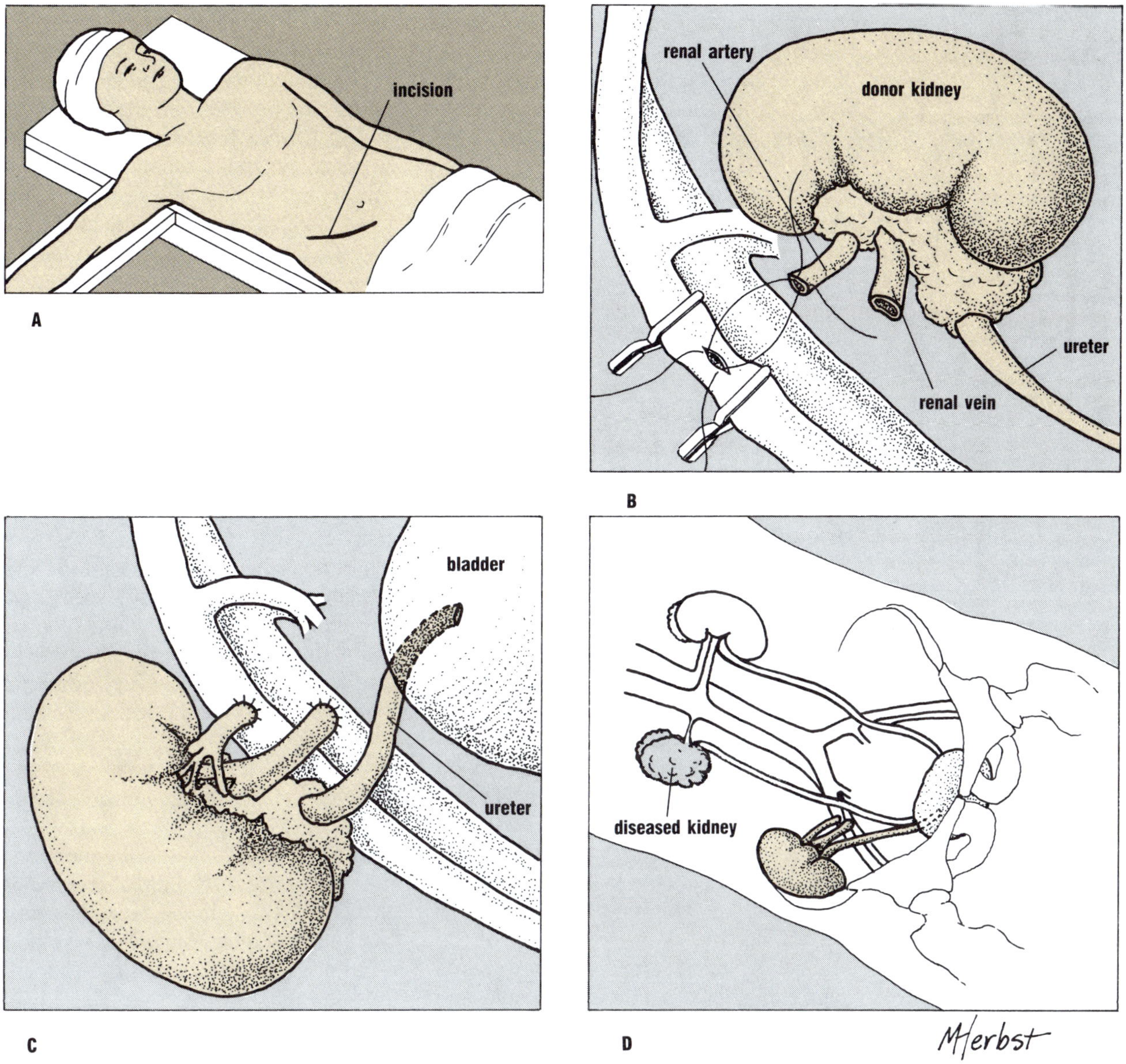

Figure 19.2
Kidney transplant. The incision is made in the lower abdomen (A). The donor kidney vein and artery are sewn in place (B), and the ureter is connected to the bladder (C). The recipient's own diseased kidneys are not removed (D).

damage from inflammation and scarring. Other causes include diabetes, high blood pressure and other vascular diseases, obstruction, drug abuse and cancer. As kidney failure progresses, there is an accumulation of fluid and toxic byproducts of metabolism which are normally eliminated by the kidneys. The artificial kidney (dialysis machine) is a life-saving process that clears these substances from the patient's blood. However, dialysis cannot correct other results of kidney failure, including problems with blood pressure control, decreased production of hemoglobin leading to anemia and weakness, and disturbances of bone formation. A successful kidney transplant can correct these abnormalities.

Kidney transplantation has become the treatment of choice for patients with chronic kidney failure. Unfortunately, less than 20 percent of all potential kidney recipients have suitable relatives who are able to donate a kidney and therefore,

Now they were waiting to find out how Caroline's surgery had gone. It had been somewhat eerie, thinking of a 19-year-old boy's kidney being transplanted into their seven-year-old daughter, but the overriding feeling was one of profound relief that now she at least had a chance. The surgeon had assured them that kidney transplants, while major surgery, were quite common now. The kidney had been flown to the hospital as soon as it was removed from the donor, since by that time they'd been able to establish that Caroline's tissue type was a close match.

Three hours had passed since the operation started. Alan had gone to the cafeteria to get them some coffee when the surgeon came out. Melanie felt her face go pale as she waited for him to speak. "She's still on the critical list, but the operation went well and the kidney seems to be working. The next forty-eight hours will tell us how she's going to do." Melanie suddenly felt very, very weak. She sat down without knowing where she was. A cup of coffee materialized in front of her, and as she took a sip, she realized that for the first time in a year, her little girl was getting better, not worse.

possible recipients must await other donor sources. There are always many patients on dialysis waiting for a transplant, so when a kidney becomes available, the best possible match is sought.

Transplantation is sometimes performed before the kidneys have deteriorated to the point that dialysis is necessary. For example, a successful kidney transplant in a diabetic with impending renal failure but not yet requiring dialysis can prevent eye damage. If the supply of donated kidneys increases, transplants could be carried out before patients require dialysis, and the expense, inconvenience and potential complications of dialysis could be avoided completely.

Although the kidneys are normally located high up in the back, protected by the rib cage, the lower abdomen is chosen as the transplant site because it is easier to connect the kidney with the bladder (Fig. 19.2). Also, the artery that supplies the pelvic organs (internal iliac artery), and the large vessels that pass to the legs (external iliac artery and vein) are readily accessible to establish blood flow to the new kidney. The renal artery and vein are usually joined end to side to the external iliac artery and vein. The tube that connects the kidney to the bladder (ureter) is trimmed and sutured to the bladder to restore continuity of the urinary system. The operation takes approximately two hours in an adult, and complications during surgery are rare. The recipient's diseased kidneys are usually not removed.

Intravenous fluids and immunosuppressive medication are continued after surgery. A catheter drains the bladder through the urethra. The urine output and other vital signs are carefully monitored, and blood tests are done each day. Special tests including ultrasound and renal isotope scans measure the flow of blood to the kidney and assess its function.

Approximately one-third of transplanted kidneys suffer from temporary loss of function (acute tubular necrosis) as a result of changes occurring in the donor kidney immediately before organ removal and/or while the kidney is stored after removal. This period of non-function varies from a few days to a couple of weeks and usually causes low urine output, a persistently high serum creatinine level (a substance that is normally eliminated from the body by the kidney) and the need for ongoing dialysis. Rarely, kidneys that appear to have acute tubular necrosis end up never functioning. Such kidneys probably suffered irreversible damage before the transplant or are damaged by rejection, which is often difficult to detect during periods of nonfunction.

Acute rejection of the new kidney often causes fever, high blood pressure, tenderness over the transplanted kidney, a falling urine output and elevated serum creatinine levels. The white blood cell count rises, reflecting the immune system's attack on the kidney. Sometimes a needle biopsy of the kidney is necessary to confirm the diagnosis. Rejection can usually be reversed by making changes in the immunosuppressive drug treatment.

Complications of the connection of the blood vessels (anastomosis) are extremely rare. If the vessels become blocked, the blood supply to the kidney is cut off, function ceases, the transplant dies and must be removed. The ureter can become obstructed, resulting in back pressure on the kidney, which is usually detected during ultrasound or renal scan. Occasionally the blood supply to the ureter is cut off, weakening the wall of the ureter and allowing urine to leak into the surrounding tissues. Severe pain occurs around the transplant and the urine must be temporarily diverted via a small tube inserted through the skin into the kidney. Once the inflammation caused by the urine leak has settled down, surgery is necessary to reconnect the bladder to a healthy part of the ureter. A collection of fluid (lymphocele) may form around the transplant and obstruct the ureter. The ureter may also kink or become narrowed by scar tissue. Surgical correction of these conditions is often necessary to restore kidney function.

The catheter is removed about five days after the operation. Most patients are discharged during the second week. Careful follow-up by physical examination and blood and urine tests is essential to ensure that the immunosuppressive medication — which must be taken for the remainder of the recipient's life — maintains optimal kidney function without causing complications such as infections.

Liver Transplants

More than 7,000 human liver transplants have been performed since the first one in 1963. Better patient selection, refinement of surgical techniques and improvements in postoperative treatment, especially immunosuppressive therapy, have contributed to the steady improvement in survival. The addition of cyclosporine to the anti-rejection therapy has increased the one-year transplant survival rate from 35 to over 75 percent.

In North America, approximately 100,000 people die each year of liver failure (most as a result of alcohol abuse), but only a small percentage are suitable for a liver transplant. Potential liver recipients may have severe liver damage caused by viral infections such as hepatitis, exposure to certain drugs or toxins, biliary cirrhosis or inflammation, and some inherited conditions in children such as biliary atresia (failure of development in the bile duct system). Since the liver is the metabolic center of the body, a damaged liver can cause severe disturbances, including generalized swelling, jaundice, spontaneous infections, and even life-threatening hemorrhage. Patients with liver failure become extremely ill and consequently are high-risk patients for major surgery.

A team of surgeons dissects the diseased liver from its normal location in the upper abdomen. Care is taken to minimize bleeding, which can occur easily because of the clotting disorders associated with liver failure. Removing the diseased liver is more difficult than implanting the new one, because of extensive scarring.

Simultaneously, another surgical team removes the donor liver. Blood is flushed out and the liver is rapidly cooled just before its removal. It is stored in a sterile plastic bag surrounded by ice in a special container and is promptly transported to the recipient center. The liver is particularly vulnerable to a lack of oxygen and nutrients, so every effort is made to transplant it within six to eight hours from the time of removal, although newer preservation solutions are being developed to extend this time limit.

The veins and arteries are reconnected during the transplant, and the bile-collecting system is reconnected. Usually a temporary tube is brought out through the skin to drain bile during the healing phase. A liver transplant takes about eight hours.

The transplanted liver usually begins functioning within minutes, and the many metabolic and blood clotting disturbances begin reversing toward normal. The patient is carefully monitored in the intensive care unit during the first few days. Signs of rejection are watched for with blood tests and liver biopsy.

When a liver transplant fails, either because of rejection or for technical reasons such as blockage of one of the vascular connections, a repeat transplant is necessary. Such patients are the highest priority on the waiting list, because they will die if a new liver is not found within two or three days. Many patients have undergone a successful second transplant under these circumstances.

The ICU nurses knew Melanie well by now. They showed her how they watched Caroline's urine output and her temperature, to check for signs of infection or rejection of the donor kidney. They always seemed to be taking her blood pressure, too. After a few days she was moved into a regular ward. Melanie knew that the first month was crucial, and that if Caroline's body were going to reject the kidney it would most likely happen then.

But three weeks passed, and Caroline steadily improved. Now she was home, returning to the hospital every two weeks to have her medication schedule and her blood checked. She was beginning to gain weight, sorely needed since the disease had arrested her growth. The surgeon was pleased with her progress, although he was careful to warn Melanie that they would always have to watch for infection, and that Caroline was at risk for other problems because of her medical history. However, Melanie felt she could cope with almost anything — now that the waiting was over.

Lung and Heart/Lung Transplants

The first human lung transplant was performed in 1963. Another 40 such transplants were done during the next 15 years. There were no long-term survivors, due to problems with rejection, infection and technical difficulties, particularly impaired healing from the use of steroids. Lung transplants were stopped for five years until cyclosporine permitted effective immunosuppression without the harmful effects on the repair process.

Single lung transplants are usually most successful for patients with end-stage fibrotic lung disease. Double lung transplants are more appropriate for patients with pulmonary emphysema or when there is infection in both lungs. When the lung disease is severe and prolonged, damage to the heart may occur, making the patient a candidate for a heart/lung transplant. These patients are respiratory cripples with shortness of breath at rest and no reserve for even minimal activity. Their life expectancy is often less than six months, and transplantation is their only hope.

Because lung infection often occurs in organ donors who are being maintained in the intensive care unit with ventilatory assist machines, fewer than 20 percent of multi-organ donors are suitable as lung donors. Special care must be taken to prevent deterioration of the respiratory tract, and careful assessment including chest X-ray and bronchoscopic examination must ensure that the lungs are transplantable. Besides the usual compatibility tests, the donor and recipient must be accurately matched for size. A large lung will not expand properly in a chest cavity that is too small.

The lungs (or heart/lungs) are removed by one team, and are stored in a sterile plastic bag on ice in a special container, where they can be kept for up to four hours. At the recipient center a second team prepares the recipient by removing the diseased lung(s) and performs the transplant. Lung transplants take approximately eight hours to complete.

Artificial ventilation is necessary for a few days after a lung transplant. Close observation is essential during the first two weeks, when signs of rejection are detected by examining the chest and/or on chest X-ray. Immunosuppressive drugs are given and include cyclosporine, anti-lymphocyte globulin and low doses of steroids later on. Physiotherapy, with exercises such as walking on a treadmill, is begun after surgery and continued after discharge from hospital.

Patients who undergo a heart/lung transplant may experience rejection in the heart and lung tissues at different times and in varying degrees. Complications include accelerated hardening of the coronary arteries (arteriosclerosis), and respiratory failure from bronchiolitis. Both of these conditions are thought to result from chronic rejection. Because of the added risks arising from heart transplantation, a combined heart/lung transplant is performed only when the heart is irreversibly damaged from lung disease.

Heart Transplants

The first human transplant was performed in 1967 by Dr. Christian Barnard in Capetown, South Africa. Several centers around the world promptly initiated cardiac transplant programs, but patient survival during these early years was dismal. Of the 20 patients receiving a heart transplant in Canada between 1968 and 1969, most had died by the end of one year as a result of infection or rejection. Only one of the patients lived longer than five years. Enthusiasm for heart transplants waned, and only a few transplant centers persevered during the 1970s. Better anti-rejection drugs and the development of a simple biopsy method to diagnose rejection contributed to steadily improving results. By 1988, over 7,000 heart transplants had been performed worldwide. Currently, 75 percent of patients are alive and well one year after heart transplantation, and by five years, the survival rate is 50 percent.

Patients suitable for heart transplants should be under age 50 with terminal heart disease and a life expectancy of less than one year. There should be no possibility of conventional medical or surgical treatment, and there should be no other major organ dysfunction. Conditions requiring a heart transplant include severe disease of the coronary vessels or heart valves, which cannot be surgically corrected, and weakness of the heart muscle caused by viral inflammation (cardiomyopathy). With improved transplant results, these criteria are being relaxed somewhat. Diabetics and some patients over age 50 are now receiving transplants.

Immediate transplantation is necessary to save the life of a patient suffering a massive heart attack. However, a suitable donor heart is often not available on such short notice. Some surgeons have implanted an artificial heart for up to two weeks in these patients until a donor heart can be found.

The donor heart must be healthy. (Because of the prevalence of asymptomatic coronary artery disease, donors over age 45 are usually excluded for heart donation, although some surgeons are performing corrective surgery on the coronary arteries as the heart is being transplanted.) The heart is quickly detached through an incision that splits the middle of the chest cavity and allows access to the large blood vessels going to and from the heart. While still in place, the heart is flushed with a cold solution. The heart is then carefully lifted out of the chest, placed in a sterile plastic bag and transferred into a cooler for transport to the recipient center. The maximum time between removal and transplant is five hours.

Meanwhile, another team prepares the recipient while waiting for the donor heart to arrive. Cardiopulmonary bypass is set up, so that machines do the work of the patient's heart and lungs while the diseased heart is removed. The donor heart is then sewn in place and the blood vessels are joined. When the clamps are released, the heart begins to beat again and the patient is taken off the bypass machine. The operation usually takes about four hours.

Close monitoring of vital signs continues in the recovery room and intensive care unit. Immunosuppressive medication is used, and signs of rejection are watched for on the electrocardiogram (ECG). Heart muscle biopsies are performed at regular intervals during recovery, and even after the patient has been discharged from hospital. A significant long-term problem is an accelerated form of arteriosclerosis of the coronary arteries, perhaps induced by chronic rejection. Also, the cyclosporine dose must be carefully monitored to prevent kidney damage.

Recent Advances

Increasingly, other organ transplants are providing a life-saving treatment for patients with various forms of organ failure. For example, over 1,000 pancreas transplants have been performed worldwide. A successful pancreas transplant appears to lessen the complications of diabetes, such as nerve deterioration, visual disturbances, accelerated hardening of the arteries and kidney failure. The one-year graft survival for pancreas transplants is currently about 40 percent.

Only a few intestinal transplants have been attempted, although none has resulted in long-term success due to technical problems such as the potential for infection, difficulties in re-establishing the blood flow to the bowel transplant, and rejection problems.

Rejection remains a central problem and is the leading cause of transplant failure. Improved techniques of matching donors with recipients, as well as new anti-rejection drugs, will lessen the tendency for rejection and improve survival rates.

The long-term hope of all physicians is that a better understanding of the disease processes leading to organ failure will result in better methods of prevention and treatment, so that one day the need for organ transplants may be virtually eliminated.

Chapter 20

Cancer Surgery

Lorne Rotstein

Assistant Professor of Surgery
University of Toronto

Chief, General Surgical Oncology
Toronto General Hospital

Almost everyone has had a relative or a friend die of cancer. Many people think that the word itself spells certain death, but far more cancer patients live out their natural life-span today. Even more live for a longer time without symptoms, thanks to newer treatment. Patients may need to have checkups every six months for the rest of their lives, but their lives will be longer because they will be treated promptly.

Surgery is the oldest form of treatment for cancer, and until recently it was the only way of curing malignant diseases. Now chemotherapy and radiation are often used to treat many types of cancer. This has led to the development of a new specialty — surgical oncology. It deals with the diagnosis and treatment of malignant diseases. The surgical oncologist tends to treat rarer cancers, cancers that may involve more than one anatomical site or system, recurrent cancer and complications arising from chemotherapy or radiation. The surgical oncologist also develops treatment schedules that coordinate surgery with other treatment.

Patients with recurrent cancer (secondary tumors) are often referred to a surgical oncologist. For example, a patient with a previous cancer of the colon who develops a tumor in the liver would usually be sent to a surgical oncologist, who would decide whether treatment should consist of surgical removal, chemotherapy or observation only.

Surgical oncologists also tend to see patients with complications arising from the other main methods of cancer therapy — radiation and chemotherapy. For example, a woman with cancer of the cervix treated with radiation may develop intestinal obstruction or bleeding as a side effect of treatment. This would likely be dealt with by a surgical oncologist. Similarly, patients on chemotherapy for long periods of time tend to develop scarring of their veins, making continuation of treatment difficult. These patients are often referred to a surgical oncologist for insertion of a permanent device giving intravenous access. Referral to the surgical oncologist may be from the family doctor, traditional surgical specialist, radiotherapist or chemotherapist/medical oncologist.

Terminology

Tumor vs. Neoplasm

The terms tumor and neoplasm are often used interchangeably by both patients and physicians. However, a tumor is actually a lump or swelling that can be due to a congenital abnormality, injury, inflammation, infection or, in some cases, a neoplasm. A neoplasm is a growth of abnormal tissue, which can be benign or malignant.

Benign vs. Malignant

All neoplasms increase in size with time. Benign neoplasms usually grow slowly and produce damage by compressing nearby structures. Malignant neoplasms grow more rapidly, and besides compressing nearby structures, they invade them. Malignant neoplasms can spread (metastasize) to distant sites, usually via the lymph glands or the blood. For example, cancers of the large intestine may spread to the liver or lungs via the bloodstream.

Malignancy vs. Cancer

The term cancer is often used interchangeably with malignancy, but this is incorrect. Malignancy implies local invasiveness and the ability to spread. There are three overall types of malignancy: carcinoma, sarcoma and lymphoma. Carcinoma is a type of malignancy arising in the skin, mucous membranes, subcutaneous glands including the breast, the gastrointestinal tract, liver and pancreas. The term "cancer" means carcinoma. Carcinomas spread directly by lymph channels to regional lymph nodes, and also to distant organs (e.g., lung, liver) via the bloodstream. The seriousness of different types of carcinoma can vary tremendously depending on the site of the organ, and the type and extent of spread at the time of diagnosis. Sarcomas are malignant growths that arise in the body's supporting tissues — muscle, ligament, bone, cartilage and fat — and tend to spread primarily via the bloodstream. Sarcomas arising in soft tissues and less than two inches in diameter are much less aggressive than larger sarcomas. In general, sarcomas arising in an arm or leg are more likely to be curable than those arising in the tissues of the trunk, head or neck. Furthermore, the seriousness of an individual sarcoma varies with its pathological type. Some, such as liposarcomas, are very slow growing while others, such as poorly differentiated fibrosarcomas, are much more aggressive.

Lymphomas are malignant growths arising in the lymph glands, spleen or tonsils. (Leukemias are closely related to lymphomas, but involve the blood or blood-forming organs.) Lymphomas tend to invade more than one site and may be associated with systemic symptoms including fever, night sweats and itchiness. The treatment of lymphoma depends on the number of sites involved, whether symptoms are present and the tissue structure of the tumor. To determine the type of tissue structure, the surgeon may remove a lymph node for dissection, but most lymphomas are treated by radiation, chemotherapy or a combination of the two. Occasionally a lymphoma that involves a site beyond the lymphatic system (such as the gastrointestinal tract) is surgically removed, and no other therapy is needed.

Biopsy

A biopsy is the removal of a tissue sample in order to make a diagnosis. Different techniques are chosen according to the site, blood supply and symptoms of a given growth. The choice of treatment will be made according to the biopsy results.

Needle Biopsies

Tissue sampling using a needle can be done in two different ways: needle aspiration biopsy and core needle biopsy. Aspiration biopsy can usually be done in the doctor's office with minimal discomfort for the patient. It tends to be most useful for superficial tumors in the thyroid gland, lymph nodes and breast. The tumor will not spread as a result of the biopsy itself.

The main problems with aspiration biopsy are sampling and interpretation errors. Sampling errors may occur because the specimen is very small and the cells removed may not be representative. Errors in interpretation may occur because only single or clumps of cells can be seen, rather than the relationship of cells to each other and the overall appearance of the tissue from which they came.

Aspiration biopsies tend to underestimate the severity of the disease in 5 to 10 percent of cases. Therefore, if a needle aspiration cytology report is positive, a malignancy is most likely present, but a report of negative does not necessarily rule out the possibility of malignancy, and further tests may still be needed.

A core needle biopsy uses a relatively large-diameter needle to remove an actual "core" or piece of tissue with the relationship of the cells intact. An anesthetic, usually local, is necessary and, depending on the site to be biopsied, there may be a risk of bleeding, or the tumor may spread because of the biopsy. Sampling errors may occur, but the likelihood of false negative reports is much lower than with aspiration biopsy. All needle biopsies are minor office or outpatient department procedures.

Open Biopsy

In some situations, needle biopsy will not be sufficient, so an "open" biopsy is done. This is actually a small operation in which the surgeon cuts through the skin and other tissues and either cuts out a portion of the tumor or, if possible, removes all of it for examination by the pathologist.

Open biopsies are used when needle biopsy is impossible due to the risk of tumor spread or bleeding, or when a larger volume of tissue is required. These procedures are usually performed in hospital or outpatient operating rooms rather than the doctor's office.

Endoscopic Biopsy

An endoscope is a flexible tube with optical systems and cutting instruments. It allows the surgeon to see the lining of the cavity into which the tube is inserted and to remove a piece of tissue. Endoscopy is a useful diagnostic tool in most areas of surgery, and endoscopic biopsy is possible at many sites such as the gastrointestinal tract or the bladder. Most endoscopic biopsy procedures require some type of anesthetic. The piece of tissue obtained is usually small.

Cancer Surgery

Cancer surgery is aimed at curing the disease, if possible. If not, it is aimed at extending survival or relieving symptoms as the disease progresses.

Curative cancer surgery often involves removing the malignant growth plus a surrounding margin of normal tissue to decrease the likelihood of recurrence. The surgeon will tie off the draining veins and lymphatic vessels and minimize handling or squeezing the growth to limit the number of malignant cells shed into the circulation during the operation. The surgeon will also remove lymph nodes from the surrounding area, so that any malignant cells that have traveled to the lymph nodes cannot grow.

This type of radical surgery may result in significant deformity or loss of function. It is usually only done when cure is a real possibility. Surgical oncologists, radiotherapists and chemotherapists have been trying to find ways of combining surgery with radiation and/or drugs to reduce the extent of the operation and therefore the associated risks.

For example, 40 years ago the accepted operation for cancer of the breast was radical mastectomy (removal of the entire breast, underlying muscles and all the lymph nodes under the arm). This has been replaced by modified radical mastectomy (removal of the breast and lymph glands) with the same cure rates. Recently we have found that for small localized malignant growths, removal of the lump (lumpectomy) plus postoperative radiation treatment results in a cure rate comparable to mastectomy, and spares the cosmetic and associated psychological disability. Similarly, radiation has decreased the need for radical removal of cancers of the anal canal. However, at many sites the best chance of a cure is still by traditional radical cancer surgery.

Oncologists have also been trying to find out if the addition to surgery of radiation and/or chemotherapy will enhance the likelihood of cure. This seems to be true for carcinomas of the breast, soft tissue sarcomas and some carcinomas of the thyroid and lung. The amount and type of radiation or chemotherapy used in these settings vary tremendously, but in general, additional treatment of this type is designed to have minimal and tolerable side effects for the patient.

Where cure is not possible, surgery may still alleviate or prevent symptoms so that the quality of the patient's remaining life is improved. This is called palliative surgery. For example, a patient may have a stomach cancer that has spread to the lymph glands or the liver. Removing the tumor would not be a cure. However, stomach cancers left in place often obstruct the stomach outlet and/or bleed intermittently, so the stomach is removed surgically if possible to improve the quality and sometimes the extent of the remaining life-span.

Obviously many factors have to be taken into account in making these decisions: the risks associated with the operation, the benefits to be derived, the extent of symptoms, the expected life-span and whether more simple non-surgical treatment might relieve the symptoms. Patients and their families should be active participants in deciding whether a palliative operation should be performed. They must be well aware of both the risks and the benefits.

Clinical Trials

Surgical oncologists are often involved in experimental studies that compare combined treatment with surgical treatment only. Patients are sometimes asked to participate as experimental subjects in "clinical trials," especially if they are being treated at a university hospital.

Clinical trials of cancer treatments are

usually referred to as Phase I, II or III. A Phase I trial studies the side effects of a given medication or treatment. This type of study usually starts out at a low dose which has proven to be non-toxic in animal studies. Subsequent patients are given higher doses based on lack of side effects in the first patients treated. A Phase I study is purely a toxicity trial, and patients with many different types of malignancies are eligible for the same study. The likelihood of benefit from the medication or treatment is essentially unknown. Therefore patients should be asked to participate in a Phase I study only when all standard means of treatment for their disease have been exhausted.

Phase II studies are basic effectiveness trials and are undertaken after Phase I toxicity studies have revealed the side effects and toxic dose of the treatment. All patients in a Phase II study must have the same type of malignancy and receive the same treatment. Results are compared to other groups of patients treated at a different institution or at the same institution at a different time by a different treatment.

These comparisons can sometimes be deceptive. First, some patients treated in the study group may be so debilitated at the time of entry that even if a treatment is potentially useful, its effect may not be seen in these patients. Second, if the patients selected are not typical of patients with that condition, or if reports of responses are overenthusiastic, the results may be misleading.

In a Phase III randomized clinical trial, all eligible patients are randomly divided into two groups. One group gets the therapy of the Phase II trial. The other groups gets the best accepted therapy known to date. Both the doctor and patient must be unaware of which group the patient will enter until the choice occurs.

In some Phase III studies, neither doctor nor patient is aware of which group an individual patient is in until the study results are analyzed. These stringent means of control help prevent errors of sampling and interpretation that sometimes occur in Phase II trials.

The treatments are compared according to overall average survival, disease-free survival, recurrence rates, and numerous other parameters. These results are then analyzed statistically so that the treatments can be compared.

The principle of a clinical trial is to treat patients in a planned manner, permitting reliable conclusions to be drawn that can benefit future patients. North American governments have adopted the view that treating a patient as part of a clinical trial may subject the physician to a conflict of interest between the best care for the patient and the best results for the trial. To protect patients from this potential conflict of interest, and to ensure that these studies are ethically and scientifically appropriate, a number of regulations are enforced by the Health Protection Branch of Health and Welfare Canada and the Food and Drug Administration of the American Department of Health, Education and Welfare. All studies must comply with these regulations, and patients should avoid involvement in any trial or form of therapy that does not meet basic criteria. First, the study must be approved by an independent ethical and scientific human experimentation review committee at the hospital or university where it is conducted. The patient must be informed of all reasonable alternative treatments and their potential side effects. The patient must agree in writing to be treated according to the study protocol, and must be able to withdraw from a trial without jeopardizing his or her subsequent treatment. Finally, there must be no additional costs to the patient as a result of experimental treatment.

Many innovative approaches to the treatment of cancer are being actively studied under these guidelines. New drugs, new methods of administering drugs, alteration of the body's immune system and new treatments such as tumor heating (hyperthermia) will undoubtedly result in improved survival for people suffering from malignant diseases.

"Five-Year Cure Rate"

Doctors and patients often loosely throw around such terms as "five-year cure rate" without understanding what this actually means in relation to the disease. Five-year survival is only one means of assessing cure rate. In some types of cancer it may be important, but in other types it is irrelevant.

For example, in cancer of the colon, the majority of recurrences happen within five years, which makes a five-year survival rate almost equivalent to cure. On the other hand, cancer of the breast carries a risk of recurrence 10 or even 15 years after initial treatment. In this disease five-year survival is obviously not synonymous with cure. Any discussion of survival and decrease of risk after a period of time must take into account the type of cancer, rather than making the overall assumption that five-year survival equals cure.

Unproven Methods of Therapy

Each year many cancer patients invest countless hours and billions of dollars exploring alternatives to scientifically proven methods of cancer diagnosis and treatment. This is not only expensive in wasted time and money, but also in terms of human life, since patients may well be beyond the scope of effective therapy by the time they seek conventional treatment.

People are afraid of cancer more than any other disease, because of associations with prolonged suffering and death. They also fear the standard accepted medical treatment. Surgery may result in permanent disfigurement; radiation is threatening because it can be neither seen nor felt; chemotherapy produces side effects such as nausea, hair loss, vomiting and diarrhea. Then there is the fear of recurrence. The responsible physician can never guarantee a cure. The conservative approach of the medical community is grounded in reality, not in false hopes or promises. Many people who seek help outside conventional medicine also tend to be suspicious of reputable methods and disillusioned with science and technology.

Unproven therapies take advantage of these fears. They usually give the individual the illusion of at least being partly in control of his or her treatment, maintaining feelings of self-sufficiency and independence. These positive feelings may well account for the improvement that some people experience after unconventional treatment.

Promoters of unconventional therapy vary greatly, with backgrounds ranging from scientific training at a university to little formal education. Despite differences in background, there are a number of similarities. Promoters often claim that the government and/or organized medicine are conspiring to keep their "cures" from the population, and that the members of the scientific establishment do not want to lose the business generated by cancer patients. Promoters are usually skilled in advertising the effectiveness of their therapy in pamphlets, books, newspapers and patient testimonials, rather than presenting information at scientific meetings or publishing in medical journals so that their claims can be scrutinized by the medical community. When promoting an unproven method, the specific "cure" is usually advertised as unique, and the theory put forward to explain the effect of the treatment is usually quite complex (as with laetrile) but not supported by scientific evidence. Unorthodox therapists are usually unwilling to disclose methods of product preparation and claim a unique ability to make the substance in question. They justify their substantial charges on this basis.

When patients do not respond to unconventional therapy, the promoter of the treatment usually lays the blame elsewhere. The patient lacked faith, failed to follow directions exactly, stopped too soon or sought the ''cure'' too late for it to be effective. In this way the failure is always the fault of the patient and not the promoter or the product.

All accepted methods of cancer treatment used by the medical community were at some stage ''unproven.'' Each one, however, has been subjected to careful scrutiny before being adopted. As potential methods of treatment become available for scientific study, those with the most potential for success receive the highest priority for further clinical testing. As new information becomes available, it is published in journals and presented at meetings, so that there are no secret or unique treatment methods that are generally unavailable because of cost. Government health protection agencies have been set up to ensure that the patient is protected from unethical, unscrupulous, costly and unscientific practices.

Chapter 21

Trauma Surgery

Robert Y. McMurtry

Professor and Head of Surgery
University of Calgary

Head, Department of Surgery
Foothills Hospital, Calgary

The word "trauma" literally means a wound or injury. In this chapter the term is being used more specifically to describe the patient who has suffered critical multiple injuries as the result of a major damaging force such as a motor vehicle accident or gunshot wound.

In the United States, about 44,000 people (about 17 out of every 100,000) die each year in motor vehicle accidents. The annual cost to society is estimated to be $36 billion. The total number of American soldiers who died in the Vietnam War approximates the average number of deaths that occur *annually* in the United States from motor vehicle accidents. In Canada, the figures are even worse: on average, about 22 people per 100,000 perish each year.

We live in a society dominated by the motor vehicle. When the energy of a motor vehicle is pitted against the human body, there is no contest. Devastating injuries occur, and death is all too common.

Among those aged one to 44, these injuries are the most common cause of death in North America. Half of all deaths in those under 35 are due to injury. Deaths due to injury cause four million work years to be lost annually. In com-

Case Study: Trauma Care

The bell jarred through the small ambulance station as a 911 call was processed and the ambulance dispatched. The police would likely reach the scene first, maybe a minute or two before the ambulance, so they'd have the highway controlled for the emergency vehicles to get through.

Friday night car accidents always seem to be the worst, thought the nurse as she raced through the hospital emergency department. This 23-year-old man had been hit by a driver coming out of a sideroad. He was lucky. Although they didn't yet know the extent of his injuries, the ambulance had reached him before he had lost too much blood. He'd probably need to be shipped out to the regional trauma center of a larger hospital some distance away, she thought. He was lucky there, too. They could get the air ambulance and the paramedics to the rural hospital within minutes. The paramedics would get the details by radio so they wouldn't lose time. They'd have the patient on his way immediately.

The emergency room doctor was with the patient. "Right, nurse, the bleeding's under control and his breathing seems okay. I'm going to call the trauma center. We'll have time to get him stabilized before the paramedics get here." The doctor went to the phone while she continued working according to the strict protocol that had been set up when their hospital staff took advanced life support training.

parison, deaths from cancer result in 1.7 million lost work years. Approximately $622 million is spent on research for cancer and heart disease, but only $112 million for injury.

Trauma Care

The first aim of trauma teams is to prevent death or disability by preventing accidents — through education programs and by advocating the use of seat belts, safer highways and lower speed limits. If an accident does happen, the aim of a trauma team is to prevent worsening of the victim's condition, by rapid recognition of injuries, immediate and appropriate first-aid, evacuation and resuscitation.

Many states and provinces have set up trauma programs to coordinate care for the patient with several different injuries. These programs require a tremendous commitment from all health-care workers involved with the care of the trauma patient and from the institutions that undertake to give this care.

Trauma programs are organized into three phases: before the victim reaches the hospital, in hospital and after discharge from hospital.

Pre-Hospital Phase

The pre-hospital phase of trauma care involves "beating the clock." Injuries treated within 30 minutes can result in a very good outcome; attempts to treat these same injuries after four hours may be completely hopeless. Lack of circulation may be irreversible. Emergency services must be organized so that they minimize the amount of time that lapses from accident to definitive care.

The first step in getting help is awareness that an accident has occurred. This is usually no problem in a populated area, but many accidents occur in remote areas. Technology exists to cope with this problem. Remote electronic warning devices could be activated by impact or by turning on a distress signal, as exists in the black box on an airplane. Such devices would be invaluable in cars, snowmobiles or even the home of an elderly person.

The next vital link in the system is communication. The 911 telephone code is becoming increasingly accepted, but still is found in a minority of states and provinces. It simply requires the existence of a functioning telephone to give the public instant access to fire, police and ambulance services. There is no need to have money in your pocket, since pay phones will activate just as they do when dialing the operator. In most metropolitan areas, all three services can reach the scene within six minutes. In small communities the response time can be up to 15 minutes, and in remote areas or the wilderness up to two hours.

The next issue in rescue is the ability to move people safely and quickly to definitive care. This function is usually handled by firefighters, who have powerful equipment that can take the roof off a car in minutes, or remove windows from an automobile safely and quickly. This is essential in winter, especially, when victims can die of exposure.

Ambulance Services and Paramedics

In Canada and the U.S. there is a wide variation in standards of training for ambulance attendants and paramedics.

Ambulance attendants staff vehicles and transport patients. Their training may vary from a first-aid course to a comprehensive one-year program. Ambulance attendants perform many life-saving procedures such as maintaining breathing, giving oxygen, stopping bleeding, splinting fractures and dressing wounds. They are also trained to cope with a wide variety of terrains, weather conditions and vehicular problems.

The air ambulance is usually a helicopter or small plane. Helicopters are most useful for trips of 10 to 100 miles, or in cases of traffic jams, floods or impassable roads. They can be invaluable in transferring seriously ill or injured patients for relatively short distances. Planes are usually used for distances of more than 100 miles. They are faster than helicopters, but require better takeoff and landing facilities.

Paramedics are usually experienced ambulance attendants with at least a further year's training, although some nurses and respiratory technicians have become paramedics. They carry out advanced life support or "delegated medical acts" — procedures that have been delegated by a physician with whom the paramedic is teamed. Paramedics can insert a tube in the patient's windpipe to maintain breathing, set up an intravenous line to replace body fluids and assess a patient's vital signs. Their role is extremely important when the victim has had a heart attack, or when accident victims have to be transported over distances longer than five miles. Paramedics are a vital link in the system, extending the emergency department's capability by hundreds of miles. Air ambulances in remote areas can communicate via satellite with metropolitan base hospitals.

The ambulance system is the lifeline that brings patients into the health-care system; it links the field to the hospital and one hospital to another.

Inter-Hospital Transfer

It is quite common for two hospitals to be involved in the care of a seriously injured patient. The patient is first taken to the nearest hospital, where life-saving stabilization is carried out. A tube is secured in the windpipe to ensure that the patient can breath, body fluids are replaced intravenously, blood transfusions are given and fractures are splinted. Once the patient's heart and lung condition is stable, transfer to a larger hospital can take place.

The hospital that initially treats the patient may very well be able to give final or definitive care. If, however, the severity and multiplicity of injuries is more than the hospital can handle with its resources, an early decision is made to transfer the patient to a hospital where all necessary services would be available, such as a university or teaching hospital. As soon as this decision is reached, communication is established between physicians in the sending and receiving hospitals.

The receiving hospital must be capable of giving complete care to the trauma victim. All major surgical specialties must be available (neurosurgeon, chest and abdominal surgeons, orthopedic, plastic, urological and vascular surgeons) plus intensive care units and anesthetists. This must all be available 24 hours a day, seven days a week.

The patient's case is discussed and an agreement reached about the best method of transfer. If an ambulance is being used, a doctor or nurse will accompany the patient. The air ambulance usually has paramedics aboard, so the presence of a doctor is not necessary — a boon to smaller hospitals that can ill afford to spare a doctor or nurse on weekends.

Ideally, the receipt of a patient, stabilization and decision for transfer should all be accomplished within an hour.

Hospital Phase

Trauma Resuscitation

The hospital phase of trauma care has four components: trauma resuscitation, operating room, intensive care unit and trauma ward.

The trauma resuscitation room is the nerve center of a regional trauma unit. The person in control is a trauma surgeon or emergency physician who has been in communication with the sending hospital and has monitored the patient's progress throughout the transport. The physician has notified all the relevant

The paramedics didn't stop for anything except the records and the X-rays — a swift transfer to the stretcher and they were off. But they already knew what they had to deal with. The emergency call had been quite specific about the possible extent of the victim's injuries, and they'd become pretty good at guessing what those injuries would be. In the air ambulance they notified their base at the trauma center that the intravenous was running okay, but they were adding whole blood. They also inflated the special suit in an attempt to maintain blood pressure. By the time they landed, their base contacts had as much idea of their patient's condition as they did.

It was early morning when they reached the trauma center, but the hospital was as busy as at midday. Another badly injured patient was just being transferred to the intensive care unit from the operating room. The waiting nurse supervisor knew that pretty soon the distraught family would arrive, and it was her job to tell them as clearly and compassionately as possible what had happened, and what would be done. Later, the senior doctor on the trauma team would come out to update her on the patient's condition, and would probably spend some time with the family, too. The hospital chaplain would be notified as well. She'd often been glad of his presence in the past. Even non-religious families seemed to find some comfort in being able to talk to someone whose concerns were spiritual rather than clinical.

As the patient was wheeled past her into the operating room, she reviewed what she knew about his case so that she'd know what to tell the family. A badly fractured leg, blood in his chest and a lacerated spleen. Bad enough, but she'd seen worse who'd pulled through. By the time the family arrived, the trauma team would have located the source of the bleeding in his chest, and would either have repaired his spleen or removed it. The fracture would be fixed that same night, not days later as had been the case when she was training.

The patient's wife arrived at the hospital, and was assured by the surgeon that her husband was holding his own. Providing he didn't have any setbacks in the next 48 hours, they expected him to pull through. He would be laid up for about six months, they said. Already the social worker had talked to her about arrangements at home, so she hoped they'd be able to get something worked out before he left the hospital.

services that must contribute to the patient's care, such as the blood bank, laboratory and radiology.

Trauma patients are met by a trauma resuscitation team, which consists of the team leader or trauma surgeon, three highly skilled registered nurses and three other doctors. In a teaching hospital, these will be residents in anesthesia, general surgery and orthopedics. Each has preassigned tasks and a routine to follow.

Although each patient is different, the fundamental principles never change. The first priority is to ensure that the patient can breathe. The second is treatment of inadequate circulation (shock). The third priority is to treat any problem of the central nervous system.

A trauma resuscitation team works like a well-oiled machine — with "unhurried haste" — to maintain the patient's vital functions. At the same time, diagnoses are made or confirmed so that a full picture of the patient's condition unfolds, and plans are made for the best treatment.

As many as 33 people may be involved in the successful resuscitation and management of a trauma patient in the first hour. Radiology technicians take X-rays. A runner transports blood samples for analysis. The blood bank matches blood for transfusions. The operating room staff prepares for the patient's arrival, and the hospital switchboard and operators keep the relevant services informed. The nurse/supervisor will come to the emergency department to ensure that vital services for other patients are protected. The chaplaincy will communicate with the patient's family as they wait in the quiet room.

One of the common emergency surgical procedures performed on trauma patients is the insertion of a chest tube. Chest tubes are inserted to relieve air and/or blood accumulating outside the lung, within the chest wall. The chest tube is inserted into the space between the chest wall and the lung. Correctly positioned, it can drain blood and air and allow the lung to expand and function better.

If there is suspicion of significant bleeding within the abdominal cavity, a "mini-laparotomy" (cutting the abdominal wall) is done. After tubes have been put in to drain the bladder beneath and the stomach above, an incision is made below the umbilicus (belly button) through to the abdominal cavity. If there is no obvious blood in the cavity, a plastic tube is inserted and sterile solution is put into the cavity from an intravenous bag. The bag is then moved to a level below the cavity and the fluid is siphoned off. The presence of blood in the fluid determines the need for abdominal surgery.

Both of these procedures can be carried out under local anesthetic within 10 minutes. Chest tubes can be life-saving, while the mini-laparotomy provides invaluable diagnostic information. Both can be done while other procedures are being carried out.

Once the injuries to the major body systems have been determined, a plan of action is formed and the patient is usually moved to the operating room, where life-saving surgery is carried out.

Operating Room

On average, the seriously injured patient has damage to two or three body systems: over 80 percent have broken bones, 70 percent have head injuries and 40 percent have abdominal injuries. If a patient has all of these injuries, the priority would be to evacuate a blood clot in the brain and control the bleeding in the abdomen. One or the other might be more urgent, but if it is impossible to decide which, simultaneous surgery is carried out. The neurosurgeon makes a hole in the skull and deepens it until the blood clot is identified. Clearing the blood clot relieves the pressure on the brain.

Meanwhile, the general surgeon will explore the abdomen and may well find bleeding from the spleen or liver that could be fatal if left uncontrolled. Until very recently a lacerated or ruptured spleen was routinely removed, but because some patients developed overwhelming infection after splenectomy, every attempt is made now to leave the spleen intact. Similarly, the surgeon may have to stitch lacerations of the liver, because only limited portions of the liver can be removed safely. The surgeon will also explore the abdominal cavity, checking for other injuries such as perforation of the intestines.

The next order of priority would be the fractures. Early treatment of fractures (within 24 hours of the injury) results in reduced disability and mortality. Orthopedic surgeons used to wait days before fixing fractures with metal plates, screws and nails, because they thought the patient would be better able to cope with the stress of surgery. However, the trend now is to do immediate fixation of the fractures if the patient's general condition permits it. Patients can become mobile earlier, and the fracture has a better chance of knitting if it is realigned and stabilized early.

The anesthetist "puts the patient to sleep" but also monitors vital signs and functions, gives fluid replacement, blood transfusion and ensures that the patient's overall condition remains stable. Many things can go wrong during surgery. It is the anesthetist who maintains the patient's vital functions while the life-saving surgery is carried out.

Intensive Care Unit

On average, patients in intensive care receive one-on-one nursing care. If a patient is critically ill, more than one nurse may be assigned. Respiratory support, support of the cardiovascular system, monitoring of the central nervous system and intravenous feeding may be some of the functions carried out. The patient will be linked to many tubes and lines, so that even the slightest change in condition will be noticed.

Occasionally, the patient does have to return to the operating room for treatment of complications, but most of the care involves adjustments that can be carried out in the intensive care unit itself.

Trauma Ward

Originally patients with multiple injuries went to neurosurgery, orthopedics or general surgery wards on leaving the intensive care unit. Now, special wards focusing on those with multiple injuries have been set up. The trauma ward is managed by a multidisciplinary team under the supervision of a trauma surgeon and involving physiotherapy, occupational therapy, social work, chaplaincy, pharmacy, nutrition, speech pathology, neuropsychology and nursing. This allows for planning of rehabilitation very early — with correspondingly improved results.

Post-Hospital Phase

Follow-up rehabilitation visits and multidisciplinary management are now a major focus of care in trauma cases. Over 80 percent of patients with multiple injuries return to work within the year, their physical injuries cured. However, depression, stress and irritability are also common in those recovering from trauma. Employers and families can be assured that these reactions are temporary. The trauma patient is "not his or herself" for six to 12 months after the event. Awareness of this hastens healing, so social workers attached to trauma teams inform both patient and family what to expect.

One of the best prevention activities that trauma units are now becoming involved in is education programs for schools, since those in their teens and early twenties are the highest-risk age group for the most common cause of trauma — motor vehicle accidents. Classes are brought into the trauma unit to see some of the consequences of, for example, drinking and driving. Young paraplegics describe what life has been like for them since their accident, all with a ''don't-let-this-happen-to-you'' focus.

Further research into the cause of accidents is also being actively pursued, so that more effective prevention programs can be carried out. At the other end of the spectrum, research into the psychosocial effects of trauma is shedding new light on the healing process, so that rehabilitation can include effective counselling.

Glossary

Abscess: A localized collection of pus.
Adenoidectomy: The surgical removal of the adenoids.
Adenoids: A soft mass of lymphoid tissues at the back of the nose; when enlarged they impede breathing and speaking.
Adhesions: An abnormal adherence of surfaces caused by inflammation and scarring.
Adrenalin: A hormone secreted by the adrenal gland, which is located near the kidney. This hormone affects circulation and muscular action, causing excitement and stimulation.
AIDS *(Acquired Immune Deficiency Syndrome)*: A disease that attacks the body's immune system so that it is unable to fight off infections.
Alveoli: The air sacs of the lungs, where the exchange of gases between the lungs and the blood takes place.
Amblyopia: Impaired vision: partial loss of sight not due to organic disease within the eye itself.
Analgesic: A drug used to relieve pain.
Anastomosis: A surgically created joining of two tubular structures (such as the ureter and colon).
Anemia: A reduction in the number of red cells in the blood, often causing paleness and tiredness.
Anesthetic: A substance or gas that produces partial or complete insensitivity to pain.
Anesthetist *(anesthesiologist)*: The person who administers the anesthetic.
Aneurysm: A ballooning of an artery due to weakness of the artery wall.
Angina pectoris: Severe constricting pain in the chest, sometimes spreading to the arms and neck; caused by coronary artery disease.
Angiogram: An X-ray of the blood vessels by injection of radio-opaque material.
Angioplasty: A technique using balloon dilatation to restore the lumen of a narrowed blood vessel.
Angioscope: An instrument inserted into a blood vessel to examine the interior.

Antibiotic: A drug that is used to destroy or inhibit the growth of bacteria.
Anticoagulant: A drug used to prevent or retard the clotting of blood.
Antigen: A substance that produces or stimulates the formation of antibodies. A vaccine would be considered an antigen.
Antihistamine: A drug used to counteract the effects of allergies.
Anvil: *See incus.*
Aorta: The major artery that carries blood from the heart to all other parts of the body.
Aortoiliac disease: Disease of the aorta and the right and left common iliac arteries (the two main branches of the aorta).
Aphasia: The loss of speech due to brain disease.
Appendectomy: The surgical removal of the appendix.
Appendicitis: Inflammation of the appendix.
Appendix: A small tube connected to the large intestine in the lower right of the abdomen.
Arteriography: The process of X-raying arteries by injection of radio-opaque dyes (*see Angiogram*).
Arteriosclerosis: A hardening and thickening of the walls of the arteries.
Artery: A tubular, thick-walled elastic vessel, through which blood is pumped throughout the body.
Arthritis: Inflammation of a joint.
Arthrodesis: The surgical stiffening, i.e., fusing of a joint.
Arthroscope: An optical instrument that is inserted into a joint to examine the interior.
Arthrotomy: Cutting into a joint.
Astigmatism: A condition where there is unequal curvature of one or more of the refractive surfaces of the eye; as a result light rays are not focused at a single point on the retina.
Atelectasis: The collapsing of a lung or part of a lung.
Atherosclerosis: A stage of arteriosclerosis characterized by irregularly distributed fatty deposits on the wall of the artery.
Atrium: The upper chamber of each half of the heart.
Atropine: A drug used to dilate the pupil of the eye and/or paralyze the focussing ability of the eye.
Audiometer: An instrument that tests hearing by producing notes of different pitch and intensity.

Bacteria: Microscopic organisms that may cause infections.
Barium: A radio-opaque solution swallowed by a patient prior to X-ray examination. It reveals any obstructions, tumors or abnormalities in the gastrointestinal tract.
Benign: A non-dangerous or non-malignant condition most commonly used to describe tumors.
Bile: Greenish-yellow fluid secreted by the liver to aid in the digestion of food.
Biliary colic: Sharp pain due to spasm of the ducts that carry bile in the cystic duct and the common bile duct. The obstruction is usually caused by stones.
Biopsy: The removal of tissue for diagnostic examination.
Blepharoplasty: Surgical correction of a defect in the eyelid.
Bone graft: A piece of fragments of bone used to stimulate new bone formation.
Brain dead: The cessation of brain activity as recorded on an EEG (electroencephalogram).
Bronchi: The two main branches of the windpipe.
Bronchiolitis: Inflammation of the fine subdivisions of the bronchi in the lungs.
Bronchitis: Inflammation of the bronchi.
Bronchoscopy: A diagnostic procedure to view the large airway connecting the nasal passages and mouth to the lungs. An instrument

called a bronchoscope is inserted into the airway via the mouth or nose.
Bypass graft: A tubular structure used to carry blood past an obstruction.

Calyces: The series of funnels that collect urine as it is filtered from the kidneys.
Capillary: One of the very small blood vessels that connects the arteries and veins to body tissues.
Carcinogenic: "Causing cancer."
Carcinoma: A malignant tumor arising in the skin, mucous membranes, and glands such as the breast, gastrointestinal tract, liver and pancreas.
Cardiac: Pertaining to the heart.
Cardiologist: A physician specializing in the diagnosis and treatment of heart disease.
Cardiovascular disease: Disease of the heart and blood vessels or circulation.
Carotid: Either of the two main arteries carrying blood to the brain.
Carotid endarterectomy: The surgical removal of an obstruction in the carotid arteries.
Carpal tunnel syndrome: The compression of the median nerve as it passes through the wrist.
Cartilage: The firm, smooth, translucent, bluish-white tissue that covers the end of bones and allows low-friction movement between the bones in a joint.
Cataract: A disease of the eye, in which the normally clear lens becomes opaque.
Catheter: A tubular instrument that passes fluid from or into a body cavity; often used to drain retained urine from the bladder.
CAT scan/CT scan *(Computerized Axial Tomography)*: The gathering of information by X-rays that photograph the body layer by layer.
Causalgia: Severe and often burning pain caused by injury to a peripheral nerve.
Cerebrospinal fluid: A colorless liquid produced by the blood, circulating between the membranes that surround the brain and spinal cord.
Cervix: The neck of the uterus (womb).
Cesarean section: A surgical operation to deliver a baby through walls of the abdomen and womb.
Chemotherapy: The treatment of disease by means of chemicals.
Chloroform: A colorless liquid used as an anesthetic.
Cholecystitis: Inflammation of the gallbladder.
Cholesterol: A fatty substance found in body cells and fluids that is produced in the liver and also consumed in fatty foods. It may be deposited in the walls of the arteries, causing hardening and thickening of the arteries.
Choroid: The vascular tissue in the eye, between the retina and sclera.
Chronic: Indicating a disease of slow progress and long duration.
Circulation: The movement of blood in the blood vessels, caused by the pumping action of the heart.
Circumcision: The surgical removal of the foreskin of the penis.
Cirrhosis: A chronic, non-infectious disease of the liver characterized by excessive scar tissue. This disease is commonly associated with alcoholism.
Claudication: Pain in the leg (often the calf) caused by reduction of blood to the muscles as a result of narrowing of the arteries.
Cleft palate: A split or opening in the roof of the mouth.
Clinical clerk: A final year medical student.
Clot: A collection of coagulated blood.
Coagulating forceps: Forceps with an electric current running through it, used in surgery to control bleeding by coagulating blood vessels.
Cochlea: The spiral part of the inner ear that receives sound vibrations and

converts it into a nervous impulse.
Codeine: A substance extracted from morphine and used for relieving pain.
Colitis: Inflammation of the colon (the major portion of the large intestine).
Collagen: A gluey protein that is the principal substance in the connecting fibers of tissues.
Collateral circulation: Referring to the side branches of larger blood vessels.
Colles' fracture: A fracture of the lower end of the radius, which is one of two bones in the forearm.
Colon: The large intestine.
Colonoscopy: A visual examination of the upper portion of the colon with a fiber-optic instrument inserted via the anus.
Colostomy: An opening in the colon that is sutured to the skin to create an artificial anus, required because of disease or blockage of the large intestine.
Coma: Prolonged loss of consciousness.
Comatose: In a state of coma.
Concussion: A jarring injury to the brain resulting in a short period of unconsciousness.
Congenital: Existing at birth.
Conjunctiva: The mucous membrane covering the outer surface of the eyeball and lining of the eyelids.
Cornea: The transparent portion of the external covering of the eyeball lying over the iris and pupil.
Coronary: Relating to the arteries of the heart.
Coronary artery disease: Disease of the arteries nourishing the heart.
Corpus luteum: A yellow glandular body formed in the ovary at the site of a ruptured ovarian follicle after ovulation.
Cortisone: A hormone secreted by the adrenal gland that affects carbohydrate metabolism and the nutritional growth of connective tissue. It is used as a drug for many medical problems and in certain types of arthritis, where it decreases inflammation.
Coumadin: A drug used to prevent blood clotting.
Craniotomy: A surgical opening of the skull.
Cryotherapy: The use of cold temperatures in the treatment of disease.
Culture: The cultivation of tissue or micro-organisms in a prepared nutritious media.
Cyclosporine: A drug used after organ transplants to suppress the body's immune system and thereby prevent rejection.
Cyst: A sac or cavity containing fluid or semisolid matter.
Cystic duct: The tube that leads from the gallbladder and joins the tube leading from the liver, to form the common bile duct that transfers bile to the intestine.
Cystitis: Inflammation of the bladder.
Cystocele: A slipping down or prolapse of the bladder into the vagina.
Cystoscope: An instrument that permits visual examination of a bladder. It is equipped with a light, observing lens and various attachments and is passed through the urethra into the bladder.
Cytology: The study of cells.

Dermis: The inner layer of skin
Detrusor: A muscle that expels a substance.
Diabetes: A disease in which sugar and starch are not properly metabolized, caused by an insulin deficiency.
Dialysis: The purification of blood by flowing through a membrane.
Diaphragm: The muscular partition that separates the chest cavity from the abdominal cavity and aids in breathing.
Dilatation and curettage *(D and C)***:** The opening of the cervix and insertion of instruments into the uterus to scrape its lining.

Disc: A flat round plate of fibrocartilage between vertebrae. It has the consistency of rubber.
Discectomy: The removal of a disc.
Doppler studies: The use of ultrasound waves to measure the blood flow through vessels.
Duodenum: The first portion of the small intestine, into which the stomach empties.
Dysfunctional menorrhagia: Abnormal or excessive menstrual bleeding in the absence of any pelvic abnormality.
Dyslexia: A nervous disorder affecting reading ability or comprehension of what is read.
Dysphasia: Lack of coordination in speech due to brain disease or injury.
Dysplasia: Abnormal tissue development.

Eardrum: *See Tympanic membrane.*
ECG *(electrocardiogram)***:** A recording of the electric currents produced by the heart; used to diagnose abnormal heart activity.
Echocardiogram: A diagnostic ultrasound of the heart.
Ectopic pregnancy: A pregnancy occurring elsewhere than in the uterus (e.g., the fallopian tubes).
Electrolytes: Chemicals found in the blood (e.g., sodium and potassium).
Embolism: Blockage of a blood vessel by a clot, air bubble or other obstruction.
Emphysema: A condition or complication of bronchitis in which the lungs and their air cells lose their elasticity and are distended with air to the point of inefficiency. It is accompanied by coughing and labored breathing, and may affect the heart.
Endocrine glands: Glands that produce hormones and secrete them into the bloodstream.
Endometrium: The mucous membrane or lining of the uterus.
Endourology: The study of certain genito-urinary structures by using small telescope-like instruments.
Enterocele: An intestinal hernia bulging against the wall of the vagina.
Epidermis: The outer layer of the skin.
Epidural block: Injection of a local anesthetic agent into the space around the spinal cord, in order to stop movement and sensation.
Esophagoscope: A hollow, rigid or flexible fiberoptic tube inserted into the esophagus, for the purpose of inspecting the esophagus.
Esophagus *(gullet)***:** The hollow tube connecting the throat to the stomach.
Estrogen: One of a group of female sex hormones that is produced by the ovaries and is responsible for the development of secondary sexual characteristics.
Eustachian tube: The tube connecting the middle ear and the back of the nose.

Fallopian tubes: The two ducts through which ova (eggs) pass from the ovaries to the uterus.
Fascia: A sheet of fibrous tissue beneath the skin, enclosing the muscles.
Femoral: Relating to or near the femur (thigh bone).
Femur: The thigh bone.
Fiberoptic: Relating to the transmission of light or images through fine glass or plastic fibers.
Fibroid tumors: A benign tumor of the wall of the uterus, resembling fibrous tissue.
Fibula: One of the two leg bones that extend from the knee to the ankle.
Flail joint: A loose, unstable joint.
Flap: A piece of tissue separated from the adjoining tissue.
Flatus: Gas or air in the gastrointestinal tract, which may be expelled through the anus.
Fracture: The breaking of a bone. Compound (open) is a fracture in which the skin is perforated and there is an open wound which may extend down to the break.

Gangrene: The death of living tissue, usually due to blockage of the artery taking blood to that part of the body.
Gastroenteritis: An inflammation of the upper intestines, causing vomiting, diarrhea and cramps.
Glaucoma: A disease of the eye, caused by an increase of pressure of the fluids within the eyeball, eventually leading to loss of vision.
Glucose: Blood sugar. It is the chief source of body energy and is the form in which carbohydrates are absorbed into the body.
Graft: A tissue transplant.
Grand mal: A severe epilepsy characterized by violent convulsions and loss of consciousness.
Gynecology: The medical specialty that deals with women and their diseases, including their sexual and reproductive functions.

Hammer: *See Malleus*
Heart attack: A lay term used to describe myocardial infarction (death of the heart muscle) due to a blockage of a coronary artery.
Heart failure: Congestion of fluids in the tissues due to failure of the heart to maintain circulation.
Hemiplegia/Hemiparesis: Paralysis on one side of the body.
Hemoglobin: An oxygen-carrying reddish protein containing iron, which is found in the red blood cells.
Hemorrhage: Uncontrolled bleeding from the blood vessels.
Heparin: An organic substance that thins the blood and prevents clotting.
Hepatitis: Inflammation of the liver.
Hernia: Protrusion of bodily organ through a wall of the cavity where it is normally contained; a rupture.
Hormones: A secretion produced by glands (such as the pituitary or adrenal), which regulates reproduction, growth and metabolism.
Hydrocele: An accumulation of fluid in the scrotum or groin.
Hydrocephalus: An excess of cerebrospinal fluid in the brain cavity, causing an enlarged skull and mental retardation.
Hyperlipidemia: The presence in the circulating blood of an abnormally large amount of a fatty substance called lipid.
Hypertension: Abnormally high blood pressure.
Hyperthyroidism: An abnormality of the thyroid gland, causing an increased rate of metabolism, loss of weight and sometimes a swollen thyroid (goiter).
Hypertrophic scar: The healing of a wound with excessive scar tissue.
Hypertrophy: An excessive growth or development of an organ or part.
Hypothermia: A body temperature significantly below normal (98.6 F/37 C).
Hysterectomy: Surgical removal of the uterus.
Hysterotomy: Surgical incision of the uterus.

ICU: Intensive care unit.
Idiopathic: Of unknown cause.
Iliac crest: A part of the pelvic bone from which bone may be taken for bone-grafting purposes.
Imbrication: The surgical overlapping of tissues to strengthen them.
Immunosuppression: The suppression or holding back of the body's immune system by use of a chemical. This is often done in graft or organ transplants to prevent rejection.
Incus *(anvil)*: The middle bone of the three small bones in the middle ear.
Inflammation: A condition marked by heat, swelling, redness and usually pain, caused by the body's action to repair damaged tissues or destroy invading organisms.
Inguinal: Relating to the groin.

Intern: A graduate of a medical school who is serving in a hospital for one year to complete his/her training before obtaining a license.
Intraocular pressure: Pressure in the eyeball.
Intravenous *(IV)*: In or into a vein (as in intravenous feeding).
In vitro fertilization *(IVF)*: Fertilization that takes place in an artificial environment such as a test tube or culture media.
Isotope scan: A procedure that determines the distribution of a specific radioactive element, administered internally for diagnostic purposes.

Jaundice: A condition caused by the blockage of bile, so that it collects in the blood, causing yellowish skin and fluids.
Joint: A place where two or more bones come together. The bone ends are lined by cartilage allowing smooth, friction-free movement.

Keloid: An overgrowth of scar tissue.

Laparoscopy: The insertion of an illuminated optical instrument through a small incision in the abdominal wall, for the purpose of viewing the abdominal cavity.
Laparotomy: A surgical incision in the abdominal wall to gain access to the cavity of the abdomen.
Laryngoscopy: Inspection of the larynx, by mirror, telescope or with the use of an illuminated tube inserted through the mouth.
Larynx: The organ of voice production situated above the windpipe (trachea). It consists of cartilage, muscle and voice box.
Laser: A device that concentrates high energy into a narrow beam of light. A laser can be used to cut, vaporize or coagulate tissue very precisely. Laser surgery is performed in cavities or tubes that would be difficult to reach with conventional instruments.
Laxative: A medicine to aid the evacuation of the bowels.
Lens: A transparent ovoid structure behind the pupil of the eye, which focuses light onto the retina.
Lesion: An abnormal change in an organ or body part, caused by injury or disease.
Ligament: A short band of fibrous tissue that connects one bone to another at a joint, or supports an organ.
Lithotripsy: The crushing of a stone.
Lobectomy: Surgical removal of part of a lung.
Lumbago: Pain in the mid and lower back.
Lumen: The cavity or passageway of a tubular organ, such as a blood vessel.
Lymph glands: A series of glands that filter impurities out of lymph, a colorless, plasma-like fluid that flows throughout the body in lymph channels that eventually drain into the venous circulation. These glands play a role in our immune defense system.
Lymphocele: Localized collection of lymph fluid, usually in the pelvis.
Lymphoma: A tumor of the lymphoid tissue.

Macula: 1) A small discolored patch or spot on skin or tissue. 2) Central portion of retina of the eye to which rays of light are focussed by the lens of the eye.
Malignant: Cancerous. The tendency to spread to other organs and tissues, and to recur after removal. If not treated, the tumor or disease could be fatal.
Malleus *(hammer)*: The outermost of the three bones in the middle ear.
Mammography: X-ray of the breast.

Marrow: The soft tissue filling up the cavities in most bones.
Mastectomy: Removal of the breast.
Mediastinum: The area between the two lungs in the center of the chest.
Meningitis: Inflammation of the membranes of the brain or spinal cord.
Meniscus: The crescent-shaped, rubbery structure that acts as a shock absorber in the knee.
Metabolic: Relating to the production of energy and the maintenance of the vital organs.
Metastasize: To spread from an orginal site to another part of the body, as with a malignant tumor.
Microvascular: Of the small veins or capillaries.
Morbidity rate: A term used to express the incidence of complications as a result of surgery.
Mortality rate: The death rate.
MRI *(Magnetic Resonance Imaging)*: an imaging technique using a static external magnetic field and radio frequency pulses to generate images of various parts of the body.
Mucous membrane: A moist sheet of tissue containing mucous glands, lining passages and cavities of the body.
Myelogram: An X-ray of the spinal cord after the injection of a radio-opaque substance.
Myocardial infarction: The death of an area of heart muscle due to insufficient blood caused by blockage of the coronary artery. Heart attack.
Myringoplasty: Surgical repair of the eardrum.
Myringotomy: A surgical incision through the eardrum into the middle ear.

Narcotic: A drug that dulls sensibility and relieves pain, e.g., morphine.
Neoplasm: A new growth of excess tissue, forming a tumor that is benign or malignant.
Nephrectomy: The surgical removal of a kidney.
Nephroscope: An instrument for inspecting the kidneys.
Nerve: A whitish cord of nerve fibers held together by an envelope of connective tissue and through which stimuli are passed to and from the nervous system.
Nervous system: The system comprising the brain, the spinal cord and the motor sensory nerves and their endings.
Neurosurgeon: A surgeon specializing in surgery of the nervous system.
Nitrous oxide: A colorless gas, with a sweetish smell, used as an anesthetic.

Obstetrics: The medical specialty dealing with childbirth.
Omentum: A fold of abdominal membrane passing from the stomach into the abdominal cavity.
Oncology: The study of tumors (cancer).
Ophthalmology: The medical specialty dealing with the complete study of the eye and its diseases, including medical and surgical treatments.
Optic nerve: The nerve located at the back of the eye which transmits information from the retina to the brain.
Optometrist: A non-physician who examines eyes for disease and prescribes corrective lenses.
Orthoptist: A paramedical who uses the technique of eye exercises designed to correct improperly coordinated eyes, and who assesses the muscle balance and coordination of the eyes, under the supervision of an ophthalmologist.
Orthotist: A specialist who deals with the support and bracing of weak joints and muscles.
Osteoarthritis: Degenerative joint disease, or wear and tear arthritis.
Osteomyelitis: Infection of a bone.
Osteoporotic: Causing a porous condition of the bones.

Osteotomy: Surgically cutting a bone.
Otolaryngology: The medical specialty concerned with diseases of the ear, nose, throat and larynx, often including the upper respiratory tract and many diseases of the head and neck.
Ovulation: The production and discharge of ova (eggs) from the ovaries.

Pacemaker: An implanted artificial device to control the rhythm of the heart.
Palliative: The alleviation of symptoms such as pain, without curing the disease.
Pancreas: A large gland behind the stomach that secretes digestive juices into the intestine and insulin into the blood.
Pancreatic duct: The tube leading from the pancreas to the intestine.
Paralytic ileus: Distension of the intestinal tract due to inactivity or paralysis of the muscles of the intestinal wall.
Paramedic: A trained medical worker (but not a medical doctor) capable of performing basic emergency medical functions.
Paraplegia: Paralysis of the lower portion of the body, including both legs.
Patella: The knee cap.
Pathologist: A specialist who studies the causes and manifestations of disease.
Pedicle: The part of a skin or tissue graft that is left attached to the original site.
Percutaneous: Performed or effected through the skin via small punctures.
Pericardium: The membrane around the heart.
Periosteum: The fibrous membrane covering the entire surface of a bone.
Peritoneum: The thin, soft sheet of tissue (membrane) lining the abdominal cavity.
Peritonitis: Inflammation of the peritoneum or lining of the abdominal cavity.
Pessary: An instrument worn in the vagina to prevent displacement of the uterus.
PET *(Positive Emission Tomography)***:** A form of brain scanning that uses isotopes.
Phlebitis: Inflammation of a vein.
Physiotherapy: The treatment of disease or injury by massage, exercise, etc., rather than by drugs.
Pinna: The broad outer upper part of the ear.
Pituitary gland: A small gland located at the base of the brain. This gland directly or indirectly controls and regulates many basic body functions.
Plasma: Blood without its cellular components.
Platelets: Microscopic discs that circulate in the bloodstream and initiate the clotting process.
Pneumonectomy: The removal of a whole lung.
Pneumonia: An inflammation of the lungs caused by a variety of chemicals, bacteria or viruses.
Polyp: A tumor or growth forming a mushroom-shaped protuberance.
Popliteal: Relating to the hollow behind the knee joint.
Progesterone: A hormone produced in the ovaries to prepare the uterus for pregnancy.
Prolapse: A slipping out of place of some internal organ.
Prostate: A muscular gland at the neck of the bladder surrounding the beginning of the urethra in males.
Prostatectomy: The surgical removal of the prostate gland.
Prosthesis: An artificial substitute for a diseased or missing part of the body such as a limb, eye, tooth or joint.
Ptosis: Drooping of the upper eyelid.
Pulmonary edema: An accumulation of excess fluid in the lungs.
Pulmonary embolism: A blood clot

in the arteries of the lungs.
Pupil: The circular opening in the center of the iris of the eye, through which light passes.
Pyloric canal: The opening at the outlet of the stomach that allows the stomach contents to move into the first part of the small intestine.
Pyloric stenosis: Narrowing of the pyloric canal.

Quadriplegia: Paralysis of all four limbs.

Radiation: The emission of energy waves or particles to treat disease (such as tumors).
Radioactive: The ability to emit radiation.
Rectocele: Protrusion of the rectum into the vagina.
Rejection: The action of the body to destroy foreign or incompatible tissue (as in organ transplants).
Renal: Pertaining to or near the kidney.
Resection arthroplasty: Removing the ends of one or more bones to form a flail joint.
Resident: A qualified physician attached to a hospital for specialist training after the intern year.
Retina: The membrane that forms the inner lining of the back wall of the eye. It responds to light and sends impulses to the brain through the optic nerve. Its central portion is the macula.
Retinopathy: Noninflammatory degenerative disease of the retina.
Retropubic urethropexy: Surgical suspension of the bladder neck to the back of the pubic bone to correct urinary stress incontinence.
Rheumatic fever: A disease characterized by fever and inflammation of the joints and heart valves.
Rhinoplasty: Plastic surgery to change the shape of the nose.
Rickets: A vitamin D deficiency.
Saline solution: A salt solution.
Saphenous: Relating to the saphenous vein, which is located in the leg.
Sarcoma: A malignant tumor arising in connective tissue such as the bones, cartilage or muscles.
Sciatica: Pain due to irritation of the sciatic nerve, which is located at the back of the thigh and leg.
Sclera: The white ''wall'' of the eye.
Sclerotherapy: A treatment involving the injection of a sclerosing or hardening solution into the veins or tissues.
Scoliosis: Curvature of the spine.
Scrotum: The pouch that contains the testes.
Sepsis: The presence of infection.
Septum: A thin wall dividing two cavities.
Shock: A condition caused by loss of blood, severe infection or inability to pump blood, characterized by cold sweats, pallor, decreased blood pressure and rapid pulse.
Shunt: A diversion or bypass by an abnormal passage or mechanical device.
Sigmoidoscopy: A visual examination of the lower portion of the colon, using an instrument inserted via the anus.
Silicone: A plastic compound that may be a liquid, gel or solid. It is sometimes used in breast enlargements.
Sinuses *(paranasal sinuses)*: Air-filled cavities within the bones of the face and skull. The maxillary sinuses lie beneath the eyes; the ethmoid sinuses lie between the eyes and the nose, and the frontal sinuses above the eyes.
Sinusitis: Inflammation of the paranasal sinuses.
Speculum: An instrument to enlarge the opening of a canal or cavity to enable viewing of the interior.
Sphincter: A ring-shaped muscle which, by its contraction, is able to close or narrow an opening.

Spinal block: Injection of a local anesthetic agent into the fluid space around the spinal cord to produce numbness and paralysis of the lower half of the body.
Spleen: A large lymphatic organ located in the upper left portion of the abdomen, which acts as a blood filter and storage organ for red blood cells.
Splenectomy: Removal of the spleen.
Sprain: An injury to a ligament.
Sputum: A sustance expelled from the respiratory passages by coughing, usually mucus.
Squint: *See Strabismus.*
Stapes *(stirrup)*: The innermost bone of the three bones in the middle ear.
Staples: Metal staples may be used instead of sutures to close the skin or other tissues, such as the bowel. When used in the skin, staples are removed, but when used in deeper layers they are left in.
Stenosis: The narrowing or constriction of the diameter of a tube or passage.
Stereopsis: A technical term describing three-dimensional vision.
Stereoscopic vision: The ability to see two images as one, in three dimensions.
Stirrup: *See Stapes.*
Stitches: *See Sutures.*
Strabismus *(squint)*: A disorder of eye alignment in which both eyes cannot be focussed on the same target at the same time.
Stress incontinence: Leakage of urine as a result of coughing, straining or sudden movement.
Stroke: Sudden neurological disability caused by blood vessel disease in the brain.
Subluxated: Partially dislocated.
Sutures *(stitches)*: A thread-like material used for closing wounds. Sutures can be biodegradable, in which case they are eventually absorbed by the body. Other types of sutures are nonabsorbable (e.g., wire, silk, nylon) and remain intact. When used in the skin, these nonabsorbable sutures must be removed.
Synovium: The internal lining membrane of the joints.

Tendon: A strong band of connective tissue joining a muscle to a bone.
Testes *(testicles)*: The male reproductive glands.
Thoracic: Relating to the chest and the upper part of the body between the neck and the abdomen.
Thrombophlebitis *(venous thrombosis)*: Inflammation of a vein with blood clot formation.
Thrombosis: Formation of a blood clot within a blood vessel.
Thyroid gland: A large gland lying in the base of the neck. The thyroid produces a hormone that has a great influence on the body's growth, development and metabolism.
Tibia: The larger of the two bones located between the ankle and the knee.
Tonsillectomy: The operation to remove the tonsils.
Tonsillitis: Inflammation of the tonsils.
Tonsils: Small lymphatic organs situated on either side of the back of the throat.
Toxicity: The state or degree of being poisonous.
Trabeculoplasty: A laser procedure that improves the drainage of fluid from the eye, to treat glaucoma.
Trachea: *See Windpipe.*
Traction: A pulling force.
Transitional epithelium: The lining of the surface of the bladder, kidneys or ureters.
Transluminal dilatation: The surgical enlarging or spreading of a blood vessel or other tubular structure by using an inserted instrument. *(See Angioplasty.)*
Trauma: A physical wound or injury.
Trigone: The triangular inner surface of the bladder bordered by the openings of the ureters and urethra.

Truss: An appliance, usually a pad with a belt or spring, to support a part of the body, as with a hernia.
Tubal ligation: The tying off or surgical closure of the fallopian tubes to prevent pregnancy.
Tumor: An abnormal growth of tissue that creates a swelling.
Tympanic membrane *(eardrum)*: A thin sheet of tissue in the ear.

Ulcer/ulceration: A circular loss of skin or mucous membrane due to injury, loss of blood supply, infection or the action of corrosive fluids such as stomach acids.
Ultrasound: The use of sound waves to obtain images for medical diagnostic purposes.
Umbilicus: The navel or belly button.
Unconscious: Without mental awareness.
Ureter: A long tube that propels urine from the kidney to the bladder.
Urethra: The duct through which urine is discharged from the bladder.
Uterus *(womb)*: The hollow muscular organ in females, in which the fetus develops and is nourished before birth.

Varicocele: Varicose veins in the scrotum.
Varicose veins: Swollen or distended veins.
Vascular: Relating to the blood vessels.
Vascular aneurysm: The ballooning or dilation of an artery or vein.
Vasectomy: Surgical excision of the vas deferens to induce sterility.
Vasovasostomy: Reversal of vasectomy in which the two ends of the vas deferens are reattached to allow the sperm to pass from the testicle to the urethra.
Vein: A tubular, thin-walled vessel that carries blood from the capillaries to the heart.
Venography: The process of X-raying a vein by injection of a radio-opaque substance.
Venous thrombosis: *See Thrombophlebitis.*
Ventricle: One of the chambers of the heart.
Venule: A minute vein.
Vitrectomy: A surgical procedure to remove all or part of the vitreous jelly from the cavity of the eye.
Vitreous: A jelly-like substance filling the cavity of the eye behind the lens.
Vocal cords: Elastic folds of thin tissue inside the larynx, which vibrate to produce voice sounds.

Windpipe *(trachea)*: The airway extending from the larynx to the lungs.

Contributors

Editors

Allan Gross, M.D., F.R.C.S. (C)
Orthopedic Surgeon
Latner Professor and Chairman
Division of Orthopedic Surgery
University of Toronto

Staff Surgeon
Mount Sinai Hospital
Toronto, Canada

Penny Gross, Ph.D.
Senior Research and Program Evaluation Analyst
Ministry of Community and Social Services
Government of Ontario
Toronto, Canada

Bernard Langer, M.D., F.R.C.S. (C), F.A.C.S.
General Surgeon
R.S. McLaughlin Professor and Chairman
Department of Surgery
University of Toronto

Staff Surgeon
Toronto General Hospital
Toronto, Canada

Authors

Peter Alberti, M.B., Ph.D., F.R.C.S. (C)
Otolaryngologist
Professor and Chairman
Department of Otolaryngology
University of Toronto

Otolaryngologist-in-Chief
Toronto General Hospital
Toronto, Canada

F. Michael Ameli, M.D., F.R.C.S. (ED) (C), F.A.C.S.
Vascular Surgeon
Associate Professor of Surgery
University of Toronto

Staff Surgeon
Wellesley Hospital
Toronto, Canada

Grant Angus Farrow, M.D., F.R.C.S. (C), F.A.C.S.
Urologic Surgeon
Assistant Professor of Surgery
University of Toronto

Staff Surgeon
Toronto General Hospital
Toronto, Canada

Robert M. Filler, M.D., F.R.C.S. (C)
Pediatric General Surgeon
Professor of Surgery and Pediatrics
University of Toronto

Surgeon-in-Chief
Hospital for Sick Children
Toronto, Canada

Robert J. Ginsberg, M.D., F.R.C.S. (C)
Thoracic Surgeon
Professor and Chairman
Division of Thoracic Surgery
University of Toronto

Surgeon-in-Chief
Mount Sinai Hospital
Toronto, Canada

Bernard Goldman, M.D., F.R.C.S. (C), F.A.C.S.
Cardiovascular Surgeon
Professor of Surgery
University of Toronto

Staff Surgeon
Toronto General Hospital
Toronto, Canada

Allan Gross, M.D., F.R.C.S. (C)
Orthopedic Surgeon
Latner Professor and Chairman
Division of Orthopedic Surgery
University of Toronto

Staff Surgeon
Mount Sinai Hospital
Toronto, Canada

Walter J. Hannah, M.D., F.R.C.S. (C)
Obstetrician and Gynecologist
Professor and Chairman
Department of Obstetrics and Gynecology
University of Toronto

Staff Surgeon
Women's College Hospital
Toronto, Canada

Alan W. Harrison, M.D., F.R.C.S. (C)
Professor of Surgery
University of Toronto

Vice-President, Medical Affairs
Sunnybrook Medical Centre
Toronto, Canada

Robert D. Henderson, M.B., F.R.C.S. (C), F.A.C.S. (Deceased)
Former Thoracic Surgeon
Professor of Surgery
University of Toronto

Former Surgeon-in-Chief
Women's College Hospital
Toronto, Canada

Ernest Hew, M.D., F.R.C.S. (C)
Anesthetist
Associate Professor of Anesthesia
University of Toronto

Staff Anesthetist and Co-Director
Intensive Care Unit, Mount Sinai Hospital
Toronto, Canada

Alan R. Hudson, M.D., M.B., F.R.C.S. (C)
Neurosurgeon
James Wallace McCutcheon Chair

Surgeon-in-Chief
Toronto Hospital Corporation and Toronto General Hospital
Toronto, Canada

Stephen P. Kraft, M.D., F.R.C.S. (C)
Ophthalmic Surgeon
Assistant Professor of Ophthalmology
University of Toronto

Staff Surgeon
Hospital for Sick Children
Toronto, Canada

Nancy H. McKee, M.D., F.R.C.S. (C), F.A.C.S.
Plastic and Microvascular Surgeon
Associate Professor of Surgery
University of Toronto

Staff Surgeon
Mount Sinai Hospital
Toronto, Canada

Robert Y. McMurtry, M.D., F.R.C.S. (C)
Orthopedic Surgeon
Professor and Head of Surgery
University of Calgary

Head, Department of Surgery
Foothills Hospital
Calgary, Canada

Clive B. Mortimer, M.A., M.D., B. Chir., F.R.C.S. (C)
Ophthalmic Surgeon
Professor of Ophthalmology
University of Toronto

Head, Division of Ophthalmology
Toronto General Hospital
Toronto, Canada

Walter J. Peters, M.D., B.Sc., Ph.D., F.R.C.S. (C)
Plastic Surgeon
Associate Professor of Plastic Surgery
University of Toronto

Medical Director,
Ross Tilley Regional Adult Burn Centre
Wellesley Hospital
Toronto, Canada

Michael A. Robinette, M.D., F.R.C.S. (C)
Urologic Surgeon
Assistant Professor of Surgery
University of Toronto

Staff Surgeon
Toronto General Hospital
Toronto, Canada

Lorne E. Rotstein, M.D., F.R.C.S. (C), F.A.C.S.
General Surgeon
Assistant Professor of Surgery
University of Toronto

Chief, General Surgical Oncology
Toronto General Hospital
Toronto, Canada

Robert B. Salter, O.C., M.D., M.S. (Tor), F.R.C.S. (C), F.A.C.S.
Orthopedic Surgeon
Professor of Surgery
University of Toronto

Staff Surgeon
Hospital for Sick Children
Toronto, Canada

Hugh E. Scully, M.D., F.R.C.S. (C), F.A.C.S.
Cardiovascular Surgeon
Associate Professor of Surgery
University of Toronto

Deputy Surgeon-in-Chief
Staff Surgeon, Toronto Hospital
Toronto, Canada

Robert M. Stone, M.D., F.R.C.S. (C), F.A.C.S.
General Surgeon
Professor of Surgery
University of Toronto

Surgeon-in-Chief
Toronto Western Hospital
Toronto, Canada

Steven M. Strasberg, M.D., F.R.C.S. (C)
General Surgeon
Professor of Surgery
University of Toronto

Head, Division of General Surgery
Mount Sinai Hospital
Toronto, Canada

Medical Art Editors

Linda Wilson-Pauwels, A.O.C.A., B.Sc., A.A.M., M.Ed.
Assistant Professor and Acting Chairman
Department of Art as Applied to Medicine
Faculty of Medicine
University of Toronto
Toronto, Canada

Margot Mackay, A.N.S.C.A.D., B.Sc., A.A.M.
Associate Professor and Course Director
Department of Art as Applied to Medicine
Faculty of Medicine
University of Toronto
Toronto, Canada

Index

A

D

E

F

G

H

I

T